Pulmonary Hypertension – Clinical Research and Challenges

Pulmonary Hypertension – Clinical Research and Challenges

Edited by **Jim Foster**

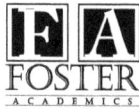

FA FOSTER ACADEMICS

New Jersey

Published by Foster Academics,
61 Van Reypen Street,
Jersey City, NJ 07306, USA
www.fosteracademics.com

Pulmonary Hypertension – Clinical Research and Challenges
Edited by Jim Foster

International Standard Book Number: 978-1-63242-340-5 (Hardback)

Printed in the United States of America.

Contents

Permissions

List of Contributors

Preface

The purpose of the book is to provide a glimpse into the dynamics and to present opinions and studies of some of the scientists engaged in the development of new ideas in the field from very different standpoints. This book will prove useful to students and researchers owing to its high content quality.

The book presents fundamental knowledge and current discoveries associated with the structure and cellular function of the pulmonary vasculature. This book elucidates the following topics: dysregulated cellular pathways observed in experimental and human pulmonary hypertension; structure and function of the normal pulmonary vasculature; introduction of numerous particular forms of this illness; clinical characteristics of the illness in general, and its management in special circumstances. It is a unique book which integrates cardiac and pulmonary physiology and pathophysiology with clinical aspects of this disease. Description of dysregulated pathways affected by pulmonary hypertension has also been provided. The book elucidates the effects of hypoxia on the pulmonary vasculature and the myocardium as well. An introduction of the techniques of assessing pulmonary hypertension has also been presented in this book. Numerous forms of pulmonary hypertension have been elucidated in this book, which are particularly challenging in clinical practice (like pulmonary arterial hypertension related to systemic sclerosis). Towards the end, the book discusses special considerations related to the management of this disease in certain clinical scenarios like pulmonary hypertension in the seriously ill.

At the end, I would like to appreciate all the efforts made by the authors in completing their chapters professionally. I express my deepest gratitude to all of them for contributing to this book by sharing their valuable works. A special thanks to my family and friends for their constant support in this journey.

Editor

Part 1

Pulmonary Vascular Function and Dysfunction

Pulmonary Hypertension: Endothelial Cell Function

Rajamma Mathew

Dept of Pediatrics, Maria Fareri Children's Hospital at Westchester Medical Center,
New York Medical College, Dept. of Physiology, New York Medical College, Valhalla, NY,
USA

1. Introduction

Pulmonary hypertension (PH) is a devastating sequel of a number of diverse systemic diseases including cardiopulmonary, autoimmune, inflammatory and myeloproliferative diseases, drug toxicity, acquired immunodeficiency syndrome, portal hypertension, sickle cell disease and thalassemia etc. Despite major advances in the field, precise mechanism/s of PH is not yet fully understood. In experimental models, endothelial dysfunction is reported to occur before the onset of PH. Therefore, it is not surprising that the clinical diagnosis is often made late during the course of the disease. The major features of PH are impaired vascular relaxation, smooth muscle cell hypertrophy and proliferation, narrowing of the lumen, elevated pulmonary artery pressure and right ventricular hypertrophy. As the disease progresses, neointima formation takes place leading to further narrowing of the lumen, worsening of the disease, right heart failure and death.

Endothelial cells (EC) maintain a balance between vasoconstriction and vasodilatation, and between cell proliferation and apoptosis. In addition, they provide barrier function, balance pro- and anticoagulation factors of the vessel wall, and participate in immune function. Plasmalemmal membrane of the EC have specialized microdomains such as caveolae, rich in cholesterol and sphingolipids that serve as a platform for a numerous signaling molecules and compartmentalize them for optimum function. Caveolin-1, a major protein constituent of caveolae maintains the shape of caveolae and interacts with numerous signaling molecules that reside in or recruited to caveolae, and stabilizes them and keeps these molecules in an inhibitory conformation. A large number of signaling pathways implicated in PH have been shown to interact with endothelial caveolin-1. Therefore, endothelial dysfunction including the loss of functional endothelial caveolin-1 induced by injury such as inflammation, toxicity, increased shear stress and hypoxia may be the initiating factor in the pathogenesis of PH and also contributing to the progression of the disease.

2. Pulmonary Hypertension

PH is a rare but a devastating disease with high mortality and morbidity rate. A large number of unrelated diseases are known to lead to PH. The current W.H.O. clinical classification of PH includes 5 groups: *Gr I:* Pulmonary arterial hypertension (PAH): This group comprises of idiopathic and heritable PAH, PAH secondary to drug toxicity and associated with congenital heart defects, connective tissue diseases, portal hypertension, infection, chronic hemolytic anemia, and persistent pulmonary hypertension of the newborn. Recently, pulmonary veno-occlusive disease and pulmonary capillary hemangiomatosis have been added to this group as a subcategory. *Gr II*: PH due to left heart diseases, *Gr III*: PH due to lung diseases and hypoxia, *Gr IV*: Chronic thromboembolic PH, and *Gr V*: PH secondary to other systemic diseases such as sarcoidosis, myeloproliferative diseases, metabolic disorders and chronic renal failure on dialysis etc. (Simonneau 2004, Hoeper 2009). Regardless of the underlying disease; the major features of PH are endothelial dysfunction, impaired vascular relaxation, smooth muscle cell proliferation and impaired apoptosis, neointima formation, narrowing of the lumen, elevated pulmonary artery pressure and right ventricular hypertrophy, subsequently leading to right heart failure and death. Early changes that occur in the vasculature are not clinically apparent. The patients usually present with vague symptoms, therefore it is not surprising that the diagnosis is often made late. By the time the diagnosis is made, extensive vascular changes have already taken place, which makes the treatment a formidable challenge.

Although major advances have been made, the precise mechanism/s leading to PH is not yet fully elucidated. Multiple signaling pathways have been implicated in the pathogenesis of PH. Loss of nitric oxide (NO), prostacyclin (PGI_2) and resulting impaired vascular relaxation is the hallmark of PH. Recent studies have revealed that certain genetic defects in humans increase the likelihood of developing PAH. Several members of transforming growth factor (TGF) β superfamily have been implicated in the pathogenesis of PAH; the most notable example being heterozygous germline mutations in bone morphogenic protein receptor type II (BMPRII). This mutation has been noted in approximately 70% of heritable PAH and 26% of idiopathic PAH. Importantly, only 20% of people with this mutation develop PAH. It has recently been shown that inflammation and serotonin increase susceptibility to develop PH in BMPRII+/- mice (Thomson 2000, Machado 2006, Long 2006, Song 2008, Mathew 2011b). Altered metabolism of estrogen resulting in low production of 2 methylestradiol is also thought to be a "second hit" for the development of PAH in females with BMPRII mutation (Austin 2009). Thus, environmental, metabolic and/or other genetic factors act as a "second hit" in the development of PAH in patients with BMPRII mutations.

Inflammation plays a significant role in the pathogenesis of clinical and experimental PH. PH has been reported in patients suffering from systemic inflammatory, autoimmune diseases and human immunodeficiency virus infection (Lespirit 1998, Dorfmüller 2003, Mathew 2010). In patients with idiopathic PAH, increased plasma levels of proinflammatory cytokines and chemokines such as interleukin (IL)-1, IL-6, fractalkine and monocyte chemoattractant protein-1 (MCP-1, currently known as CCL2) have been documented. Perivascular inflammatory cells, chiefly macrophages and monocytes, and regulated upon activation normal T-cell expressed and secreted (RANTES) have also been reported in the lungs of these patients [Tuder 1994, Humbert 1995, Dorfmüller 2002, Balabanian 2002, Itoh 2006, Sanchez 2007, Mathew 2010). In the monocrotaline (MCT) model, early and progressive upregulation of IL-6 mRNA with increased IL-6 bioactivity, progressive loss of endothelial caveolin-1 coupled with activation (tyrosine phosphorylation, PY) of signal transducer and the activator of transcription (STAT) 3 have been shown to occur before the onset of PH; and the rescue of endothelial caveolin-1 inhibits PY-STAT3 activation and attenuates PH (Mathew 2007, Huang 2008). These observations not only underscore a role for inflammation in the pathogenesis of PH but also show the importance of endothelial cell membrane integrity in vascular health.

BMPRII is predominantly expressed in endothelial cells (EC). A part of BMPRII has been shown to colocalize with caveolin-1 in caveolar microdomain and also in golgi bodies. BMPRII signaling is essential for BMP-mediated regulation of vascular smooth muscle cell (SMC) growth and differentiation, and it also protects EC from apoptosis (Yu 2008, Teichert-Kuliszewska 2006). In some cell systems, persistent activation of PY-STAT3 leads to a reduction in the BMPRII protein expression, and BMP2 induces apoptosis by inhibiting PY-STAT3 activation and by down-regulating Bcl-xL, a downstream mediator of PY-STAT3 (Brock 2009, Kawamura 2000). In addition, the loss of BMPRII in in-vivo and in-vitro studies has been shown to increase the production of cytokines such as IL-6, MCP-1 and TGFβ; and exogenous BMP ligand decreases these cytokines. Interestingly, reduction in the expression of BMPRII has been reported in patients with idiopathic PAH without BMPRII mutation and to a lesser extent in patients with secondary PH (Atkinson 2002, Mathew 2010). Furthermore, both MCT and hypoxia models of PH exhibit reduction in the expression of BMPRII (Murakami 2010, Reynolds 2009). Since there is a significant interaction and crosstalk between the BMP system and IL-6/STAT3 pathway, a reduction in the expression of BMPRII may exacerbate inflammatory response in PH.

3. Endothelial cell function

Endothelium, a monolayer lining the cardiovascular system, is a critical interface between circulating blood on one side, and tissues and organs on the other. EC form a non-thrombogenic and a selective barrier to circulating macromolecules and other elements. Vascular EC subjected to blood flow-induced shear stress transform mechanical stimuli into biological signaling. EC are a group of heterogeneous cells adapted to function for the underlying organs. They have numerous metabolic functions. Depending on the stimuli they are capable of secreting several transducing molecules for participation in vascular tone and structure, inflammation, thrombosis, barrier function, cell proliferation and apoptosis. The dominance of these various factors, determines whether the effect would be cytoprotective or cytotoxic. EC have specialized microdomains on the plasmalemmal membrane. Caveolae, a subset of these specialized microdomains are omega shaped invaginations (50-100 nm) found on a variety of cells including EC, SMC and epithelial cells. Caveolae serve as a platform and compartmentalize a number of signaling molecules that reside in or are recruited to caveolae. Caveolae are also involved in transcytosis, endocytosis and potocytosis. Three isoforms of caveolin proteins have been identified. Caveolin-1 (22kD) is the major scaffolding protein that supports and maintains the structure of caveolae. It interacts with numerous transducing molecules that reside in or are recruited to caveolae, and it regulates cell proliferation, differentiation and apoptosis via a number of diverse signaling pathways. Caveolin-2 requires caveolin-1 for its membrane localization and functions as an anti-proliferative molecule. However, unlike caveolin-1, caveolin-2 has no effect on vascular tone. Caveolin-3 is a muscle specific protein found predominantly in cardiac and skeletal muscle (Razani 2002, Mathew 2011b).

Caveolin-1 interacts, regulates and stabilizes several proteins including Src family of kinases, G-proteins (α subunits), G protein-coupled receptors, H-Ras, PKC, eNOS, integrins and growth factor receptors such as VEGF-R, EGF-R. Caveolin-1 exerts negative regulation of the target protein within caveolae, through caveolin-1-scaffolding domain (CSD, residue 82-101). Major ion channels such as Ca^{2+}-dependent potassium channels and voltage-dependent K^+ channels (Kv1.5), and a number of molecules responsible for Ca^{2+} handling such as inositol triphosphate receptor (IP_3R), heterodimeric GTP binding protein, Ca^{2+}

ATPase and several transient receptor potential channels localize in caveolae, and interact with caveolin-1. Production of vasodilators such as nitric oxide (NO), prostacyclin (PGI$_2$) and endothelium-derived hyperpolarizing factor [EDHF] within caveolae are dependent on caveolin-1-mediated regulation of Ca^{2+} entry (Mathew 2011b).

EC have important cytoplasmic organelles such as Weibel Palade bodies, initially formed in trans-golgi network; as these organelles mature they become responsive to secretagogues such as thrombin and histamine. Weibel Palade bodies store a number of molecules that are necessary for hemostasis, inflammation, vascular proliferation and angiogenesis. These molecules including vWF, P-selectin, angiopoietin 2, ET-1 and endothelin converting enzyme, IL-8, calcitonin gene-related peptide and osteoprotegerin are readily available for the designated function (Metcalf 2008).

3.1 Vasomotor tone

3.1.1 Endothelial nitric oxide synthase (eNOS)/cyclic guanosine monophosphate (cGMP) pathway

eNOS/cGMP pathway plays a major role in vascular tone and structure. In addition to vasodilatory function, it inhibits cell proliferation, DNA synthesis, platelet aggregation, and it modulates inflammatory responses. eNOS is tightly regulated by a variety of intracellular processes, post-translational modification and protein-protein interaction with caveolin-1 and Ca^{2+}/calmodulin. For efficient synthesis, eNOS is associated with golgi bodies, and for optimum activation, eNOS is targeted to caveolae. An increase in intracellular Ca^{2+} induced by shear stress and varying oxygen tension activate eNOS (Sessa 1995, Shaul 1996). NO, a short lived free radical gas is synthesized by the catalytic activity of eNOS on L-arginine in the vascular EC. NO activates the enzyme, soluble guanylate cyclase (sGC) that converts guanosine triphosphate (GTP) to cGMP.

cGMP through its protein kinase (PKG) causes vascular relaxation, inhibits cell proliferation and inflammation. It is thought that the extracellular L-arginine and its transport through cationic amino acid transporter-1 (CAT-1), localized in the caveolae, are available for eNOS activity. L-arginine found in different intracellular compartments may not be readily available for eNOS activity. This dependence on extracellular L-arginine for NO production has been termed "L-arginine paradox" (McDonald 1997, Zharikov 1998). In addition to CAT-1, tetrahydrobiopterin (BH4) and sGC are compartmentalized in caveolae with eNOS for optimum activation. BH4 is an essential cofactor required for the activity of eNOS and is synthesized from GTP by a rate limiting enzyme, guanosine triphosphate cyclohydrolase 1 (GTPCH-1). Interestingly, GTPCH-1 also localizes in caveolar microdomain with caveolin-1 and eNOS. This spatial colocalization with eNOS may ensure NO synthesis (Peterson 2009). Caveolin-1 inhibits eNOS through protein-protein interaction, but it also facilitates the increase in intracellular Ca^{2+}. HSP90 binds to eNOS away from caveolin-1 in Ca^{2+}-calmodulin-depedent manner and reduces the inhibitory influence of caveolin-1 to increase eNOS activity. Thus, caveolin-1 and eNOS have a dynamic interrelationship (Gratton 2000, Mathew 2007).

3.1.2 Prostacyclin (PGI$_2$)/cyclic adenosine monophosphate (cAMP) pathway

PGI$_2$, a potent vasodilator produced by EC is formed from arachidonic acid by the enzymatic activity of PGI$_2$ synthase, catalyzed by cyclooxygenase 2. PGI$_2$ synthase belongs to a family of G-protein coupled receptors and it colocalizes with endothelial caveolin-1. PGI_2 binds to the receptor resulting in the stimulation of adenylyl cyclase which catalyzes the conversion of ATP to second messenger cAMP. In vascular system, PGI_2 via cAMP and cAMP-dependent protein kinase (PKA) promotes vascular relaxation, inhibits platelet aggregation, inflammation and cell proliferation. In addition, cAMP/PKA pathway activates NO production via phosphorylation of eNOS (Stitham 2011, Kawabe 2010, Zhang 2006). Unlike eNOS, PGI_2 synthase remains enzymatically active even when bound to caveolin-1. Furthermore, eNOS, PGI_2 synthase and vascular endothelial growth factor receptor (VEGFR) 2 colocalize with caveolin-1 suggesting a role for caveolin-1 in angiogenesis signaling pathways (Spisni 2001).

3.1.3 Endothelium-derived hyperpolarizing factor (EDHF)

An elevation of intracellular Ca^{2+} is essential for EDHF-mediated responses; and the family of transient receptor potential cation (TRPC) channels participates in Ca^{2+} entry. TRPC1 is associated with caveolae and a direct interaction with caveolin-1 is necessary for TRPC membrane localization, and Ca^{2+} influx. Ca^{2+} influx also occurs via TRPV4 channel that belongs to a subfamily of TRPC. TRPV4 channel is expressed in a variety of cells including EC, and is also linked to caveolin-1. Interestingly, arachidonic acid metabolites epoxyeicosatrienoic acids (5, 6-EET and 8, 9-EET) act as direct TRPV4 channel activators in EC. Furthermore, genetic deletion of caveolin-1 has been shown to abrogate EDHF-induced hyperpolarization by altering Ca^{2+} entry, thus highlighting the role of caveolin-1 in EDHF regulation (Rath 2009, Vriens 2005, Saliez 2008).

3.2 Barrier function

Endothelial cytoskeleton maintains barrier integrity, and EC are linked with each other through tight junctions (TJ) and adherens junctions (AJ). EC control the passage of blood constituents to the underlying tissue. The solutes pass through transcellular or paracellular pathway. Transcellular permeability is regulated by signaling pathways responsible for endocytosis and vesicular trafficking. Paracellular permeability is the result of opening and closing of the endothelial cellular junction; it is governed by a complex arrangement of adhesion proteins and related cytoskeleton proteins organized in distinct structures such as TJ and AJ. Vascular endothelial (VE)-cadherin plays a critical role in integrating spatial signals into cell behavior. VE-cadherin interacts with β-catenin, p120 and plakoglobulin, and binds to α-catenin. Association of VE-cadherin with catenins is required for cellular control of endothelial permeability and junction stabilization. It is believed that the tyrosine phosphorylation of VE-cadherin and other components of AJ results in a weak junction and impaired barrier function (Dejana 2008, Mahta 2006). Furthermore, VE-cadherin is a link between AJ and TJ; it upregulates the gene encoding for the protein claudin-5, a TJ adhesive protein (Taddei 2008). RhoA is considered crucial for the endothelial contractile machinery. Basal activity of RhoA maintains EC junctions, but the induced activity mediates cell contraction, AJ destabilization, barrier disruption and increased permeability. Suppression of RhoA by the activation of p190RhoGAP (GTPase activating protein) reverses permeability. Interestingly, caveolin-1 deficiency impairs AJ integrity and reduces the expression of VE-cadherin and β-catenin. In caveolin-1 deficient EC, increased activity of eNOS accompanied by reactive oxygen species (ROS) generation leads to nitration; the consequent inactivation of p190RhoGAP-A results in RhoA activation and increased permeability. Inhibition of RhoA or eNOS reduces hyper-permeability in caveolin-1$^{-/-}$ mice (van Nieuw Amerongen 2007, Siddiqui 2011, Schubert 2002). It has also been shown that NO-mediated s-nitrosylation of β-catenin is involved in the VEGF-induced permeability. Interestingly, blocking sGC improves high tidal volume ventilator-induced endothelial barrier function. These mice with ventilator-induced lung injury exhibit high cGMP and low cAMP levels, and treatment with iloprost improves vascular leak (Thibeau 2010, Schmidt 2008, Birukova 2010). Thus, cGMP and cAMP levels appear to have opposing effects on endothelial barrier function.

Activated protein C (APC), a plasma serine protease that forms a complex with EC protein C receptor (EPCR) is a cytoprotective agent functioning as an anticoagulant and profibrinolytic factor, and it participates in anti-inflammatory responses. In addition, EPCR has been shown to support APC-induced protease-activated receptor (PAR)-1-mediated cell signaling. APC via EPCR inhibits RhoA activation, increases Rac1 expression and inhibits vascular permeability. In support of this view, recent studies have shown reduced expression of EPCR and reciprocal increase in the expression of Rho associated kinase (ROCK)1 in a mouse model of ventilation-induced lung injury; and the treatment with APC restored the EPCR expression, attenuated ROCK1 expression and inhibited capillary leak (Baes 2007, Sen 2011, Finigan 2009). Interestingly, both thrombin and APC activate PAR1 with opposing effects. APC-induced PAR1 is cytoprotective whereas thrombin-induced PAR1 activation stimulates RhoA/ROCK, actin stress fiber formation, and alters the integrity of EC layer. Localization of APC-activated PAR1 and EPCR in caveolae is essential for the cytoprotective effects, but for thrombin-activated PAR1 caveolar localization is not necessary. APC treatment inhibits thrombin-induced activation of ERK1/2, whereas in caveolin-1-deficient EC, APC treatment does not prevent thrombin-induced ERK1/2 activation (Russo 2009, Carlisle-Klusack 2007). These studies underscore the importance of EC including endothelial caveolin-1 in maintaining vascular health.

3.3 Inflammation

It is well established that inflammation plays a significant role in the pathogenesis of PH. Inflammation is an orchestrated process designed to combat injury/infection. The relevance of endothelium in controlling and modulating inflammatory responses in general is accepted. Under normal conditions, the apoptosis rate in EC is extremely low. Activated EC exhibit a reduction in the endothelial surface layer, glycocalyx, and increased rate of apoptosis. EC detached from the basement membrane appear in blood circulation. Therefore, it is not surprising that increased circulating endothelial cell levels in PH are indicative of poor prognosis (Grange 2010, Jones 2005, Smadja 2010). Both NO and ROS are implicated in the EC response to inflammation. Increased NO levels compared to ROS results in anti-inflammatory response via cGMP pathway, whereas, increased levels of ROS and/or the presence of reactive NO species activate proinflammatory transcription factors (Grange 2010).

In response to infection and inflammatory mediators, EC secrete increased amounts of Interleukin (IL)-6, and upregulate intracellular adhesion molecule (ICAM) and vascular adhesion molecule (VCAM), which spread over the surface of EC. ICAM, VCAM and also P-selectin released from Weibel Palade bodies allow rapid rolling and adhesion of leukocytes on the EC surface; and biosynthesized E-selectin maintains this process. Interaction of leukocyte platelet endothelial cell adhesion molecule-1 (PECAM-1) and EC PECAM-1 leads to transmigration of leukocytes through the inter EC junction and possibly through EC as well. Furthermore, stimulation of ICAM leads to VE-cadherin phosphorylation resulting in destabilization of AJ, thus further facilitating transmigration of leukocytes (Jirik 1989, Grange 2010, Muller 2009, van Buul 2007). IL-6 plays an important role in inflammatory response, thus, is critical for the acute phase response. It is believed that IL-6 resolves acute phase response and promotes acquired immune responses, which is controlled by chemokine-directed leukocyte recruitment but also by efficient activation of leukocyte apoptosis. IL-6-driven STAT3 activation is thought to limit the recruitment of neutrophils as well as pro-inflammatory cytokine. However, IL-6 also rescues cells from apoptosis via the activation of STAT3, and increased expression of anti-apoptotic factors such as Bcl-xL and Bcl2 (Jones 2005, Fielding 2008). In addition, the expression of isoforms of ROCK is increased. Inhibition of ROCK is thought to impair IL-6-mediated resolution of neutrophils-dependent acute inflammation (Mong 2009). Thus, IL-6 can function as an anti-inflammatory or a pro-inflammatory factor.

Deregulated IL-6/STAT3 pathway underlies a number of vascular diseases including PH, autoimmune diseases and cancer (Mathew 2004, Huang 2008, Hirano 2010, Yu 2009). In addition, the loss of caveolin-1 has been reported in theses cases. Caveolin-1 is known to inhibit PY-STAT3 activation as well as the expression of Bcl-xL and Bcl2. Caveolin-1 also inhibits and degrades inflammatory and pro-neoplastic protein COX2 (Mathew 2004, Huang 2010, Mathew 2011b, Mathew 2007). Caveolin-1 modulates inflammatory processes via its regulatory effect on eNOS, and depending on the cell type and context of the disease, the effect can be positive or negative.

Hemoxygenase (HO)-1, one of the isoenzymes has emerged as an important player in cellular defense mechanism. HO-1 catalyzes the metabolism of free heme into equimolar ferrous iron, carbon monoxide (CO) and biliverdin. The latter is converted to bilirubin by biliverdin reducatse. HO-1 suppresses inflammation by removing pro-inflammatory molecule, heme, and by generating CO. CO, biliverdin and bilirubin have cytoprotective function. HO-1/CO inhibits pro-inflammatory cytokines such as CCL2 and IL-6, and increases the production of IL-10 an anti-inflammatory cytokine. Interestingly, HO-1 and biliverdin reducatse are compartmentalized in endothelial caveolae; and similar to eNOS, HO-1 activity is inhibited by caveolin-1. CO has been shown also to activate sGC (Durante 2011, Pae 2009, Liang 2011).

3.4 Coagulation and thrombosis

In health, endothelium prevents thrombosis via a number of endothelium-derived inhibitors of coagulation such as thrombomodulin, protein S, heparin sulfate proteoglycans and tissue plasminogen activator (tPA). In addition, PGI$_2$, NO and CD39 inhibit platelet aggregation. Released tPA catalyzes the conversion of plasminogen to plasmin thus, facilitating proteolytic degradation of thrombus (Oliver 2005). Activation of coagulation cascade is necessary for normal hemostasis. Tissue factor (TF) is a transmembrane glycoprotein that initiates coagulation cascade; and thrombin is the key effector enzyme for the clotting process. The coagulation cascade is activated to stop the blood loss by forming a clot (Shovlin 2010). TF, a member of cytokine superfamily that functions as high affinity receptor and a cofactor for plasma factors VII/VIIa, the initiator of blood coagulation. TF is not expressed in EC, but it is rapidly induced by infection and inflammatory cytokines (TNFα, IL-1β). VEGF, a major stimulator of angiogenesis, is known to upregulate TF expression in EC (Mechtcheriakova 1999). Following injury/infection, Weibel Palade bodies fuse with endothelial cell membrane and release vWF, P-selectin and IL-8. Interestingly, capillary EC lack Weibel Palade bodies but they do express vWF, P-selectin, thus, are capable of participating in coagulation process. The inter-activation of vWF multimers with exposed subintimal matrix results in adherence to activated platelets and participation in clot formation. The release of P-selectin facilitates neutrophil adherence to EC and transmigration (Ochoa 2010).

It is well accepted that there are cross-talks between inflammatory responses and thrombosis. Coagulation has been shown to augment inflammatory responses, and anticoagulants blunt the coagulation-induced inflammatory responses. Furthermore, PGI2 and APC inhibit injury-induced Ca^{2+} flux and NFκB activation, and reduce significantly the expression of proinflammatory cytokines such as TNFα, IL-6 and IL-8. EPCR augments APC by thrombin/thrombomodulin complex; but EPCR is shed from EC by inflammatory mediators and thrombin, thus favoring thrombosis (Esmon 2001).

Under physiological state, circulating platelets are in a quiescent state, and the activation is inhibited by endothelium-derived NO and PGI_2. Platelets are recruited early to the site of inflammation/injury to provide rapid protection from bleeding; however, they contribute both to coagulation and inflammation. Platelets form a layer, and vWF plays a critical role in the adherence of platelets to the injury site. At the site of adherence, platelets release platelet activating factors such as adenosine diphosphate (ADP), thromboxane A2 (TxA2), serotonin, collagen and thrombin. Thrombin is the most potent thrombogenic factor. In addition, release of ADP and TxA2 from platelets increases the expression of P-selectin and CD40 ligand (Angeolillo 2010). CD40, the receptor for CD40 ligand, is found on a number of cells including EC, macrophages, B-cells and vascular SMC. The interaction between CD40 and its ligand causes severe inflammatory responses, matrix degradation and thrombus formation; and it has been implicated in the pathogenesis of PH. Platelet-derived member of TNF superfamily "lymphotoxin-like inducible protein that competes with glycoprotein D for herpes virus entry mediator on T lymphocytes" (LIGHT) levels in serum are increased in patients with PAH; interestingly, LIGHT levels are not altered in PH secondary to left heart failure. LIGHT increases the expression of TF and plasminogen activator inhibitor (PAI)-1, and decreases thrombomodulin levels, thus, making EC pro-thrombogenic (Otterdal 2008). PAI-1, a potent endogenous inhibitor of fibrinolysis, is produced by several cells including EC. ROS has been shown to have a significant role in cytokine-induced increase in PAI-1 expression. Increased levels of PAI-1 enhance thrombosis and impair fibrinolysis. Recent studies suggest that PAI-1 regulates EC integrity and cell death. Increased levels are thought to confer resistance to apoptosis and facilitate cell proliferation (Jaulmes 2009, Balsara 2008, Schneider 2008).

3.5 Angiogenesis

The formation of new capillaries from a preexisting vessel is called angiogenesis. Angiogenesis plays a pivotal role in a numerous physiological and pathological processes such as organ development, tissue repair and carcinogenesis. Angiogenesis is controlled by opposing angiogenic and angiostatic factors. Some of the angiogenic factors are VEGFs, fibroblast growth factor (FGF)s, angiopoietins, PECAM-1, integrins, and VE-cadherin, and the angiostatic factors are angiostatin, endosatstin and thrombospondin (Distler 2003). Angiogenic factors such as angiopoietins 1 and 2 (Ang 1 and Ang 2), and VEGF orchestrate EC proliferation, migration and new blood vessel formation. These angiogenic factors also participate in inflammatory responses and barrier function. VEGFA is a major regulator of angiogenic signaling and functions through a tyrosine kinase receptor, VEGFR-2, found on the surface of EC. Downstream effector of VEGF-induced angiogenesis is eNOS. Not surprisingly, angiogenesis is impaired in eNOS knockout mice and the inhibition of eNOS antagonizes VEGF-induced angiogenesis. NO induces the expression of $\alpha v \beta 3$ integrin, and the synthesis and release of collagen IV (a major component of endothelial basement membrane) from EC. Binding of these two molecules leads to the activation of integrin, facilitating cell adhesion, migration, cell proliferation and protection of EC from apoptosis (Ziche 1997, Wang 2011). vWF modulates angiogenesis via multiple pathways involving $\alpha v \beta 3$ integrin (a receptor for vWF on EC), VEGFR-2 signaling and Ang2. Inhibition of vWF in-vitro has been shown to increase angiogenesis, to increase VEGFR-2-dependent cell proliferation and migration associated with reduction in $\alpha v \beta 3$ integrin and increased Ang2 levels (Starke 2011). VE-cadherin not only mediates inter-endothelial cell adhesion but also controls VEGF-mediated EC survival and angiogenesis via pathways involving β-catenin, PI3 kinase and VEGFR-2. Deficiency of VE-cadherin results in the failure of transmission of VEGF-induced survival signaling to Akt kinase and Bcl$_2$, resulting in apoptosis of EC (Carmeliet 1999).

Tie2, an endothelium-specific tyrosine kinase receptor and its ligand Ang1 and Ang2 are modulators of vascular development and angiogenesis. Ang1 does not promote EC proliferation but supports EC survival, maturation and stabilization of the new vessels formed by the activity of VEGF. In addition, Ang1 administration protects adult vasculature from leakage and Ang1 over-expressing mice are resistant to VEGF-induced vascular leak (Thurston 2000). Although Ang2 has been thought to counteract Ang1 and Tie2 activity, the recent studies show that Ang2 in the presence of VEGF supports EC survival and angiogenesis. EC death increases when Ang2 is injected with VEGF blocker (Lobov 2002). Thus, the presence or the absence of VEGF determines how Ang2 modulates EC survival. Recent studies show that both Ang1 and Ang2 have similar agonistic capacity to mediate endothelial P-selectin translocation, neutrophils adhesion and inflammatory response. Furthermore, both can activate Tie2 receptor on neutrophils (Lemieux 2005).

Interestingly, caveolin-1 deficient mice exhibit increased microvascular permeability and angiogenesis. EC from caveolin-1 null mice show increased tyrosine phosphorylation of VEGFR-2 and decreased association with VE-cadherin. The increased permeability and angiogenesis in caveolin-1 null cells may also be related to increased eNOS activity (Lin 2007, Chang 2009). Thus, the loss of inhibitory function of caveolin-1 on VEGFR-2 phosphorylation coupled with increased eNOS activity may accentuate permeability and angiogenesis.

4. Endothelial injury and pulmonary hypertension

From the foregoing sections, it is clear that EC orchestrates a complex metabolic machinery involving a number of signaling molecules to maintain vascular health. These multiple signaling pathways cross talk at different levels to preserve normal function and cell survival. Dysregulation of one signaling pathway has a profound effect on the other pathways, resulting in a cascade of events including deregulation of multiple pathways, impaired vascular relaxation, and the loss of barrier function, transmigration of neutrophils, thrombo-embolic phenomenon, cell proliferation and anti-apoptosis leading to vascular diseases including PH. Injurious stimuli such as inflammatory cytokines, increased shear stress, drug toxicity, hypoxia and exposure to reactive oxygen species, ventilation-induced lung injury lead to the loss of protective function of EC. The end results are an imbalance between vasodilatation and vasoconstriction, coagulation and fibrinolysis, and between cell proliferation and apoptosis.

In response to infection, inflammatory mediators or oxidant stress, EC lose barrier function, develop coagulation abnormities, secrete increased amounts of IL-6 and RANTES, express adhesion molecules and chemokines that promote adhesion and transmigration of leukocytes, and activate pro-proliferative and anti-apoptotic pathways. IL-6, a 20-30 kD glycoprotein, produced by several types of cells including macrophages, EC, vascular SMC, is induced in response to stress. It is a potent, inflammatory cytokine that plays a central role in host-defense mechanisms. IL-6 has been shown to induce proliferation of SMCs in a dose dependent manner. Increased levels of IL-6 have been reported in clinical and experimental forms of PH. Furthermore, IL-6 is also thought to contribute to PH complicating chronic obstructive pulmonary disease. Recent studies show that the increased levels of IL-6 portend poor prognosis in patients with PAH (Humbert 1995, Mathew 2010, Soon 2010). During the inflammatory response, upregulated IL-6 binds to gp130, a plasma membrane receptor complex that colocalizes with caveolin-1, to activate Janus kinase (JAK), a tyrosine kinase family member leading to PY-STAT3 activation, a downstream effector of IL-6. The downstream signaling molecules of PY-STAT3 such as Bcl-xL, survivin and cyclin D1 are implicated in PAH. In addition, pulmonary EC obtained from patients with idiopathic PAH show activation of STAT3. Recent studies have shown that caveolin-1 inhibits STAT3 activation, and the rescue of caveolin-1 not only inhibits PY-STAT3 activation but also attenuates MCT-induced PH (Mathew 2010, Huang 2010, Masri 2007, Mathew 2007, Huang 2008). The initial inflammatory response is an attempt to repair the injury. But as IL-6/STAT3 pathway becomes deregulated, the results are further EC damage, increased cell proliferation and disruption of barrier function leading to vascular remodeling and PH.

Depending on the type of injury, the major effect on EC is either a progressive loss of cell membrane integrity coupled with the loss of endothelial caveolin-1 and other EC proteins, or caveolin-1 dysfunction without any protein loss. In either case the end results are impaired endothelium-dependent vascular relaxation, medial hypertrophy, narrowing of the lumen, elevated pulmonary artery pressure and right ventricular hypertrophy.

4.1 Endothelial cell disruption

4.1.1 Loss of endothelial caveolin-1

Injury such as inflammation, chemical/drug toxicity, ventilation-induced lung injury and cyclic shear stress disrupt endothelial membrane integrity. Monocrotaline (MCT), an inflammatory model of PH has been extensively studied. Although this model is not exactly akin to the human from of PH, nevertheless, it has provided valuable information. In this model, disruption of caveolae, progressive loss of caveolin-1, reciprocal activation of PY-STAT3 and upregulation of Bcl-xL are observed within 48 hrs of MCT injection, i.e. before the onset of PH. Other EC membrane proteins such as PECAM-1 and Tie2 are lost in tandem with caveolin-1. At 2 wks post-MCT, with the onset of PH, there is a further loss of proteins such as HSP90, Akt, and IκB-α. The eNOS expression is relatively well preserved, but with transient eNOS uncoupling as indicated by increased ROS generation. Furthermore, at this stage, impaired NO bioavailability, low cGMP and sulfhydryl levels have been observed. By 3-4 wks post-MCT, there is a significant reduction in the expression of eNOS protein, and ROS generation returns to normal level. Early treatment with anti-inflammatory agents prevents the loss of endothelial caveolin-1, inhibits the activation of proliferative pathways and attenuates PH; however, once the PH is established, these agents are not effective (Mathew 2007, Huang 2008, Huang 2010). Caveolin-1 null mice exhibit vascular defect and cardiomyopathy with a propensity to develop PH; rescue of caveolin-1 ameliorates cardiovascular function and attenuates PH (Murata 2007). Loss of endothelial caveolin-1 has also been reported in idiopathic PAH (Achcar 2006, Patel 2007, Mathew 2011a). Thus, there is a strong evidence that endothelial caveolin-1 has a pivotal role in PH. Endothelial caveolin-1 regulates inflammatory response, proinflammatory cytokines, inhibits a number of mitogens implicated in PH, and it controls cell proliferation and apoptosis. Thus, the loss of endothelial caveolin-1 is sufficient to initiate PH and facilitate the progression of the disease.

4.1.2 Enhanced expression of caveolin-1 in SMC

Recently it was reported that in addition to the loss of endothelial caveolin-1, pulmonary arterial SMC from patients with idiopathic PAH exhibited enhanced expression of caveolin-1. These SMC with enhanced expression of caveolin-1 exhibited altered Ca^{2+} handling, increased cytosolic $[Ca^{2+}]_i$ and increased DNA synthesis. Increased $[Ca^{2+}]_i$ is a trigger for DNA synthesis and cell proliferation (Patel 2007). In patients with chronic obstructive pulmonary disease (COPD), enhanced expression of caveolin-1 in SMC correlates with the presence of PH (Huber 2009). Recently it was reported that a child developed PH about 2 years after having completely recovered from acute respiratory distress syndrome (ARDS). It is well established that underlying pathology of ARDS is pulmonary vascular endothelial damage. At the time of the diagnosis of PH, pulmonary arteries exhibited loss of endothelial caveolin-1 and medial wall thickening. Importantly, the arteries that exhibited loss of endothelial caveolin-1 coupled with the loss of vWF had robust expression of caveolin-1 in SMC; whereas, the arteries that exhibited endothelial caveolin-1 loss alone did not have enhanced expression of caveolin-1 in SMC. Second lung biopsy done 3 years later exhibited neointima formation and by then the vasculature had become unresponsive to therapy (Mathew 2011a). These results suggest that the initial EC injury during ARDS was progressive although not clinically apparent. Since vWF is stored in Weibel Palade bodies within the EC, the loss of vWF is indicative of an extensive endothelial damage and/or loss. Therefore, it is not surprising that increased plasma levels of vWF and Ang2, and circulating endothelial cells in PAH are considered markers of poor prognosis (Kawut 2005, Kümpers 2010, Smadja 2010). It is worth noting here that both vWF and Ang2 are stored in Weibel Palade bodies and during stress/activation, these bodies deliver their cargo at the endothelial cell surface.

Caveolin-1 is essential for normal functioning of SMC. Under normal circumstances, caveolin-1 inhibits receptor and non-receptor tyrosine kinases by sequestering them to caveolae and prevents cell proliferation. Disruption of caveolin-1 has been shown to increase cell proliferation in airway and vascular SMC. Caveolin-1 keeps mitogens inactive in caveolae; however, under increased mechanical stress/strain, caveolin-1 translocates from caveolae to non-caveolar sites within the plasma membrane of cultured SMC, and translocated caveolin-1 triggers cell cycle progression and cell proliferation (Gosens 2006, Hassan 2006, Kawabe 2004, Mathew 2011b). It has also been shown that cultured cells (murine lung endothelial and HeLa cells) exposed to mechanical stress exhibit reduction in caveolin-1 and cavin-1 (also known as polymerase 1 and transcript release factor) interaction, disappearance of caveolae and increased expression of caveolin-1 at the plasma membrane. Importantly, caveolin-1 requires cavin for caveolae formation [Sinha 2011, Mathew 2011b). From these studies it appears that the progressive EC damage and the eventual loss expose underlying SMC to blood elements and cyclic shear stress, leading to enhanced expression of caveolin-1 and its translocation from caveolae. It is worth noting here that the activation of matrix metalloproteinases (MMP) 2 is a critical step in the migration of SMC through the basement barrier, which facilitates neointima formation. Increased expression and activity of MMP2 has been reported in SMC from patients with idiopathic PAH. MMP2 and its physiologic activator MT1-MMP colocalize in caveolae and are negatively regulated by caveolin-1 [Mathew 2011b). These observations further support the view that SMC exposed to increased shear stress may translocate caveolin-1 from caveolae to other plasma membrane sites, thus losing its inhibitory activity on MT1-MMP and MMP2, thus, facilitating cell migration via MMP2.

Increased eNOS expression and PKG nitration have been shown in caveolin-1 null mice and also in the lungs of patients with idiopathic PAH contributing to the worsening of the disease. The expression of eNOS is reported to be either low or increased in the lungs of patients with PH. This is not surprising because the disease does not progress uniformly, the expression of eNOS depends on the stage of disease in a given lung section. In PH, the initial loss of EC is followed by the appearance of apoptosis resistant EC. These neointimal EC have increased expression of eNOS and reduced expression of caveolin-1, thus, resulting in uncoupling of eNOS, oxidant and nitration injury [Mathew 2011b).

As shown in Figure 1, the sequel of EC injury (shear stress, drug toxicity, inflammation) can be summarized as follows: *1)* a progressive disruption of EC membrane integrity and the loss of endothelial caveolin-1, *2)* impaired Ca^{2+} entry into EC resulting in reduced production of NO, PGI_2 and EDHF leading to impaired vascular relaxation, *3)* activation of proliferative and antiapoptotic pathways leading to vascular cell proliferation, medial wall thickening and PH. As the disease progresses, further loss of proteins occurs indicating extensive EC damage/loss. This is followed by enhanced expression of cav-1 in SMC, where cav-1 facilitates cell proliferation and migration leading to neointima formation. Thus, the translocated caveolin-1 in SMC not only loses its ability to inhibit proliferative pathways but also switches from being antiproliferative to proproliferative that may eventually lead to SMC phenotype change from contractile to synthetic. Recent studies indicate that there is increased expression of eNOS in neointimal EC; but eNOS is dysfunctional, resulting in oxidant/nitration injury thus further aggravating PH (Mathew 2011b).

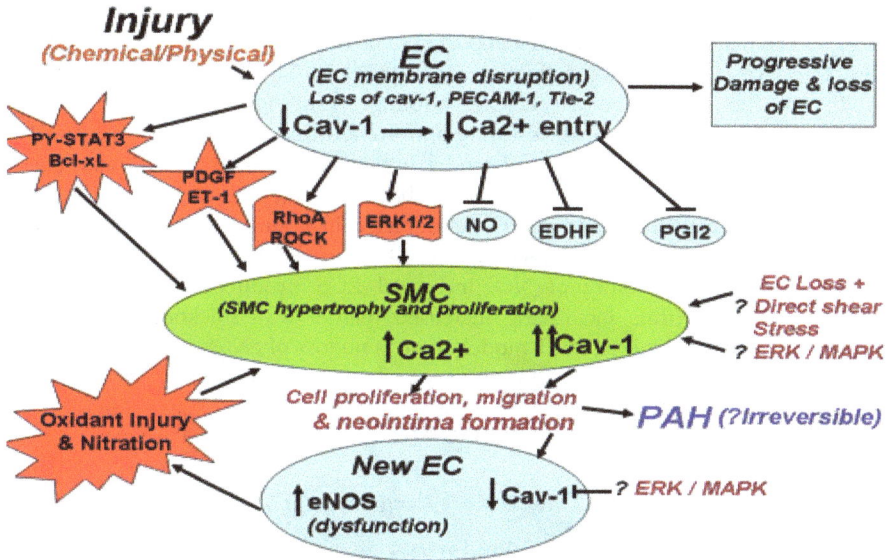

Fig. 1. *Adapted from Mathew R, Pulmonary Medicine 2011; 2011:57432.* A proposed model for PH associated with disruption of endothelial caveolin-1 resulting in the loss of vasodilators, and the activation of proliferative and anti-apoptotic pathways leading to pulmonary vascular remodeling. EC disruption is progressive and extensive damage/ loss of EC exposes SMC to direct shear stress leading to enhanced expression of caveolin-1 in SMC which participates in further cell proliferation and cell migration resulting in neointima formation. Newly formed EC in neointima express increased eNOS; low caveolin-1 expression in these cells may in part be responsible for the observed dysfunctional eNOS. Resulting oxidant/nitration injury may further influence SMC adversely leading to irreversible PH.

4.2 Endothelial dysfunction without caveolin-1 loss

PH is an important cause of increased mortality in patients suffering from chronic heart diseases associated with hypoxia. Acute hypoxia causes reversible pulmonary vasoconstriction and PH. Chronic hypoxia causes vasoconstriction with subsequent vascular remodeling and sustained PH. Not unlike MCT-induced PH, hypoxia-induced PH is associated with low bioavailability of NO and impaired endothelium-dependent pulmonary vascular relaxation. In contrast to the MCT model, in the hypoxia model there is no loss of eNOS, caveolin-1 or HSP90 proteins (Huang 2010, Mathew 2011b). Pulmonary arteries of rats with hypoxia-induced PH reveal that eNOS forms a tight complex with caveolin-1, and becomes dissociated from HSP90 and calmodulin, resulting in eNOS dysfunction. Bovine pulmonary artery EC exposed to hypoxia also exhibit tight coupling of eNOS and caveolin-1 accompanied by PY-STAT3 activation. Since caveolin-1 inhibits PY-STAT3 activation, the activation of PY-STAT3 in hypoxia-induced PH despite the unaltered expression of caveolin-1 protein indicates that caveolin-1 has lost its inhibitory function (Huang 2008, Mathew 2011b, Murata 2002). Thus, this complex formation renders both eNOS and caveolin-1 dysfunctional. Statins therapy has shown to protect eNOS function in hypoxia-induced PH. The major effect of statins is reported to be the uncoupling of eNOS/caveolin-1 complex, thus, freeing eNOS for activation (Murata 2005). Therefore, it is likely that the statins disrupt the tight cavolin-1/eNOS coupling, resulting from hypoxia- induced perturbation of EC membrane, thus, restoring antiproliferative properties of caveolin-1 and NO production by eNOS. Unlike the MCT model, hypoxia does not appear to cause physical disruption of EC membrane, but causes perturbation of the EC membrane leading to "mislocalization" of caveolin-1 and eNOS. As depicted in Figure 2, hypoxia induces tight complex formation of eNOS and caveolin-1 resulting in dysfunction of both molecules leading to impaired availability of NO, increased ROS production and activation of proliferative pathways, thus facilitating increased medial wall thickness and PH. It is important to note that unlike the MCT model, there is no loss of eNOS or caveolin-1 protein in the hypoxia model.

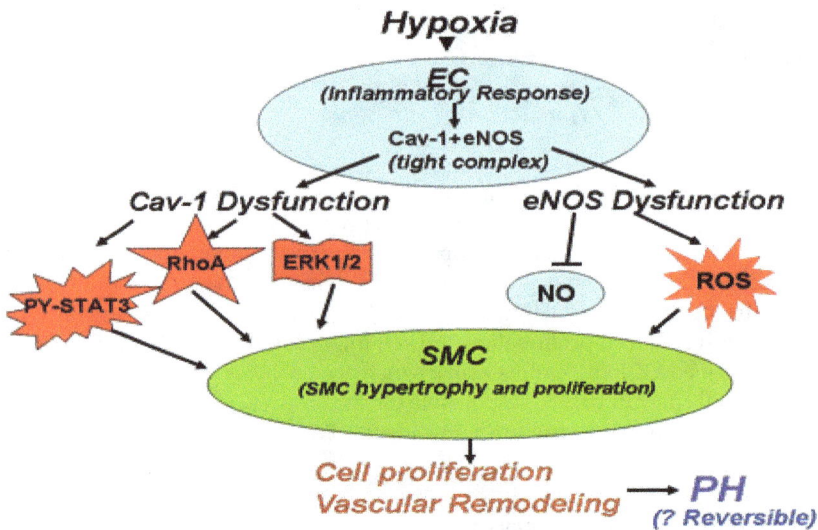

Fig. 2. *Adapted from Mathew R, Pulmonary Medicine 2011; 2011:57432.* Hypoxia-induced perturbation of endothelial cell membrane results in a tight complex formation of caveolin-1 and eNOS, rendering both molecules dysfunctional leading to low NO bioavailability and superoxide generation; and the loss of ability of caveolin-1 to inhibit proliferative pathways.

5. Therapeutic potential

Since the introduction of vasodilators and anti-mitogenic therapy, there has been a significant improvement in exercise tolerance and life expectancy in patients with PH compared with the historical controls. However, there is no cure; the disease is progresses albeit at a slower rate. Currently approved therapy belongs to 3 major groups: 1) PGI_2 analogues: PGI_2 remains the mainstay in the treatment of PH. Synthetic PGI_2 used as continuous infusion has been found to be efficacious in several forms of PH. Other synthetic analogues for use via oral and subcutaneous routes are available. 2) ET-1 blockers: ET-1 is a potent vasoconstrictor with mitogenic and inflammatory properties; and it functions both in paracrine and autocrine fashion. The effects of ET-1 are mediated through ETA and ETB receptors. Bosentan, a sulfonamide-based dual endothelin receptor antagonist has been in use for the treatment of PH. Several studies have shown improvement in hemodynamic parameters, exercise tolerance and the time to clinical worsening in patients with PAH. One of the important side effects of bosentan is abnormal liver function tests. Ambrisentan, a propanoic-based ET-1 receptor blocker seems to have much lower incidence of liver function abnormalities. 3) PDE5 inhibitors: PDE5 inhibitors block the conversion of cGMP to 5' GMP. Sildenafil is the most commonly used drug in this group. These drugs are used as monotherapy or in combination. Newer drugs such as soluble guanylate cyclase activators, tyrosine kinase inhibitors are being tested (Rhodes 2009, Stenmark 2009).

Endothelial progenitor cells (EPC) and gene therapy are being actively pursued. However, the vectors and gene delivery systems still need to be refined (Reynolds 2011). Several experimental studies with EPC/gene therapy have shown encouraging results. Administration of bone-derived EPC transduced with eNOS was found to be effective in reversing the disease process in established MCT-induced PH, but EPC administration had no effect on hypoxia-induced PH (Zhao 2005, Raoul 2007). In contrast, BMPRII gene therapy attenuated hypoxia-induced PH but had no effect on MCT-induced PH (Reynolds 2009, McMurtry 2007). The MCT model is associated with progressive loss of endothelial cell membrane integrity leading to extensive EC damage and/or loss; whereas, hypoxia does not cause EC loss. These studies raise important questions: 1) whether the state of native EC is important in selecting EPC transduced with the desired gene or the vector-driven gene therapy, or 2) these results are simply related to the efficacy of the genes in question. An ideal treatment would be to tailor the EPC/gene therapy for individual patients. A combination of gene therapy and pharmacological agents may be able to reverse the disease or at least halt the progression.

6. Summary

EC with specialized membrane rafts and organelles conduct a fine orchestra with multiple interacting sections (signaling pathways) to produce harmonious music (vascular health). Events such as injury/inflammation/shear stress leading to one false note, if not repaired early, leads to utter chaos, and the recovery becomes almost impossible. In response to injury, several signaling pathways are activated in an attempt to repair the damage. However, these pathways do become deregulated and the cytoprotective molecules become cytotoxic leading to the loss of barrier function, vasodilatation mechanisms, and the activation of cell proliferative and antiapoptotic pathways. Current therapy is based on individual signaling pathways. A holistic approach to recover EC function may be an attractive strategy to pursue for the treatment of PH.

7. References

Achcar RO, Demura Y, Rai PR, Taraseviciene-Stewart L, Kasper M et al. Loss of caveolin and heme oxygenase expression in severe pulmonary hypertension. *Chest* 2006; 129:696-705.

Angiolillo DJ, Ueno M, Goto S. Basic principles of platelet biology and clinical implications. *Circ J* 2010; 74:597-607.

Atkinson C, Stewart S, Upton PD, Machado R, Thomson JR et al. Primary pulmonary hypertension is associated with reduced pulmonary vascular expression of type II bone morphogenic protein receptor. *Circulation* 2002; 105:1672-1678.

Austin ED, Cogan JD, West JD, Hedges LK, Hamid R et al. Alterations in oestrogen metabolism: Implications for higher penetrance of familial pulmonary arterial hypertension in females. *Eur Respir J* 2009; 34:1093-1099.

Baes JS, Yang L, Manithody C, Rezaie AR. The ligand occupancy of endothelial protein C receptor switches the protease activated receptor-dependent signaling specificity of thrombin from a permeability-enhancing to a barrier –protective response in endothelial cells. *Blood* 2007; 110:3909-3916.

Balabanian K, Foussat A, Dorfmüller P, Durand-Gasselin I, Capel F et al. CX$_3$C chemokine fractalkine in pulmonary arterial hypertension. *Am J Respir Crit Care Med* 2002; 165:1419-1425.

Balsara RD, Ploplis VA. Plasminogen activator inhibitor-1: the double edged sword in apoptosis. *Thromb Haemost* 2008: 100:1029-1036.

Birukova AA, Fu P, Xing J, Cokie I, Birukov KG. Lung endothelial barrier protection by iloprost in the two-hit models of ventilator-induced lung injury (VILI) involves inhibition of Rho signaling. *Transl Res* 2010; 155:44-54.

Brock M, Trenkmann M, Gay RE, Michel BA, Gay S et al. Interleukin 6 modulates the expression of the bone morphogenic protein receptor type II through a novel STAT3 micro RNA cluster 17/29 pathway. *Circ Res* 2009;104:1184-1191.

Carlisle-Klusack ME, Rizzo V. Endothelial cytoskeleton reorganization in response to PAR1 stimulation is mediated by membrane rafts but not caveolae. *Am J Physiol* 2007; 293:H366-H375.

Carmeliet P, Lampugnani MG, Moons L, Breviario F, Compernolle V et al. Targeted deficiency or cytosolic truncation of the VE-cadherin gene in mice impairs VEGF-mediated endothelial survival and angiogenesis. *Cell* 1999; 98:147-157.

Chang SH, Feng D, Nagy JA, Sciuto TE, Dvorak AM et al. Vascular permeability and pathological angiogenesis in caveolin-1-null mice. *Am J Pathol* 2009; 175:1768-1776.

Dejana E, Orsenigo F, Lamugnani MG. The role of adherens junctions and VE-cadherin in control of vascular permeability. *J Cell Sci* 2008; 121:2115-2122.

Distler JH, Hirth A, Kurowska-Stolarska M, Gay RE, Gay S et al. Angiogenic and angiostatic factors in the molecular control of angiogenesis. *Q J Nuc Med* 2003; 47:149-161.

Dorfmuller P, Perros F, Balabanian K, Humbert M. Inflammation in pulmonary arterial hypertension. *Eur Respir J* 2003; 22:358-363.

Dorfmüller P, Zarka V, Durand-Gasselin J, Monti G, Balabanian K et al. Chemokine RANTES in severe pulmonary arterial hypertension. *Am J Respir Crit Care Med* 2002;165:534-539.

Durante W. Protective role of hemoxygenase-1 against inflammation in atherosclerosis. *Front Biosci* 2011; 17:2372-2388.

Esmon CT. Role of coagulation inhibitors in inflammation. *Thromb Hemost* 2001; 86:51-56.

Fielding CA, McLoughlin RM, McLeod L, Colmont CS, Najdovska M et al. IL-6 regulates neutrophils trafficking during acute inflammation via STAT3. *J Immunol* 2008; 181:2189-2195.

Finigan JH, Boueiz A, Wilkinson A, Damico R, Skirball J et al. Activated protein C protects against ventilator-induced pulmonary vascular leak. *Am J Physiol* 2009;296 L1002-L1011.

Gosens R, Stelmark GL, Dueck G , McNeill KD, Yamasaki A et al. Role of caveolin-1 in p42/p44 Map kinase activation and proliferation of human airway smooth muscle. *Am J Physiol* 2006; 291:L523-L534.

Grange DN, Senchenkova E. Inflammation and microcirculation. *Integrated system physiology: From cell to function.* 2010 San Rafael (CA), Morgan Claypool Life Sciences.

Gratton JP, Fontana J, O'Connor DS, Garcia-Cardena G, McCabe TJ et al. Reconstitution of an endothelial nitric oxide synthase (eNOS), hsp90 and caveolin-1 complex in vitro. Evidence that hsp90 facilitates calmodulin stimulated displacement of eNOS from caveolin-1. *J Biol Chem* 2000; 275:22268-22272.

Hassan GS, Williams TM, Frank PG, Lisanti MP. Caveolin-1-deficient aortic smooth muscle cells show cell autonomous abnormalities in proliferation, migration, and endothelin-based signal transduction. *Am J Physiol* 2006; 290:H2393-H2401.

Hirano T. IL-6 in autoimmune and inflammatory diseases: A personal memoir. *Proc Jpn Acad Ser B Phys Biol Sci* 2010; 86:717-730.

Hoeper MM. Definition, classification, and epidemiology of pulmonary arterial hypertension. *Semin Respir Crit Care Med.* 2009; 30:369-375.

Huang J, Kaminski PM, Edwards JG, Yeh A, Wolin-MS et al. Pyrrolidine dithiocarbamate restores endothelial cell membrane integrity and attenuates monocrotaline-induced pulmonary artery hypertension. *Am J Physiol* 2008; 294:L-1250-L1259

Huang J, Wolk J, Gewitz MH, Mathew R. Progressive Endothelial Cell Damage in an Inflammatory Model of Pulmonary Hypertension. *Exp Lung Res* 2010; 36:57-66.

Huber LC, Soltermann A, Fischler M, Gay S, Weder W et al. Caveolin-1 expression and hemodynamics in COPD patients. *Open Respir Med J* 2009; 3:73-78.

Humbert M, Monti G, Brenot F, Sitbon O, Portier A et al. Increased interleukin-1 and interleukin-6 serum concentrations in severe primary pulmonary hypertension. *Am J Respir Crit Care Med* 1995; 151:1628-1631.

Itoh T, Nagaya N, Ishibashi-Ueda-H, Kyotani S, Oya H et al. Increased plasma monocyte chemoattractant protein-1 level in idiopathic pulmonary arterial hypertension. *Respirology* 2006;11:158-163.

Jaulmes A, Sansilvestri-Morel P, Rolland-Volognes G, Bernhardt F, Gaertner R et al. NOX4 mediates the expression of plasminogen activator inhibitor-1 via p38MAPK pathway in cultured endothelial cells. *Thromb Res* 2009; 124:439-446.

Jirik FR, Podor TJ, Hirano T, Kishimoto T, Loskutoff DJ et al. Bacterial lipopolysaccharide and inflammatory mediators augment IL-6 secretion by human endothelial cells. *J Immunol* 1989;142:144-147.

Jones SA, Directing transition from innate to acquired immunity: defining a role for IL-6. *J Immunol* 2005; 175:3463-3468.

Kawabe J, Okumura S, Lee MC, Sadoshima J, Ishikawa Y. Translocation of caveolin regulates stretch-induced ERK activity in vascular smooth muscle cells. *Am J Physiol* 2004; 286:H1845-H1852.

Kawabe J, Ushikubi F, Hasebe N. Prostacyclin in vascular diseases: Recent insight and future perspectives. *Circ J* 2010; 74:936-943.

Kawamura C, Kizaki M, Yamato K, Uchida H, Fukuchi Y et al. Bone Morphogenic protein-2 induces apoptosis in human myeloma cells with modulation of STAT3. *Blood* 2000; 96:2005-2011.

Kawut SM, Horn EM, Berekashvili KK, Widitz AC, Rosezweig EB et al. von Willebrand factor independently predicts long-term survival in patients with pulmonary arterial hypertension. *Chest* 2005; 128:2355-2362

Kümpers P, Nickel N. Lukasz A, Golpon H, Westerkamp V et al. Circulating angiopoietins in idiopathic pulmonary arterial hypertension. *Eur Heart J* 2010; 31:2291-2230.

Lemieux C, Maliba R, Favier J, Théorêt JF, Merhi Y et al. Angiopoietins can directly activate endothelial cells and neutrophils to promote proinflammatory responses. *Blood* 2005; 105:1523-1530.

Lesprit P, Godeau B, Authier FJ, Soubrier M, Zuber M et al. Pulmonary hypertension in POEMS syndrome: a new feature mediated by cytokines. *Am J Respir Crit care Med* 1998; 157:907-911.

Liang OD, Mistialis SA, Chang MS, Vergadi E, Lee C et al. Mesenchymal stromal cells expressing heme oxygensase-1 reverses pulmonary hypertension. *Stem Cells* 2011; 29:99-107.

Lin MI, Yu J, Murata T, Sessa WC. Caveolin-1-deficient mice have increased tumor microvascular permeability, angiogenesis, and growth. *Cancer Res* 2007; 67:2849-2856.

Lobov IB, Brooks PC, Lang RA. Angiopoietin-2 displays VEGF-dependent modulation of capillary structure and endothelial cell survival in vivo. *Proc Natl Acd Sci* 2002; 99:11205-11210.

Long L, MacLean MR, Jeffery TK, Morecroft I, Yang X et al. Serotonin increases susceptibility to pulmonary hypertension in BMPR2-deficeint mice. *Circ Res* 2006; 98:818-827.

Machado R, Aldred MA, James V, Harrison RE, Patel B et al. Mutations of the TGF-β type II receptor BMPR2 in pulmonary arterial hypertension. *Hum Mutation* 2006; 27:121-132.

Masri FA, Xu W, Combair SA, Asosingh K, Koo M et al. Hyperproliferative apoptosis-resistant endothelial cells in idiopathic pulmonary artery hypertension. *Am J Physiol* 2007; 293:L548-L554.

Mathew R, Huang J, Gewitz MH. Hypertension: caveolin-1 and eNOS Interrelationship: a new perspective. *Cardiol Rev* 2007; 15:143-149

Mathew R, Huang J, Katta UD, Krishnan U, Sandoval S et al. Immunosuppressant- induced endothelial damage and pulmonary arterial hypertension. *J Ped Hem Onc* 2011a; 33:55-58.

Mathew R, Huang J, Shah M, Patel K, Gewitz MH et al. Disruption of endothelial cells raft scaffolding during the development of monocrotaline-induced pulmonary hypertension. *Circulation* 101:1499-1506, 2004.

Mathew R. Cell specific dual role of caveolin-1 in pulmonary hypertension. *Pulm Med* 2011b; 2011: 573432

Mathew R. Inflammation and Pulmonary Hypertension. *Cardiol Rev* 2010; 18:67-72, 2010.

McDonald KK, Zharkovit S, Block ER, Kilberg MS. A caveolar complex between the cationic amino acid transporter 1 and endothelial nitric oxide synthase may explain the "arginine paradox". *J Biol Chem* 272:31213-31216, 1997.

McMurtry MS, Moudgil R, Hashimoto K, Bonnet S, Michelakis ED et al. Overexpression of human bone morphogenetic protein receptor 2 does not ameliorate monocrotaline pulmonary arterial hypertension. *Am J Physiol* 2007; 292:L872-L828.

Mechtcheriakova D, Wlachos A, Holzmüller H, Binder BR, Hofer E. Vascular endothelial growth factor–induced tissue factor expression in endothelial cells is modulated by EGR-1. *Blood* 1999; 93:3811-3823.

Mehta D, Malik AB. Signaling mechanisms regulating endothelial permeability. *Physiol Rev* 2006; 86:279-367.

Metcalf DJ, Nightingale TD, Zenner H, Lui-Roberts WW, Cutler DF. Formation and function of Weibel Palade bodies. *J Cell Sci* 2008; 121:19-27.

Mong PY, Wang Q. Activation of Rho Kinase isoforms in lung endothelial cells during inflammation. *J Immunol* 2009; 182:2385-2394.

Muller WA. Mechanisms of trans-endothelial migration of leukocytes. *Circ Res* 2009; 105: 223-230.

Murakami K, Mathew R, Huang J, Farahani R, Peng H et al. Smurf-1 ubiquitin ligase causes downregulation of BMP receptors and is induced in monocrotaline and hypoxia models of pulmonary arterial hypertension. *Expt Biol Med* 2010; 235:805-813.

Murata T, Kinoshita K, Hori M, Kuwahara M, Tsubone H et al. Statin protects endothelial nitric oxide synthase activity in hypoxia-induced pulmonary hypertension. *Arterioscler Thromb Vasc Biol* 2005; 25:2335-2342.

Murata T, Lin MI, Huang Y, Yu J, Bauer PM et al. Reexpression of caveolin-1 in endothelium rescues the vascular, cardiac, and pulmonary defect in global caveolin-1 knockout mice. *J Exp Med* 2007; 204:2373-2382.

Murata T, Sato K, Hori M, Ozaki H, Karaki H. Decreased endothelial nitric oxide synthase (eNOS) activity resulting from abnormal interaction between eNOS and its regulatory proteins in hypoxia induced pulmonary hypertension. *J Biol Chem* 2002; 277:44085-44092.

Ochoa CD, Wu S, Stevens T. New developments in lung endothelial heterogeneity: von Willebrand factor, P-selectin and Weibel Palade body. *Semin Thromb Hemost* 2010; 36:301-308.

Oliver JJ, Webb DJ, Newby DE. Stimulated plasminogen activator release as a marker of endothelial function in humans. *Arterioscl Thromb Vasc Biol* 2005; 25:2470-2479.

Otterdal K, Andreassen AK, Yndestad A, Oie E, Sandberg WJ et al. Raised LIGHT levels in pulmonary arterial hypertension: potential role in thrombus formation. *Am J Respir Crit Care Med* 2008; 117:202-207.

Pae HO, Chung HT. Heme oxygenase -1: its therapeutic roles in inflammatory diseases. *Immune Netw* 2009; 9:12-19.

Patel HH, Zhang S, Murray F, Suda RY, Head BP et al. Increased smooth muscle cell expression of caveolin-1 and caveolae contribute to the pathophysiology of idiopathic pulmonary arterial hypertension. *FASEB J* 2007; 21:2970-2979.

Peterson TE, d'Uscio LV, Cao S, Wang XL, Katusic ZS. Guanosine triphosphate cyclohydrolase 1 expression and enzymatic activity are present in caveolae of endothelial cells. *Hypertension* 2009; 53:189-195.

Raoul W, Wagner-Ballon O, Saber G, Hulin A, Marcos E et al. Effects of bone marrow-derived cells on monocrotaline- and hypoxia-induced pulmonary hypertension in mice. *Respir Res* 2007, 8:8

Rath G, Dessy C, Feron O. Caveolae, caveolin and control of vascular tone: nitric oxide (NO) and endothelium-derived hyperpolarizing factor (EDHF) regulation. *J Physiol Pharmacol* 2009; 60 (suppl 4): 105-109.

Razani B, Wang XB, Engelman JA, Battista M, Lagaud G et al. Caveolin-2 deficient mice show evidence of severe pulmonary dysfunction without disruption of caveolae. *Mol Cell Biol* 2002; 22:2329-2344.

Reynolds AM, Xia W, Holmes MD, Hodges SJ, Danilov S et al. Bone morphogenetic protein type 2 receptor gene therapy attenuates hypoxia pulmonary hypertension. *Am J Physiol* 2009; 292:L1182-L1192.

Reynolds PN. Gene therapy for pulmonary hypertension: prospects and challenges. *Expert Opin Biol Ther* 2011; 11:133-143.

Rhodes CJ, Davidson A, Gibbs JS, Wharton J, Wilkins MR. Therapeutic targets in pulmonary hypertension. *Pharmacol Therap* 2009; 121:69-88.

Russo A, Soh UJ, Paing MM, Arora P, Trejo J. Caveolae are required for protease-selective signaling by protease-activated receptor-1. *Proc Natl Acad Sci* 2009; 106:6393-6397.

Saliez J, Bouzin C, Rath G, Ghisdal P, Desjardin F et al. Role of caveolar compartmentation in endothelium-derived hyperpolarizing factor-mediated relaxation: Ca^{2+} signals and gap junction function are regulated by caveolin in endothelial cells. *Circulation* 2008; 117:1065-1074.

Sanchez O, Marcos E, Perros F, Fadel E, Tu L et al. Role of endothelium–derived CC chemokine ligand 2 in idiopathic pulmonary arterial hypertension. *Am J Resp Crit care Med.* 2007; 176:1041-1047.

Schmidt EP, Damarla M, Rentsendorj O, Servinsky LE, Zhu B et al. Soluble guanylate cyclase contributes to ventilator-induced lung injury in mice. *Am J Physiol* 2008; 295:L1059-L1065.

Schneider DJ, Chen Y, Sobel BE. The effect of plasminogen activator inhibitor type-1 on apoptosis. *Thromb Haemost* 2008; 100:1037-1040.

Schubert W, Frank PG, Woodman SE, Hyogo H, Cohen DE et al. Microvascular hyperpermeability in caveolin-1 (-/-) knockout mice: Treatment with a specific nitric oxide synthase inhibitor L-NAME restores normal microvascular permeability in caveolin-1 null mice. *J Biol Chem* 2002; 277:40091-40098

Sen P, Gopalkrishnan R, Kothari H, Keshava S, Clark CA et al. Factor VIIa bound to endothelial cell protein C receptor activates protease activated receptor-1 and mediates cell signaling and barrier function. *Blood* 2011; 117:3199-3208.

Sessa WC, Garcia-Cardena G, Liu J, Keh A, Pollock JS et al. The golgi association of endothelial nitric oxide synthase is necessary for the efficient synthesis of nitric oxide. *J Biol Chem* 1995; 270:17641-17644.

Shaul PW, Smart EJ, Robinson LJ, Guzman Z, Yuhanna IS et al. Acylation targets eNOS to plasmalemmal caveolae. *J Biol Chem* 1996; 271:6518-6522.

Shovlin CL, Angus G, Manning RA, Okoli GN, Govani S et al. Endothelial cell processing and alternately spliced transcripts of factor VIII: potential implications for coagulation cascade and pulmonary hypertension. *PLoS One* 2010; 5:e9154.

Siddiqui MR, Kamarova YA, Vogel SM, Gao X, Bonini MG et al. Caveolin-1-eNOS signaling promotes p190RhoGAP-A nitration and endothelial permeability. *J Cell Biol* 2011; 193:841-850.

Simonneau G, Galie N, Rubin LJ, Langleben D, Seeger et al. Clinical classification of pulmonary hypertension. *J Am Coll Cardiol* 2004:43:5S-12S.

Sinha B, Köster D, Ruez R , Gonnord P, Bastiani M et al. Cells respond to mechanical stress by rapid disassembly of caveolae. *Cell* 2011; 144:402-413.

Smadja DM, Gaussem P, Mauge L, Lacroix R, Gandrille S et al. Comparison of endothelial biomarkers according to reversibility of pulmonary hypertension secondary to congenital heart disease. *Ped Cardiol* 2010; 31:657-662.

Song Y, Coleman L, Shi J, Beppu H, Sato K et al. Inflammation, endothelial injury and persistent pulmonary hypertension in heterozygous BMPR2 mutant mice. *Am J Physiol* 2008; 295:H677-H690.

Soon E, Holmes AM, Treacy CM, Doughty NJ, Southgate L et al. Elevated levels of inflammatory cytokines predict survival in idiopathic and familial pulmonary arterial hypertension. *Circulation* 2010; 122:920-927.

Spisni E, Griffoni C, Santi S, Riccio M, Marulli R et al. Colocalization of prostacyclin (PGI2) synthase-caveolin-1 in endothelial cells and new roles for PGI2 an angiogenesis. *Expt Cell Res* 2001; 266:31-43.

Starke RD, Ferraro F, Paschalaki KE, Dryden NH, McKinnon TA et al. Endothelial von Willebrand factor regulates angiogenesis. *Blood* 2011; 117:1071-1080.

Stenmark KR, Rabinovitch M. Emerging therapy for the treatment of pulmonary hypertension. *Pediatr Crit Care Med* 2010; 11:S85-S90.

Stitham J, Midgett C, Martin KA, Hwa J. Prostacyclin: an inflammatory paradox. *Front Pharmacol* 2011; 2:24

Taddei A, Giampietro C, Conti A, Orsengo F, Brevario F et al. Endothelial adherens junctions control tight junctions by VE-cadherin-mediated upregulation of claudin-5. *Nat Cell Biol* 2008; 10:923-934.

Teichert-Kuliszewska K, Kutryk MJ, Kuliszewski MA, Karoubi G, Courtman DW et al. Bone morphogenetic protein receptor-2 signaling promotes pulmonary arterial endothelial cell survival. Implication for loss-of-function mutations in the pathogenesis of pulmonary hypertension. *Circ Res* 2006; 98:209-217.

Thibeault S, Rautureau Y, Oubaha M, Faubert D, Wilkes BC et al. S-nitrosylation of β-catenin by eNOS-derived NO promotes VEGF-induced endothelial cell permeability. *Mol Cell* 2010; 39:468-476.

Thomson JR, Machado RD, Pauciulo MW, Morgan NV, Humbert M et al, Sporadic primary pulmonary hypertension is associated with germline mutations of the gene encoding BMPR-II, a receptor member of the TGF-beta family. *J Med Genet* 2000; 37:741-745.

Thurston G, Rudge JS, Ioff E, Zhou H, Ross L et al Angiopoietin-1 protects the adult vasculature against plasma leakage. *Nat Med* 2000; 6:460-463.

Tuder RM, Groves B, Badesch DB, Voelkel NF. Exuberant endothelial cell growth and elements of inflammation are present in plexiform lesions of pulmonary hypertension. *Am J Path* 1994; 144:275-285.

van Buul JD, Kanters E, Hordjik PL. Endothelial signaling by Ig-like cell adhesion molecules. *Arterioscl Thromb Vasc Biol* 2007; 27:1870-1876. .

van Nieuw Amerongen GP, Beckers CM, Achekar ID, Zeeman S, Musters RJ et al. Involvement of Rho kinase in endothelial barrier maintenance. *Arterioscler Thromb Vasc Biol* 2007; 27:2332-2339.

Vriens J, Owsiank G, Fisslthaler B Suzuki M, Janssens A et al. Modulation of Ca^2 permeable cation channel TRPV4 by cytochrome P450 epoxygenases in vascular endothelium. *Circ Res* 2005; 97:908-915.

Wang H, Su Y. Collagen IV contributes to nitric oxide-induced angiogenesis of lung. *Am J Physiol* 2011; 300:C979-C988.

Yu H, Pardoll D, Jove R. STAT3 in cancer, inflammation and immunity: A leading role for STAT3. *Nat Rev Cancer* 2009; 9:798-809.

Yu PB, Deng DY, Beppu H, Hong CC, Lai C et al. Bone morphogenic protein (BMP) type II receptor is required for BMP-mediated growth arrest and differentiation in pulmonary artery smooth muscle cells. *J Biol Chem* 2008; 283:3877-3888.

Zhang XP, Hintze TH. cAMP signal transduction induces eNOS activation by promoting PKB phosphorylation. *Am J Physiol* 2006; 290:H2376-H2384.

Zhao YD, Courtman DW, Deng Y, Kugathasan L, Zhang Q et al. Rescue of monocrotaline-induced pulmonary arterial hypertension using bone marrow-derived endothelial-like progenitor cells. Efficacy of combined cell and eNOS gene therapy in established disease. *Circ Res* 2005; 96:442-450.

Zharikov SI, Block ER. Characterization of L-arginine uptake by plasma membrane vesicles isolated from cultured pulmonary arterial endothelial cells. *Biochim biophys Acta* 1369:173-183, 1998.

Ziche M, Morbidelli L, Choudhari R, Zhang HT, Donnini S et al. Nitric oxide synthase lies downstream from vascular endothelial growth factor-induced but not fibroblast growth factor-induced-angiogenesis. *J Clin Invest* 1997; 99:2625-2634.

2

Interplay Between Serotonin Transporter Signaling and Voltage-Gated Potassium Channel (Kv) 1.5 Expression

Christophe Guignabert
INSERM UMR 999, "Pulmonary Hypertension: Physiopathology and Novel Therapies", Le Plessis-Robinson, France

1. Introduction

The exact mechanisms of pulmonary arterial remodeling that lead to the onset and progression of pulmonary arterial hypertension (PAH) are still largely unclear. However, many disease-predisposing factors and/or contributing factors have been identified, including inflammation, endothelial cell dysfunction, aberrant vascular wall cell proliferation and mutations in the *bone morphogenetic protein receptor type II (BMPRII)* gene (Humbert *et al.*, 2004; Mandegar *et al.*, 2004; Chapman *et al.*, 2008; Rabinovitch, 2008; Hassoun *et al.*, 2009; Morrell *et al.*, 2009). During the last few years, the serotoninergic system and voltage-gated potassium (Kv) channels have attracted special attention and substantial evidence now supports a close relationship between them in the physiopathology of PAH.

2. The serotoninergic system in the pathogenesis of PAH

Serotonin (5-hydroxytryptamine or 5-HT) and its transporter (SERT or 5-HTT) have long been suspected of playing important roles in the pathogenesis of idiopathic PAH and have, for several reasons, been tightly linked to its etiology. 5-HT is an endogenous vasoactive indolamine found mainly in enterochromaffin tissue, brain and blood platelets. It promotes pulmonary arterial smooth muscle cell (PA-SMC) proliferation, pulmonary arterial vasoconstriction and local microthrombosis. Plasma 5-HT levels are elevated in patients with PAH and remain high even after lung transplantation, indicating that this condition is not secondary to the disease (Herve *et al.*, 1995). 5-HTT belongs to a large family of integral membrane proteins and is responsible for 5-HT uptake (e.g., by platelets, endothelial and vascular SMCs). Analysis of distal pulmonary arteries of patients with PAH and their cultured PA-SMCs indicates that 5-HTT is overexpressed and that the level of expression correlates with PAH severity (Eddahibi *et al.*, 2001; Eddahibi *et al.*, 2002; Marcos *et al.*, 2004; Marcos *et al.*, 2005). Tryptophan hydroxylase (TPH), the rate-limiting enzyme in 5-HT biosynthesis, is also expressed at abnormally high levels in pulmonary endothelial cells from patients with idiopathic PAH, and therefore raises 5-HT levels locally (Eddahibi *et al.*, 2006). There is evidence that alterations in platelet 5-HT storage and/or increased platelet consumption by the lung may trigger the development of PAH (Herve *et al.*, 1990; Herve *et al.*, 1995; Breuer *et al.*, 1996; Eddahibi *et al.*, 2000b; Kereveur *et al.*, 2000; Morecroft *et al.*, 2005). Furthermore, serotoninergic appetite suppressant drugs have been associated with an increased risk of developing PAH (Douglas *et al.*, 1981; Gurtner, 1985; Loogen *et al.*, 1985; Brenot *et al.*, 1993; Abenhaim *et al.*, 1996; Souza *et al.*, 2008). Additionally, studies on animal models of pulmonary hypertension consolidate all these observations obtained from human subjects. Plasma 5-HT levels are elevated not only in rodents treated with the anorectic agent dexfenfluramine (Eddahibi *et al.*, 1998), but also in the progression of monocrotaline- and chronic hypoxia-induced pulmonary hypertension. The chronic infusion of exogenous 5-HT via osmotic pumps can potentiate the development of PH in rats exposed to chronic hypoxia (Eddahibi *et al.*, 1997). A bone morphogenetic protein type II receptor (BMPR-II) deficiency increases susceptibility to PH induced by 5-HT in mice (Long *et al.*, 2006). In the fawn-hooded rat, a strain with a genetic deficit in platelet 5-HT storage that causes elevated plasma 5-HT concentrations, PH develops when the animals are exposed to mild hypoxia but not in control rats (Sato *et al.*, 1992). An abnormally high level of 5-HTT in the lungs was reported for fawn-hooded rats (Sato *et al.*, 1992; Morecroft *et al.*, 2005). Furthermore, rodents engineered to constitutively express angiopoietin 1 in the lung develop PH. This effect was found to be directly related to the elevated production and secretion of 5-HT by stimulated pulmonary endothelial cells (Sullivan *et al.*, 2003). It has also been shown in the monocrotaline model that 5-HTT expression levels increased prior to the onset of PH, which strongly supports a role for 5-HTT overexpression in disease development (Guignabert *et al.*, 2005). Treatment with selective serotonin reuptake inhibitors (e.g. fluoxetine) abrogates the disease in chronically hypoxic mice and rats with monocrotaline-induced PH (Li *et al.*, ; Wang *et al.*, ; Marcos *et al.*, 2003; Guignabert *et al.*, 2005; Guignabert *et al.*, 2009; Zhai *et al.*, 2009; Zhu *et al.*, 2009). Furthermore, mice carrying null mutations at the 5-HTT locus are protected from developing PH induced by prolonged hypoxia (Eddahibi *et al.*, 2000a). Similarly, hypoxia-induced PH in mice lacking the *tph1* gene, which exhibit marked reductions in 5-HT synthesis rates and contents in their peripheral organs, was less severe than in wild-type mice (Izikki *et al.*, 2007).

More recently, direct evidence that elevated levels of *5-HTT* gene expression can promote pulmonary vascular remodeling and spontaneous PH was obtained with the creation of two different types of transgenic mice: (1) SM22 5-HTT+ mice that selectively express the human *5-HTT* gene in smooth muscle at levels close to that found in human idiopathic PAH; and (2) SERT+ mice that ubiquitously express high levels of the human *5-HTT* gene from a yeast artificial chromosome (YAC) construct. SM22 5-HTT+ mice undergo pulmonary vascular remodeling, develop PH and exhibit marked increases in right ventricular systolic pressures (RVSPs), right ventricular hypertrophy (RVH), and muscularization of pulmonary arterioles (Figure 1). One major point is that PH in these mice developed without any alterations in 5-HT bioavailibility, and therefore occurred as a sole consequence of the increased 5-HTT protein levels in SMCs. Compared to wild-type mice, SM22 5-HTT+ mice exhibited increases of three- to four-fold in lung 5-HTT mRNA & protein, together with increased lung 5-HT uptake activity. However, there were no changes in platelet 5-HTT activity or blood 5-HT levels. PH worsened as the SM22 5-HTT+ mice grew older (Guignabert *et al.*, 2006). Consistent with these observations, female SERT+ mice housed in normoxic conditions developed a three-fold increase in RVSP values compared to those of their wild-type controls (MacLean *et al.*, 2004).

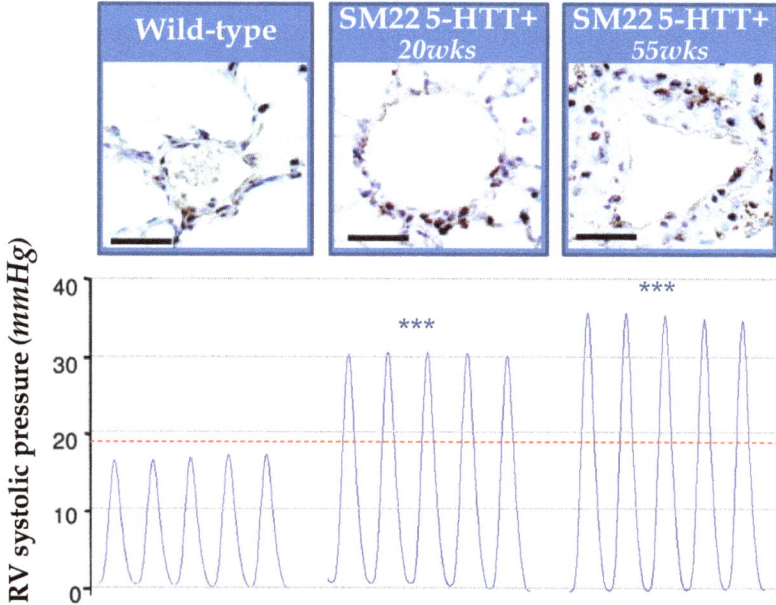

Fig. 1. Development of pulmonary hypertension and vascular remodeling in SM22 5-HTT+ mice versus wild-type mice at 20 and 55 weeks of age under normoxic conditions. Right ventricular systolic pressure and representative pictures of in situ cell proliferation in muscularized vessels, shown by proliferating cell nuclear antigen (PCNA) immunohistochemistry.
Scale bar = 50 μm.

Of the fourteen distinct 5-HT receptors, the 5-HT-2A, -2B, and -1B receptors are particularly relevant to the pathogenesis of PAH. High levels of 5-HT-1B, -2A, and -2B receptor immunoreactivity were reported in remodeled pulmonary arteries from patients with various forms of pulmonary hypertension, but only the 5-HTT was found to be overexpressed in pulmonary artery smooth muscle cells (Marcos *et al.*, 2005). Several lines of evidence support the notion that functional interactions exist between some of these 5-HT receptors and 5-HTT, and thus have encouraged studies to better understand these complex relationships (Lawrie *et al.*, 2005; Launay *et al.*, 2006). Antagonism of the 5-HT-2A receptor inhibits not only monocrotaline-induced pulmonary ypertension in mice (Hironaka *et al.*, 2003) but also the 5-HT-induced pulmonary vasoconstriction in vessels from normoxic and hypoxic rats (Morecroft *et al.*, 2005; Cogolludo *et al.*, 2006). However, the 5HT-2A receptor antagonist ketanserin is not specific for pulmonary circulation, and systemic effects have limited its use in PAH (Frishman *et al.*, 1995). 5-HT-2B knockout mice are resistant to hypoxia-induced pulmonary hypertension and administration of the specific 5-HT-2B receptor antagonist RS-127445 prevented an increase in pulmonary arterial pressure in mice challenged with hypoxia (Launay *et al.*, 2002). Furthermore, the 5-HT-2B receptor may control 5-HT plasma levels *in vivo* (Callebert *et al.*, 2006), and its functional loss may predispose humans to fenfluramine-associated PAH (Blanpain *et al.*, 2003). A very recent study showed that terguride, a potent 5-HT-2A/5-HT-2B receptor antagonist, inhibits the proliferative effects of 5-HT on PA-SMCs and prevents the development and progression of monocrotaline-induced PH in rats (Dumitrascu *et al.*). The 5-HT-1B receptor mediates 5-HT-induced constriction in human pulmonary arteries (Morecroft *et al.*, 1999), and has been shown to be involved in the development of PH in rodents exposed to chronic hypoxia (Keegan *et al.*, 2001). Recently, Morecroft et al. have reported that co-inhibition of the 5-HT-1B receptor and 5-HTT with a combined 5-HT-1B receptor/5-HTT antagonist (LY393558) is effective at preventing and reversing experimental PH in animal models and 5-HT-induced proliferation in PA-SMCs derived from idiopathic PAH patients.

3. Expression and activity of the Kv1.5 channel in the pathogenesis of PAH

Potassium ion (K[+]) channels play a crucial role in the immediate and long-term regulation of vascular smooth muscle function. They are integral membrane proteins that allow the selective passage of K[+] across biological membranes. Their activity determines and regulates cell membrane potential, which in turn, regulates the open state probability of voltage-gated calcium ion (Ca[2+]) channels, Ca[2+] influx, and intracellular Ca[2+] levels. The increase in cytoplasmic free Ca[2+] concentration in SMCs is an important trigger for cell contraction but also a stimulus for pulmonary SMC proliferation. Among the different types of K[+] channels, Kv channels are expressed at high levels in most vascular SMCs and are regarded as a major determinant of vascular tone and resting membrane potential (Post *et al.*, 1995; Yuan, 1995; Evans *et al.*, 1996; Ko *et al.*, 2008). There are four major families of Kv channels, Kv1.x to Kv4.x, with two to eight members in each family. Differential distribution of Kv channels exists in several types of SMCs and this contributes to the large functional diversity that has been noted for native Kv currents in different myocytes (Archer *et al.*, 1996; Coppock & Tamkun, 2001). Although Kv1.2, Kv1.5, Kv2.1, Kv3.1b and Kv9.3 play important roles in the hypoxia-inhibited K+ current found in PA-SMCs, much attention has been attracted by the Kv1.5 channel (Archer *et al.*, 1993; Archer *et al.*, 1996; Patel *et al.*, 1997; Archer *et al.*, 1998; Osipenko *et al.*, 2000; Archer *et al.*, 2001; Coppock *et al.*, 2001; Coppock & Tamkun, 2001; Archer & Michelakis, 2002; Archer *et al.*, 2004a; Guignabert *et al.*, 2009). In addition to hypoxia, endothelin-1, thromboxane A2, 5-HT, and anorectic drugs have been shown to inhibit Kv currents in PA-SMCs (Weir *et al.*, 1996; Archer *et al.*, 1998; Cogolludo *et al.*, 2003; Cogolludo *et al.*, 2006). Kv1.5 is widely represented in the cardiovascular system (Overturf *et al.*, 1994). In the human heart, the Kv1.5 channel is expressed predominantly in the atrial myocardium and is responsible for the ultra-rapid component of the delayed rectifier K[+] current, IKur (Fedida *et al.*, 1993; Wang *et al.*, 1993; Gaborit *et al.*, 2007). A familial form of atrial fibrillation has been attributed to a loss-of-function mutation in the *Kv1.5* gene (Olson *et al.*, 2006). It is also expressed in the human ventricle where it possibly contributes to the K[+] current through formation of hetero-multimeric K+ channels with other Kv-alpha subunits (Mays *et al.*, 1995). In the human lung, Kv1.5 was shown to be expressed in SMCs, endothelial cells, macrophages, and dendritic cells. Importantly, the expression levels of Kv1.5 channel proteins are higher in distal pulmonary arteries than in proximal pulmonary arteries, thus making its involvement in PAH disease an attractive possibility (Archer *et al.*, 2004b).

Low levels of *Kv1.5* gene expression and channel activity are hallmarks of human and experimental PH, including the chronic-hypoxia and monocrotaline models (Yuan *et al.*, 1998a; Yuan *et al.*, 1998b; Reeve *et al.*, 2001; McMurtry *et al.*, 2004; McMurtry *et al.*, 2005; Bonnet *et al.*, 2006; Guignabert *et al.*, 2006; Young *et al.*, 2006; Remillard *et al.*, 2007; Archer *et al.*, 2008; Guignabert *et al.*, 2009). However, the underlying mechanism of Kv1.5 in PH pathology remains unclear even though there has been significant progress made in understanding how the expression of its gene is regulated. A variety of transcriptional factors, such as HIF-1α (Bonnet *et al.*, 2006), c-Jun (Yu *et al.*, 2001), a signal-transducing transcription factor of the AP-1 family, and nuclear factor of activated T cells (NFAT) (Guignabert *et al.*, 2009) are involved in *Kv1.5* gene regulation. Several single nucleotide polymorphisms (SNPs) in the *Kv1.5* gene of idiopathic PAH patients have been reported, and these SNPs may correlate with altered *Kv1.5* gene expression or protein function in PA-SMCs (Remillard *et al.*, 2007). Restoring *Kv1.5* gene expression to normal levels in rats reduces PH induced by chronic hypoxia and restores hypoxic pulmonary vasoconstriction (Pozeg *et al.*, 2003). Taken together, all these observations strongly support the hypothesis that Kv1.5 channel dysfunction and gene down-regulation represent predisposing factors that may operate in conjunction with other factors and/or genetic defects.

4. Connections between serotonin transporter signaling and Kv1.5 channel expression

During the last few years, direct evidence for a molecular interplay between 5-HTT signaling and Kv1.5 expression/activity has emerged. Exogenous 5-HT has been shown to reduce Kv1.5 mRNA levels in cultured human PA-SMCs, an effect totally abolished by a selective 5-HTT antagonist fluoxetine (Guignabert *et al.*, 2006). In normal rat PA-SMCs and in Ltk− cells stably transfected with the human *Kv1.5* gene, Kv currents were inhibited by 5-HT via activation of the 5-HT-2A receptor (Cogolludo *et al.*, 2006). Compared to wild-type mice, SM22 5-HTT+ mice exhibited a marked decrease in the levels of the Kv1.5 channel protein in the lung (Figure 2), but no changes in the levels of expression in the lung were detected for endothelin-1, Tie2 receptor, prostacyclin synthase, or members of the bone morphogenetic protein (BMP) pathway (BMP-RII, BMP-RIA, BMP-RIB, BMP-2, and BMP-4). Furthermore, SM22 5-HTT+ mice show depressed hypoxic pulmonary vasoconstriction and greater severity to hypoxia- or monocrotaline-induced PH (Guignabert *et al.*, 2006). In contrast, 5-HTT knockout mice exhibit a potentiation of acute hypoxic hypoxic pulmonary vasoconstriction (Eddahibi *et al.*, 2000a).

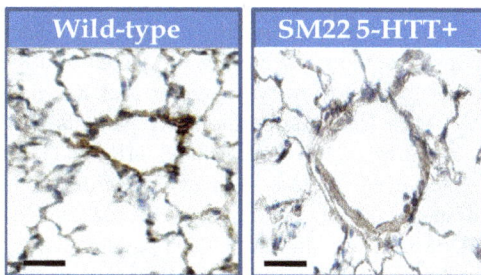

Fig. 2. Kv1.5 expression is lower in the lung tissues of SM22 5-HTT+ mice than in the lungs of wild-type mice.
A representative immunohistochemistry slide shows strong Kv1.5 staining in the SMCs of distal pulmonary arteries from wild-type mice and weak staining in the arterial SMCs of SM22 5-HTT+ mice.
Scale bar= 50 μm.

A recent study has provided the first evidence that 5-HT, via 5-HTT, decreases Kv1.5 expression by inhibiting nuclear NFATc2 translocation *in vitro* & *in vivo* (Guignabert et al., 2009). In the first part of this study, chronic dichloroacetate administration (an inducer of Kv1.5 expression, apoptosis, and depolarization of mitochondrial membranes) vs. saline limited the progression of pulmonary vascular remodeling and PH in SM22 5-HTT+ mice by progressively and markedly reducing hemodynamic values, right ventricular hypertrophy and the pulmonary vessel remodeling. Furthermore, oral fluoxetine (a selective 5-HTT antagonist) therapy totally reversed the established PH in these mice. Interestingly, the authors found that Kv1.5 expression progressively normalized in the lungs of SM22 5-HTT+ mice treated with either dichloroacetate or fluoxetine, which contrasted with the persistently low levels of Kv1.5 expression detected in control SM22 5-HTT+ mice treated with vehicle (Figure 3).

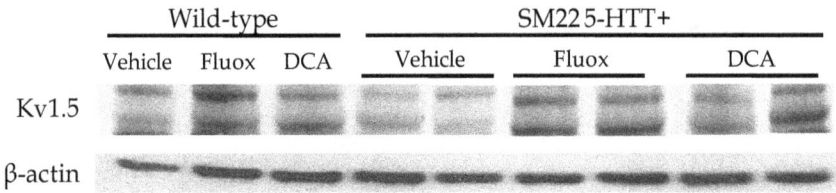

Fig. 3. Changes in Kv1.5 expression in the lungs of SM22 5-HTT+ and wild-type mice treated for 21 days with dichloroacetate (DCA; 80 mg/kg/day) or fluoxetine (Fluox; 10 mg/kg/day) or vehicle (saline).
Representative western blots of Kv1.5 and β-actin proteins in SM22 5-HTT+ and wild-type mice treated with an active drug or vehicle.

Due to the finding that dichloroacetate upregulated Kv1.5 expression by an NFAT-dependent mechanism (Bonnet et al., 2007b) and to the demonstrated interrelationships between 5-HT signaling, Ca^{2+}/calcineurin signaling activation, and cardiac muscle cell hypertrophy (Bush et al., 2004), the hypothesis that NFAT may be a major molecular link between 5-HTT signalling and Kv1.5 expression/activity was tested. Consistent with this theory, 5-HT treatment of human PA-SMCs *in vitro* induced significant nuclear translocation of NFATc2, which led to a subsequent and significant decrease in Kv1.5 protein expression (Figure 4). NFATc2 nuclear translocation was greater and Kv1.5 protein expression was significantly lower in PA-SMCs from idiopathic PAH patients than in control PA-SMCs under basal conditions. In addition, dichloroacetate, 11R-VIVIT (a selective inhibitor of NFAT translocation), cycloporine A (an indirect inhibitor of NFAT activation) and fluoxetine markedly inhibited the elevated nuclear NFATc2 translocation and normalized the low Kv1.5 levels in PA-SMCs from idiopathic PAH patients (Guignabert et al., 2009).

In addition, Guignabert et al. also clearly showed by [^{3}H]-thymidine incorporation that dichloroacetate (5×10^{-4} M), 11R-VIVIT (4×10^{-6} M), cycloporine A (10^{-6} M) and fluoxetine (10^{-6} M) markedly inhibited the growth of PA-SMCs from idiopathic PAH patients and the growth of normal PA-SMCs treated with the highest dose of 5-HT (10^{-6} M). All these *in vitro* findings confirm and extend previous evidence obtained by Bonnet et al. (Bonnet et al., 2007b) and clearly demonstrated that NFAT serves as a link between 5-HTT activation and Kv1.5 downregulation.

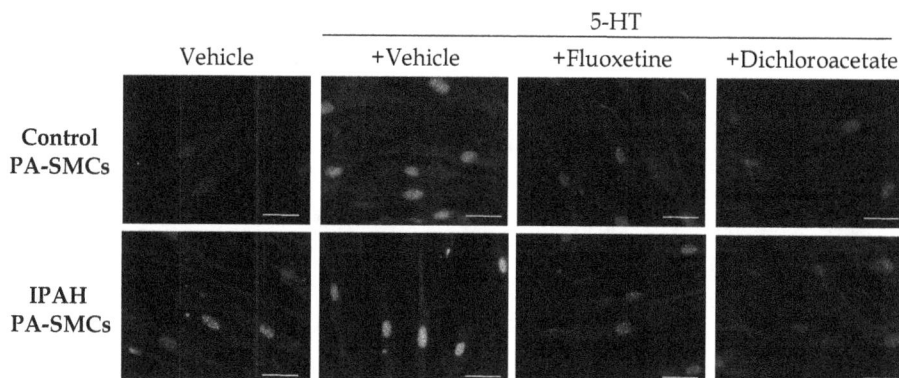

Fig. 4. Representative micrographs showing immunoreactivity for the active form of NFAT in cultured PA-SMCs isolated from patients with idiopathic PAH (IPAH PA-SMCs) and normal subjects (Control PA-SMCs) treated with serotonin (10^{-6} M) or vehicle (phosphate buffered saline or PBS) with or without one of the following: PBS, fluoxetine (10^{-6} M), or dichloroacetate (5×10^{-4} M).
Scale bar= 20 μm.

Furthermore, an abnormal level of activated NFAT was found in the lungs of SM22 5-HTT+ mice, which gradually decreased over time with oral dichloroacetate and fluoxetine therapy. To further study the importance of NFAT activation and its downstream effects on disease progression, separate experiments were performed in SM22 5-HTT+ and wild-type mice with an indirect inhibitor of NFAT, the calcineurin inhibitor: cyclosporine A (1 mg/kg/day, *per os*, daily for three weeks). Cyclosporine A treatment reduced the pulmonary levels of active NFAT and increased Kv1.5 protein levels in SM22 5-HTT+ mice, but yielded no beneficial effects on pulmonary hemodynamics or arterial structures. In contrast, a similar cyclosporine A treatment for two weeks partially reversed monocrotaline-induced PH in rats (Bonnet *et al.*, 2007b). Several possible explanations have been proposed for this discrepancy. First, NFAT regulates many cytokines known to be central in the pathogenesis of PAH (Macian, 2005), and inflammation is an important component of PAH in the monocrotaline rat model but not in SM22 5-HTT+ mice. Second, normalization of Kv1.5 expression in vitro neither completely inhibited PA-SMC proliferation induced by 5-HT nor completely abolished the differences between idiopathic PAH and control PA-SMCs. These observations suggest that inhibition of NFAT activation alone was not sufficient to counteract all the effects induced by 5-HT via its transporter in SM22 5-HTT+ mice, which exhibit constant and sustained 5-HTT activation in SMCs. Such activation induces cellular proliferation by activating several other intracellular signal transduction pathways (Figure 5), including: tyrosine phosphorylation of GTPase-activating protein (Lee *et al.*, 1997), rapid formation of superoxide (O); and activation of Rho/Rho kinase (ROCK) (Liu *et al.*, 2004; Guilluy *et al.*, 2009), extracellular signal-regulated kinase 1 (ERK1)/ERK2, and mitogen-activated protein (MAP) kinase (Lee *et al.*, 1998; Lee *et al.*, 2001). Intracellular accumulation of 5-HT has also been found to interact with other intracellular signal transduction pathways including the transcription factor GATA-4 (Suzuki *et al.*, 2003; Lawrie *et al.*, 2005), the platelet-derived growth factor receptor (PDGF-R) (Ren *et al.*, ; Liu *et al.*, 2007), and the serine/threonine protein kinase, Akt (Liu & Fanburg, 2006).

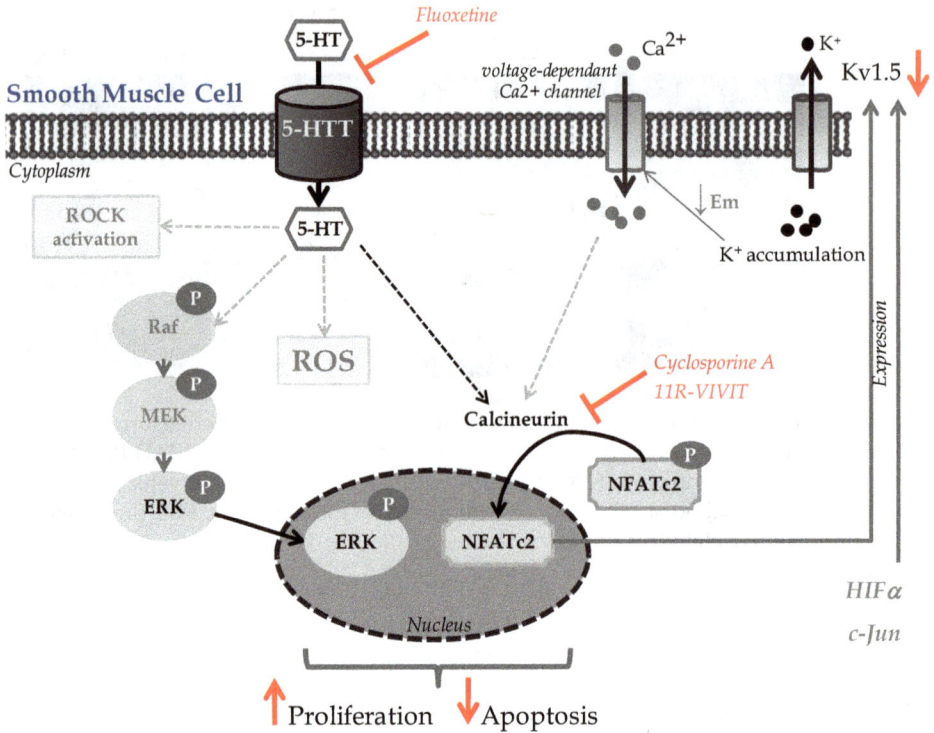

Fig. 5. Diagram of the link between 5-HTT activation and Kv1.5 downregulation. Intracellular accumulation of 5-HT induces arterial SMC proliferation via activation of several intracellular signal transduction pathways, including reactive oxygen species (ROS) production and activation of Rho-kinase (ROCK), which lead to phosphorylation and nuclear translocation of extracellular-regulated kinase 1 (ERK1)/2 and to dephosphorylation and nuclear translocation of NFATc2. NFATc2 remains in the cytoplasm when phosphorylated. Following intracellular accumulation of 5-HT or activation by calcium (Ca^{2+}), NFAT is dephosphorylated by the phosphatase calcineurin. Once in the nucleus, NFATc2 can regulate gene expression in coordination with ERK, leading to Kv1.5 downregulation and changes in the balance between proliferation and apoptosis.

In contrast to cyclosporine A, dichloroacetate elicits a wide spectrum of beneficial effects able to ameliorate dysfunctions related to abnormal NFAT activation, production of reactive oxygen species, fragmentation and/or hyperpolarization of the mitochondrial reticulum, and changes in the apoptosis/proliferation ratio (Bonnet et al., 2007a; Archer et al., 2008; Michelakis et al., 2008). In addition, dichloroacetate treatment led to rapid and marked decreases in anti-apoptotic factor B-Cell Lymphoma 2 (BCL2) expression and in the BCL2/Bax ratio compared to vehicle, which suggests that down-regulation of BCL2 by dichloroacetate might be an important mechanism in the reversal of pulmonary vascular remodeling in SM22 5-HTT+ mice and chronic hypoxia- or monocrotaline-induced pulmonary hypertension.

In addition to the effects of intracellular accumulation of 5-HT, activation of HIF-1α and c-Jun are two other major drivers of Kv1.5 down-regulation (Yu *et al.*, 2001; Bonnet *et al.*, 2006). c-Jun is a nuclear protein that serves as a nuclear signal transduction intermediate in cell growth and differentiation. Overexpression of c-Jun downregulates expression of Kv1.5 and upregulates expression of the β-subunit (Kvß2) in PA-SMCs (Yu *et al.*, 2001). Thus, c-Jun modulates Kv current, influences the resting membrane potential and affects the SMC proliferation. Abnormal activation of HIF-1α has been reported in the PA-SMCs of patients with idiopathic PAH and in those from fawn-hooded rats. Inhibition of HIF-1α restores Kv1.5 expression and normalizes Kv current in experimental PH (Bonnet *et al.*, 2006). The presence of an evolutionarily conserved and functional consensus NFAT binding site in the HIF-1α promoter at position 728 bp suggests that NFAT and HIF-1α, either individually or via cooperative effects, are also two key players in Kv1.5 down-regulation (Walczak-Drzewiecka *et al.*, 2008). In addition to the serotoninergic system, other NFAT activators have been identified that include the transcription factor signal transducer and activator of transcription 3 (STAT3), peroxisome proliferator-activated receptor γ (PPARγ), Pim1, vasoactive intestinal peptide (VIP) and miR-204 (Courboulin *et al.*, ; Paulin *et al.*, ; Bao *et al.*, 2008; Said, 2008).

5. Conclusion

In summary, multiple downstream signaling pathways are activated following 5-HTT activation and a better understanding of this complex network of interactions will be crucial for developing methods to limit its potential pathogenic role. Recent evidence has demonstrated that 5-HTT activation and Kv1.5 downregulation are connected via a NFAT-dependent mechanism (Guignabert *et al.*, 2009). Although chronic dichloroacetate, cyclosporine A or fluoxetine administration returned the Kv1.5 level to normal in SM22 5-HTT+ mice, only dichloroacetate and fluoxetine treatments substantially diminished pulmonary artery pressure, right ventricular hypertrophy, and pulmonary arterial muscularization in this experimental model. These findings suggest that inhibition of NFAT alone with cyclosporine A is not sufficient to counteract all the effects induced by 5-HT via its transporter. Thus, pharmacological inhibition of the upstream components of the serotoninergic pathway or the use of dichloroacetate with pleiotropic effects are very attractive as therapeutic strategies for treating pulmonary hypertension.

6. Acknowledgments

The author thanks Saadia Eddahibi, Marc Humbert, Elie Fadel, Michel Hamon, Serge Adnot, Bernard Maître, Gerald Simonneau, and Phillipe Hervé for valuable discussions.

7. References

Abenhaim L, Moride Y, Brenot F, Rich S, Benichou J, Kurz X, Higenbottam T, Oakley C, Wouters E, Aubier M, Simonneau G & Begaud B (1996) Appetite-suppressant drugs and the risk of primary pulmonary hypertension. International Primary Pulmonary Hypertension Study Group. *N Engl J Med* 335, 609-616.

Archer S & Michelakis E (2002) The mechanism(s) of hypoxic pulmonary vasoconstriction: potassium channels, redox O(2) sensors, and controversies. *News Physiol Sci* 17, 131-137.

Archer SL, Gomberg-Maitland M, Maitland ML, Rich S, Garcia JG & Weir EK (2008) Mitochondrial metabolism, redox signaling, and fusion: a mitochondria-ROS-HIF-1alpha-Kv1.5 O2-sensing pathway at the intersection of pulmonary hypertension and cancer. *Am J Physiol Heart Circ Physiol* 294, H570-578.

Archer SL, Huang J, Henry T, Peterson D & Weir EK (1993) A redox-based O2 sensor in rat pulmonary vasculature. *Circ Res* 73, 1100-1112.

Archer SL, Huang JM, Reeve HL, Hampl V, Tolarova S, Michelakis E & Weir EK (1996) Differential distribution of electrophysiologically distinct myocytes in conduit and resistance arteries determines their response to nitric oxide and hypoxia. *Circ Res* 78, 431-442.

Archer SL, London B, Hampl V, Wu X, Nsair A, Puttagunta L, Hashimoto K, Waite RE & Michelakis ED (2001) Impairment of hypoxic pulmonary vasoconstriction in mice lacking the voltage-gated potassium channel Kv1.5. *Faseb J* 15, 1801-1803.

Archer SL, Souil E, Dinh-Xuan AT, Schremmer B, Mercier JC, El Yaagoubi A, Nguyen-Huu L, Reeve HL & Hampl V (1998) Molecular identification of the role of voltage-gated K+ channels, Kv1.5 and Kv2.1, in hypoxic pulmonary vasoconstriction and control of resting membrane potential in rat pulmonary artery myocytes. *J Clin Invest* 101, 2319-2330.

Archer SL, Wu XC, Thebaud B, Moudgil R, Hashimoto K & Michelakis ED (2004a) O2 sensing in the human ductus arteriosus: redox-sensitive K+ channels are regulated by mitochondria-derived hydrogen peroxide. *Biol Chem* 385, 205-216.

Archer SL, Wu XC, Thebaud B, Nsair A, Bonnet S, Tyrrell B, McMurtry MS, Hashimoto K, Harry G & Michelakis ED (2004b) Preferential expression and function of voltage-gated, O2-sensitive K+ channels in resistance pulmonary arteries explains regional heterogeneity in hypoxic pulmonary vasoconstriction: ionic diversity in smooth muscle cells. *Circ Res* 95, 308-318.

Bao Y, Li R, Jiang J, Cai B, Gao J, Le K, Zhang F, Chen S & Liu P (2008) Activation of peroxisome proliferator-activated receptor gamma inhibits endothelin-1-induced cardiac hypertrophy via the calcineurin/NFAT signaling pathway. *Mol Cell Biochem* 317, 189-196.

Blanpain C, Le Poul E, Parma J, Knoop C, Detheux M, Parmentier M, Vassart G & Abramowicz MJ (2003) Serotonin 5-HT(2B) receptor loss of function mutation in a patient with fenfluramine-associated primary pulmonary hypertension. *Cardiovasc Res* 60, 518-528.

Bonnet S, Archer SL, Allalunis-Turner J, Haromy A, Beaulieu C, Thompson R, Lee CT, Lopaschuk GD, Puttagunta L, Bonnet S, Harry G, Hashimoto K, Porter CJ, Andrade MA, Thebaud B & Michelakis ED (2007a) A mitochondria-K+ channel axis is suppressed in cancer and its normalization promotes apoptosis and inhibits cancer growth. *Cancer Cell* 11, 37-51.

Bonnet S, Michelakis ED, Porter CJ, Andrade-Navarro MA, Thebaud B, Bonnet S, Haromy A, Harry G, Moudgil R, McMurtry MS, Weir EK & Archer SL (2006) An abnormal mitochondrial-hypoxia inducible factor-1alpha-Kv channel pathway disrupts oxygen sensing and triggers pulmonary arterial hypertension in fawn hooded rats: similarities to human pulmonary arterial hypertension. *Circulation* 113, 2630-2641.

Bonnet S, Rochefort G, Sutendra G, Archer SL, Haromy A, Webster L, Hashimoto K, Bonnet SN & Michelakis ED (2007b) The nuclear factor of activated T cells in pulmonary arterial hypertension can be therapeutically targeted. *Proc Natl Acad Sci U S A* 104, 11418-11423.

Brenot F, Herve P, Petitpretz P, Parent F, Duroux P & Simonneau G (1993) Primary pulmonary hypertension and fenfluramine use. *Br Heart J* 70, 537-541.

Breuer J, Georgaraki A, Sieverding L, Baden W & Apitz J (1996) Increased turnover of serotonin in children with pulmonary hypertension secondary to congenital heart disease. *Pediatr Cardiol* 17, 214-219.

Bush E, Fielitz J, Melvin L, Martinez-Arnold M, McKinsey TA, Plichta R & Olson EN (2004) A small molecular activator of cardiac hypertrophy uncovered in a chemical screen for modifiers of the calcineurin signaling pathway. *Proc Natl Acad Sci U S A* 101, 2870-2875.

Callebert J, Esteve JM, Herve P, Peoc'h K, Tournois C, Drouet L, Launay JM & Maroteaux L (2006) Evidence for a control of plasma serotonin levels by 5-hydroxytryptamine(2B) receptors in mice. *J Pharmacol Exp Ther* 317, 724-731.

Chapman ME, Taylor RL & Wideman RF, Jr. (2008) Analysis of plasma serotonin levels and hemodynamic responses following chronic serotonin infusion in broilers challenged with bacterial lipopolysaccharide and microparticles. *Poult Sci* 87, 116-124.

Cogolludo A, Moreno L, Bosca L, Tamargo J & Perez-Vizcaino F (2003) Thromboxane A2-induced inhibition of voltage-gated K+ channels and pulmonary vasoconstriction: role of protein kinase Czeta. *Circ Res* 93, 656-663.

Cogolludo A, Moreno L, Lodi F, Frazziano G, Cobeno L, Tamargo J & Perez-Vizcaino F (2006) Serotonin inhibits voltage-gated K+ currents in pulmonary artery smooth muscle cells: role of 5-HT2A receptors, caveolin-1, and KV1.5 channel internalization. *Circ Res* 98, 931-938.

Coppock EA, Martens JR & Tamkun MM (2001) Molecular basis of hypoxia-induced pulmonary vasoconstriction: role of voltage-gated K+ channels. *Am J Physiol Lung Cell Mol Physiol* 281, L1-12.

Coppock EA & Tamkun MM (2001) Differential expression of K(V) channel alpha- and beta-subunits in the bovine pulmonary arterial circulation. *Am J Physiol Lung Cell Mol Physiol* 281, L1350-1360.

Courboulin A, Paulin R, Giguere NJ, Saksouk N, Perreault T, Meloche J, Paquet ER, Biardel S, Provencher S, Cote J, Simard MJ & Bonnet S Role for miR-204 in human pulmonary arterial hypertension. *J Exp Med* 208, 535-548.

Douglas JG, Munro JF, Kitchin AH, Muir AL & Proudfoot AT (1981) Pulmonary hypertension and fenfluramine. *Br Med J (Clin Res Ed)* 283, 881-883.

Dumitrascu R, Kulcke C, Konigshoff M, Kouri F, Yang X, Morrell N, Ghofrani HA, Weissmann N, Reiter R, Seeger W, Grimminger F, Eickelberg O, Schermuly RT & Pullamsetti SS Terguride ameliorates monocrotaline induced pulmonary hypertension in rats. *Eur Respir J*.

Eddahibi S, Guignabert C, Barlier-Mur AM, Dewachter L, Fadel E, Dartevelle P, Humbert M, Simonneau G, Hanoun N, Saurini F, Hamon M & Adnot S (2006) Cross talk between endothelial and smooth muscle cells in pulmonary hypertension: critical role for serotonin-induced smooth muscle hyperplasia. *Circulation* 113, 1857-1864.

Eddahibi S, Hanoun N, Lanfumey L, Lesch KP, Raffestin B, Hamon M & Adnot S (2000a) Attenuated hypoxic pulmonary hypertension in mice lacking the 5-hydroxytryptamine transporter gene. *J Clin Invest* 105, 1555-1562.

Eddahibi S, Humbert M, Fadel E, Raffestin B, Darmon M, Capron F, Simonneau G, Dartevelle P, Hamon M & Adnot S (2001) Serotonin transporter overexpression is responsible for pulmonary artery smooth muscle hyperplasia in primary pulmonary hypertension. *J Clin Invest* 108, 1141-1150.

Eddahibi S, Humbert M, Fadel E, Raffestin B, Darmon M, Capron F, Simonneau G, Dartevelle P, Hamon M & Adnot S (2002) Hyperplasia of pulmonary artery smooth muscle cells is causally related to overexpression of the serotonin transporter in primary pulmonary hypertension. *Chest* 121, 97S-98S.

Eddahibi S, Humbert M, Sediame S, Chouaid C, Partovian C, Maitre B, Teiger E, Rideau D, Simonneau G, Sitbon O & Adnot S (2000b) Imbalance between platelet vascular endothelial growth factor and platelet-derived growth factor in pulmonary hypertension. Effect of prostacyclin therapy. *Am J Respir Crit Care Med* 162, 1493-1499.

Eddahibi S, Raffestin B, Launay JM, Sitbon M & Adnot S (1998) Effect of dexfenfluramine treatment in rats exposed to acute and chronic hypoxia. *Am J Respir Crit Care Med* 157, 1111-1119.

Eddahibi S, Raffestin B, Pham I, Launay JM, Aegerter P, Sitbon M & Adnot S (1997) Treatment with 5-HT potentiates development of pulmonary hypertension in chronically hypoxic rats. *Am J Physiol* 272, H1173-1181.

Evans AM, Osipenko ON & Gurney AM (1996) Properties of a novel K+ current that is active at resting potential in rabbit pulmonary artery smooth muscle cells. *J Physiol* 496 (Pt 2), 407-420.

Fedida D, Wible B, Wang Z, Fermini B, Faust F, Nattel S & Brown AM (1993) Identity of a novel delayed rectifier current from human heart with a cloned K+ channel current. *Circ Res* 73, 210-216.

Frishman WH, Huberfeld S, Okin S, Wang YH, Kumar A & Shareef B (1995) Serotonin and serotonin antagonism in cardiovascular and non-cardiovascular disease. *J Clin Pharmacol* 35, 541-572.

Gaborit N, Le Bouter S, Szuts V, Varro A, Escande D, Nattel S & Demolombe S (2007) Regional and tissue specific transcript signatures of ion channel genes in the non-diseased human heart. *J Physiol* 582, 675-693.

Guignabert C, Izikki M, Tu LI, Li Z, Zadigue P, Barlier-Mur AM, Hanoun N, Rodman D, Hamon M, Adnot S & Eddahibi S (2006) Transgenic mice overexpressing the 5-hydroxytryptamine transporter gene in smooth muscle develop pulmonary hypertension. *Circ Res* 98, 1323-1330.

Guignabert C, Raffestin B, Benferhat R, Raoul W, Zadigue P, Rideau D, Hamon M, Adnot S & Eddahibi S (2005) Serotonin transporter inhibition prevents and reverses monocrotaline-induced pulmonary hypertension in rats. *Circulation* 111, 2812-2819.

Guignabert C, Tu L, Izikki M, Dewachter L, Zadigue P, Humbert M, Adnot S, Fadel E & Eddahibi S (2009) Dichloroacetate treatment partially regresses established pulmonary hypertension in mice with SM22alpha-targeted overexpression of the serotonin transporter. *Faseb J* 23, 4135-4147.

Guilluy C, Eddahibi S, Agard C, Guignabert C, Izikki M, Tu L, Savale L, Humbert M, Fadel E, Adnot S, Loirand G & Pacaud P (2009) RhoA and Rho kinase activation in human pulmonary hypertension: role of 5-HT signaling. *Am J Respir Crit Care Med* 179, 1151-1158.

Gurtner HP (1985) Aminorex and pulmonary hypertension. A review. *Cor Vasa* 27, 160-171.

Hassoun PM, Mouthon L, Barbera JA, Eddahibi S, Flores SC, Grimminger F, Jones PL, Maitland ML, Michelakis ED, Morrell NW, Newman JH, Rabinovitch M, Schermuly R, Stenmark KR, Voelkel NF, Yuan JX & Humbert M (2009) Inflammation, growth factors, and pulmonary vascular remodeling. *J Am Coll Cardiol* 54, S10-19.

Herve P, Drouet L, Dosquet C, Launay JM, Rain B, Simonneau G, Caen J & Duroux P (1990) Primary pulmonary hypertension in a patient with a familial platelet storage pool disease: role of serotonin. *Am J Med* 89, 117-120.

Herve P, Launay JM, Scrobohaci ML, Brenot F, Simonneau G, Petitpretz P, Poubeau P, Cerrina J, Duroux P & Drouet L (1995) Increased plasma serotonin in primary pulmonary hypertension. *Am J Med* 99, 249-254.

Hironaka E, Hongo M, Sakai A, Mawatari E, Terasawa F, Okumura N, Yamazaki A, Ushiyama Y, Yazaki Y & Kinoshita O (2003) Serotonin receptor antagonist inhibits monocrotaline-induced pulmonary hypertension and prolongs survival in rats. *Cardiovasc Res* 60, 692-699.

Humbert M, Morrell NW, Archer SL, Stenmark KR, MacLean MR, Lang IM, Christman BW, Weir EK, Eickelberg O, Voelkel NF & Rabinovitch M (2004) Cellular and molecular pathobiology of pulmonary arterial hypertension. *J Am Coll Cardiol* 43, 13S-24S.

Izikki M, Hanoun N, Marcos E, Savale L, Barlier-Mur AM, Saurini F, Eddahibi S, Hamon M & Adnot S (2007) Tryptophan hydroxylase 1 knockout and tryptophan hydroxylase 2 polymorphism: effects on hypoxic pulmonary hypertension in mice. *Am J Physiol Lung Cell Mol Physiol* 293, L1045-1052.

Keegan A, Morecroft I, Smillie D, Hicks MN & MacLean MR (2001) Contribution of the 5-HT(1B) receptor to hypoxia-induced pulmonary hypertension: converging evidence using 5-HT(1B)-receptor knockout mice and the 5-HT(1B/1D)-receptor antagonist GR127935. *Circ Res* 89, 1231-1239.

Kereveur A, Callebert J, Humbert M, Herve P, Simonneau G, Launay JM & Drouet L (2000) High plasma serotonin levels in primary pulmonary hypertension. Effect of long-term epoprostenol (prostacyclin) therapy. *Arterioscler Thromb Vasc Biol* 20, 2233-2239.

Ko EA, Han J, Jung ID & Park WS (2008) Physiological roles of K+ channels in vascular smooth muscle cells. *J Smooth Muscle Res* 44, 65-81.

Launay JM, Herve P, Peoc'h K, Tournois C, Callebert J, Nebigil CG, Etienne N, Drouet L, Humbert M, Simonneau G & Maroteaux L (2002) Function of the serotonin 5-hydroxytryptamine 2B receptor in pulmonary hypertension. *Nat Med* 8, 1129-1135.

Launay JM, Schneider B, Loric S, Da Prada M & Kellermann O (2006) Serotonin transport and serotonin transporter-mediated antidepressant recognition are controlled by 5-HT2B receptor signaling in serotonergic neuronal cells. *Faseb J* 20, 1843-1854.

Lawrie A, Spiekerkoetter E, Martinez EC, Ambartsumian N, Sheward WJ, MacLean MR, Harmar AJ, Schmidt AM, Lukanidin E & Rabinovitch M (2005) Interdependent serotonin transporter and receptor pathways regulate S100A4/Mts1, a gene associated with pulmonary vascular disease. *Circ Res* 97, 227-235.

Lee SD, Shroyer KR, Markham NE, Cool CD, Voelkel NF & Tuder RM (1998) Monoclonal endothelial cell proliferation is present in primary but not secondary pulmonary hypertension. *J Clin Invest* 101, 927-934.

Lee SL, Simon AR, Wang WW & Fanburg BL (2001) H(2)O(2) signals 5-HT-induced ERK MAP kinase activation and mitogenesis of smooth muscle cells. *Am J Physiol Lung Cell Mol Physiol* 281, L646-652.

Lee SL, Wang WW & Fanburg BL (1997) Association of Tyr phosphorylation of GTPase-activating protein with mitogenic action of serotonin. *Am J Physiol* 272, C223-230.

Li XQ, Wang HM, Yang CG, Zhang XH, Han DD & Wang HL Fluoxetine inhibited extracellular matrix of pulmonary artery and inflammation of lungs in monocrotaline-treated rats. *Acta Pharmacol Sin* 32, 217-222.

Liu Y & Fanburg BL (2006) Serotonin-induced growth of pulmonary artery smooth muscle requires activation of phosphatidylinositol 3-kinase/serine-threonine protein kinase B/mammalian target of rapamycin/p70 ribosomal S6 kinase 1. *Am J Respir Cell Mol Biol* 34, 182-191.

Liu Y, Li M, Warburton RR, Hill NS & Fanburg BL (2007) The 5-HT transporter transactivates the PDGFbeta receptor in pulmonary artery smooth muscle cells. *Faseb J* 21, 2725-2734.

Liu Y, Suzuki YJ, Day RM & Fanburg BL (2004) Rho kinase-induced nuclear translocation of ERK1/ERK2 in smooth muscle cell mitogenesis caused by serotonin. *Circ Res* 95, 579-586.

Long L, MacLean MR, Jeffery TK, Morecroft I, Yang X, Rudarakanchana N, Southwood M, James V, Trembath RC & Morrell NW (2006) Serotonin increases susceptibility to pulmonary hypertension in BMPR2-deficient mice. *Circ Res* 98, 818-827.

Loogen F, Worth H, Schwan G, Goeckenjan G, Losse B & Horstkotte D (1985) Long-term follow-up of pulmonary hypertension in patients with and without anorectic drug intake. *Cor Vasa* 27, 111-124.

Macian F (2005) NFAT proteins: key regulators of T-cell development and function. *Nat Rev Immunol* 5, 472-484.

MacLean MR, Deuchar GA, Hicks MN, Morecroft I, Shen S, Sheward J, Colston J, Loughlin L, Nilsen M, Dempsie Y & Harmar A (2004) Overexpression of the 5-hydroxytryptamine transporter gene: effect on pulmonary hemodynamics and hypoxia-induced pulmonary hypertension. *Circulation* 109, 2150-2155.

Mandegar M, Fung YC, Huang W, Remillard CV, Rubin LJ & Yuan JX (2004) Cellular and molecular mechanisms of pulmonary vascular remodeling: role in the development of pulmonary hypertension. *Microvasc Res* 68, 75-103.

Marcos E, Adnot S, Pham MH, Nosjean A, Raffestin B, Hamon M & Eddahibi S (2003) Serotonin transporter inhibitors protect against hypoxic pulmonary hypertension. *Am J Respir Crit Care Med* 168, 487-493.

Marcos E, Fadel E, Sanchez O, Humbert M, Dartevelle P, Simonneau G, Hamon M, Adnot S & Eddahibi S (2004) Serotonin-induced smooth muscle hyperplasia in various forms of human pulmonary hypertension. *Circ Res* 94, 1263-1270.

Marcos E, Fadel E, Sanchez O, Humbert M, Dartevelle P, Simonneau G, Hamon M, Adnot S & Eddahibi S (2005) Serotonin transporter and receptors in various forms of human pulmonary hypertension. *Chest* 128, 552S-553S.

Mays DJ, Foose JM, Philipson LH & Tamkun MM (1995) Localization of the Kv1.5 K+ channel protein in explanted cardiac tissue. *J Clin Invest* 96, 282-292.

McMurtry MS, Archer SL, Altieri DC, Bonnet S, Haromy A, Harry G, Bonnet S, Puttagunta L & Michelakis ED (2005) Gene therapy targeting survivin selectively induces pulmonary vascular apoptosis and reverses pulmonary arterial hypertension. *J Clin Invest* 115, 1479-1491.

McMurtry MS, Bonnet S, Wu X, Dyck JR, Haromy A, Hashimoto K & Michelakis ED (2004) Dichloroacetate prevents and reverses pulmonary hypertension by inducing pulmonary artery smooth muscle cell apoptosis. *Circ Res* 95, 830-840.

Michelakis ED, Webster L & Mackey JR (2008) Dichloroacetate (DCA) as a potential metabolic-targeting therapy for cancer. *Br J Cancer* 99, 989-994.

Morecroft I, Heeley RP, Prentice HM, Kirk A & MacLean MR (1999) 5-hydroxytryptamine receptors mediating contraction in human small muscular pulmonary arteries: importance of the 5-HT1B receptor. *Br J Pharmacol* 128, 730-734.

Morecroft I, Loughlin L, Nilsen M, Colston J, Dempsie Y, Sheward J, Harmar A & MacLean MR (2005) Functional interactions between 5-hydroxytryptamine receptors and the serotonin transporter in pulmonary arteries. *J Pharmacol Exp Ther* 313, 539-548.

Morrell NW, Adnot S, Archer SL, Dupuis J, Jones PL, MacLean MR, McMurtry IF, Stenmark KR, Thistlethwaite PA, Weissmann N, Yuan JX & Weir EK (2009)

Cellular and molecular basis of pulmonary arterial hypertension. *J Am Coll Cardiol* 54, S20-31.

Olson TM, Alekseev AE, Liu XK, Park S, Zingman LV, Bienengraeber M, Sattiraju S, Ballew JD, Jahangir A & Terzic A (2006) Kv1.5 channelopathy due to KCNA5 loss-of-function mutation causes human atrial fibrillation. *Hum Mol Genet* 15, 2185-2191.

Osipenko ON, Tate RJ & Gurney AM (2000) Potential role for kv3.1b channels as oxygen sensors. *Circ Res* 86, 534-540.

Overturf KE, Russell SN, Carl A, Vogalis F, Hart PJ, Hume JR, Sanders KM & Horowitz B (1994) Cloning and characterization of a Kv1.5 delayed rectifier K+ channel from vascular and visceral smooth muscles. *Am J Physiol* 267, C1231-1238.

Patel AJ, Lazdunski M & Honore E (1997) Kv2.1/Kv9.3, a novel ATP-dependent delayed-rectifier K+ channel in oxygen-sensitive pulmonary artery myocytes. *Embo J* 16, 6615-6625.

Paulin R, Courboulin A, Meloche J, Mainguy V, Dumas de la Roque E, Saksouk N, Cote J, Provencher S, Sussman MA & Bonnet S Signal transducers and activators of transcription-3/pim1 axis plays a critical role in the pathogenesis of human pulmonary arterial hypertension. *Circulation* 123, 1205-1215.

Post JM, Gelband CH & Hume JR (1995) [Ca2+]i inhibition of K+ channels in canine pulmonary artery. Novel mechanism for hypoxia-induced membrane depolarization. *Circ Res* 77, 131-139.

Pozeg ZI, Michelakis ED, McMurtry MS, Thebaud B, Wu XC, Dyck JR, Hashimoto K, Wang S, Moudgil R, Harry G, Sultanian R, Koshal A & Archer SL (2003) In vivo gene transfer of the O2-sensitive potassium channel Kv1.5 reduces pulmonary hypertension and restores hypoxic pulmonary vasoconstriction in chronically hypoxic rats. *Circulation* 107, 2037-2044.

Rabinovitch M (2008) Molecular pathogenesis of pulmonary arterial hypertension. *J Clin Invest* 118, 2372-2379.

Reeve HL, Michelakis E, Nelson DP, Weir EK & Archer SL (2001) Alterations in a redox oxygen sensing mechanism in chronic hypoxia. *J Appl Physiol* 90, 2249-2256.

Remillard CV, Tigno DD, Platoshyn O, Burg ED, Brevnova EE, Conger D, Nicholson A, Rana BK, Channick RN, Rubin LJ, O'Connor D T & Yuan JX (2007) Function of Kv1.5 channels and genetic variations of KCNA5 in patients with idiopathic pulmonary arterial hypertension. *Am J Physiol Cell Physiol* 292, C1837-1853.

Ren W, Watts SW & Fanburg BL Serotonin transporter interacts with the PDGFbeta receptor in PDGF-BB-induced signaling and mitogenesis in pulmonary artery smooth muscle cells. *Am J Physiol Lung Cell Mol Physiol* 300, L486-497.

Said SI (2008) The vasoactive intestinal peptide gene is a key modulator of pulmonary vascular remodeling and inflammation. *Ann N Y Acad Sci* 1144, 148-153.

Sato K, Webb S, Tucker A, Rabinovitch M, O'Brien RF, McMurtry IF & Stelzner TJ (1992) Factors influencing the idiopathic development of pulmonary hypertension in the fawn hooded rat. *Am Rev Respir Dis* 145, 793-797.

Souza R, Humbert M, Sztrymf B, Jais X, Yaici A, Le Pavec J, Parent F, Herve P, Soubrier F, Sitbon O & Simonneau G (2008) Pulmonary arterial hypertension associated with fenfluramine exposure: report of 109 cases. *Eur Respir J* 31, 343-348.

Sullivan CC, Du L, Chu D, Cho AJ, Kido M, Wolf PL, Jamieson SW & Thistlethwaite PA (2003) Induction of pulmonary hypertension by an angiopoietin 1/TIE2/serotonin pathway. *Proc Natl Acad Sci U S A* 100, 12331-12336.

Suzuki YJ, Day RM, Tan CC, Sandven TH, Liang Q, Molkentin JD & Fanburg BL (2003) Activation of GATA-4 by serotonin in pulmonary artery smooth muscle cells. *J Biol Chem* 278, 17525-17531.

Walczak-Drzewiecka A, Ratajewski M, Wagner W & Dastych J (2008) HIF-1alpha is up-regulated in activated mast cells by a process that involves calcineurin and NFAT. *J Immunol* 181, 1665-1672.

Wang Y, Han DD, Wang HM, Liu M, Zhang XH & Wang HL Downregulation of Osteopontin Is Associated with Fluoxetine Amelioration of Monocrotaline-Induced Pulmonary Inflammation and Vascular Remodelling. *Clin Exp Pharmacol Physiol*.

Wang Z, Fermini B & Nattel S (1993) Sustained depolarization-induced outward current in human atrial myocytes. Evidence for a novel delayed rectifier K+ current similar to Kv1.5 cloned channel currents. *Circ Res* 73, 1061-1076.

Weir EK, Reeve HL, Huang JM, Michelakis E, Nelson DP, Hampl V & Archer SL (1996) Anorexic agents aminorex, fenfluramine, and dexfenfluramine inhibit potassium current in rat pulmonary vascular smooth muscle and cause pulmonary vasoconstriction. *Circulation* 94, 2216-2220.

Young KA, Ivester C, West J, Carr M & Rodman DM (2006) BMP signaling controls PASMC KV channel expression in vitro and in vivo. *Am J Physiol Lung Cell Mol Physiol* 290, L841-848.

Yu Y, Platoshyn O, Zhang J, Krick S, Zhao Y, Rubin LJ, Rothman A & Yuan JX (2001) c-Jun decreases voltage-gated K(+) channel activity in pulmonary artery smooth muscle cells. *Circulation* 104, 1557-1563.

Yuan JX, Aldinger AM, Juhaszova M, Wang J, Conte JV, Jr., Gaine SP, Orens JB & Rubin LJ (1998a) Dysfunctional voltage-gated K+ channels in pulmonary artery smooth muscle cells of patients with primary pulmonary hypertension. *Circulation* 98, 1400-1406.

Yuan XJ (1995) Voltage-gated K+ currents regulate resting membrane potential and [Ca2+]i in pulmonary arterial myocytes. *Circ Res* 77, 370-378.

Yuan XJ, Wang J, Juhaszova M, Gaine SP & Rubin LJ (1998b) Attenuated K+ channel gene transcription in primary pulmonary hypertension. *Lancet* 351, 726-727.

Zhai FG, Zhang XH & Wang HL (2009) Fluoxetine protects against monocrotaline-induced pulmonary arterial hypertension: potential roles of induction of apoptosis and upregulation of Kv1.5 channels in rats. *Clin Exp Pharmacol Physiol* 36, 850-856.

Zhu SP, Mao ZF, Huang J & Wang JY (2009) Continuous fluoxetine administration prevents recurrence of pulmonary arterial hypertension and prolongs survival in rats. *Clin Exp Pharmacol Physiol* 36, e1-5.

Integrin-Mediated Endothelial Cell Adhesion and Activation of c-Src, EGFR and ErbB2 are Required for Endothelial-Mesenchymal Transition

Enrique Arciniegas[1], Luz Marina Carrillo[2], Héctor Rojas[3] and José Cardier[4]
[1]*Instituto de Biomedicina, Facultad de Medicina, Universidad Central de Venezuela*
[2]*Servicio Autónomo Instituto de Biomedicina*
[3]*Instituto de Inmunología, Facultad de Medicina, Universidad Central de Venezuela*
[4]*Instituto Venezolano de Investigaciones Científicas, Centro de Medicina Experimental*
Venezuela

1. Introduction

The adhesion of cells to the extracellular matrix (ECM) is a critical requisite to generate cell shape, migration, proliferation, differentiation, and gene expression (Geiger & Yamada, 2011; Papusheva & Heisenberg, 2010). Beyond this role, cell-ECM adhesion promotes various intracellular signalling pathways and effectors modulating cell survival or apoptosis and tumor growth (Geiger & Yamada, 2011). Cells use a number of different cell surface receptors that mediate cell-ECM adhesion, being one of the best studied the integrins (Jean et al., 2011; Schwartz, 2010). It is known that binding of integrins to their ligands is dependent on the presence of divalent cations including Ca^{2+}, Mg^{2+}, and Mn^{2+} (Cierniewska-Cieslak et al., 2002; Cluzel et al., 2005; Leitinger et al., 2000; Luo & Springer, 2006). These heterodimeric transmembrane proteins which lack intrinsic enzymatic activity, in addition to being considered as indispensable to mediate cell-ECM adhesion, promote the assembly of cell-to-cell adhesion also promote receptor tyrosine kinase (RTK) activation triggering signalling cascades that regulate cell growth, proliferation and control cell death. Of note, growth factors that activate RTK may also modulate some of the cellular events that are mediated by integrins (Streuli & Akhtar, 2009). Now, it is clear that binding of certain integrins to their ligands as well as mechanical stimuli including shear stress, compression and tensile forces, promotes integrin clustering and that clustered integrins provoke recruitment and activation of other signalling molecules, including the RTKs, and therefore controlling cell survival, proliferation and migration (Guo & Giancotti, 2004; Ivaska and Heino, 2010; Streuli & Akhtar, 2009; Yamada & Even-Ram, 2002). Interestingly, functional cooperation between integrins and RTKs is actually considered as critical during normal vascular development and in vascular and inflammatory diseases (Eliceiri, 2001; Streuli & Akhtar, 2009) as well as in tumor progression and metastasis (Desgrosellier & Cheresh, 2010; Guo & Giancotti, 2004). In this context, studies have demonstrated that during cell-ECM adhesion some members of the epidermal growth factor (EGF) receptor family such as

EGFR/ErbB1 and ErbB2/Neu which has no known ligand, may be partially activated by association with particular integrins regulating important cellular functions including adhesion, proliferation, differentiation, survival, and migration in the absence of their ligands (Bill et al., 2004; Moro et al., 1998). These functions are mediated via upstream and downstream signalling pathways. However, the implications of the interactions between integrins and RTKs need further investigation.

Cell-ECM adhesion also involves various signalling intermediates including non-receptor tyrosine kinases (non-RTK) such as c-Src, focal adhesion kinase (FAK) and paxillin (Geiger & Yamada, 2011; Huveneers & Danen, 2010). c-Src may regulate not only increased cell growth and survival, but also it may promote cytoskeletal reorganization and decreased cell-ECM adhesion and cell-to-cell adhesion, facilitating cell spreading, migration, differentiation and transcription (Alper & Bowden, 2005; Guarino, 2010). Importantly, studies in diverse human cancer cells have revealed overexpression and /or overactivation of EGFRs and c-Src in the absence of ligands (Alper, & Bowden, 2005; Donepudi & Resh, 2008; Guarino, 2010; Marcotte et al., 2009). Also, increasing evidence indicates that in the absence of growth factors the activation of c-Src and tyrosine phosphorylation at 416-419 residues occurs by direct interaction with the cytoplasmic tail of integrins and that activated c-Src phosphorylates EGFR at Tyr845 residue and ErbB2 at Tyr877 residue (Bill et al., 2004; Cabodi et al., 2004; Desgrosellier & Cheresh, 2010; Guarino, 2010; Guo et al., 2006; Kim et al., 2005; Marcotte et al., 2009; Moro et al., 2002; Streuli & Akhtar, 2009). Interestingly, these patterns of phosphorylation in response to adhesion are different from those triggered by the binding of EGF (Bill et al., 2004; Cabodi et al., 2004; Moro et al., 2002). However, mechanisms involved in c-Src, EGFR and ErbB2 interactions as well as their implications have not being completely understood.

Growth factors can also indirectly influence integrin function by disrupting cell-to-cell contacts modulating cell-ECM interaction and therefore facilitating cell migration and invasion. Outstandingly, overstimulation signalling of growth factors or aberrant activation tyrosine kinases that lead to loss of epithelial apico-basal polarity and cell-to-cell contacts have been consistently reported during the epithelial mesenchymal transition (EMT) (Baum et al., 2008; Guarino, 2007). Nevertheless, the molecular, cellular, and mechanical aspects by which EGF and their receptors exert these actions remain to be elucidated. In the context of endothelial cells, there are reports showing that disruption of endothelial cell-cell contacts or adherens junctions (AJs) and changes in the reorganization of microtubules (MTs) and actin cytoskeleton may occur in response to mechanical injury, shear stress and / or cross talk of a variety of growth factors including transforming growth factor-β (TGFβ), insulin-like growth factor II (IGFII), and fibroblast growth factor-2 (FGF-2), and that such events are necessary in the transition of endothelial cells to a mesenchymal phenotype (EndoMT) (Arciniegas et al., 2007). However, how these factors and intracellular signals induce the endothelial transformation is still matter of debate (Arciniegas & Candelle, 2008). Recent evidence from studies on EGF and their receptors indicate that ErbB2, which has no known ligand, may form heterodimer with EGFR in response to ligands including EGF and TGF-α and that this heterodimer is essential during cardiovascular development and angiogenesis (Camenisch et al., 2002; Dreux et al., 2006; Fuller et al., 2008; Mukherjee et al., 2006; Negro et al., 2004). Moreover, expression of EGF, TGF-α and heparin binding- EGF (HB-EGF) as well as their respective receptors EGFR and ErbB2, have been detected in the intimal thickening and medial smooth muscle cells (SMCs) of atherosclerotic lesions, whereas little or no presence of these molecules is observed in the cells of healthy vessels (Dreux et al., 2006). EndoMT is not only recognized as a phenomenon that occurs during cardiac fibrosis and intimal thickening formation observed in atherosclerosis and restenosis but also in heart and vascular development (Arciniegas et al., 2000; Mironov et al., 2005), pulmonary arterial hypertension (Arciniegas et al., 2007; Morrell et al., 2009; Sakao et al., 2010), cardiac (Goumans et al., 2008) and kidney fibrosis (Zeisberg et al., 2008), hyperthrophic scarring (Xi-Qiao et al., 2009), diabetic nephropathy (Li & Bertram, 2010), and during cancer progression (Potenta et al., 2008). However, there are no studies about the specific role of EGF signalling pathway in the EndoMT process.

In view of the above observations, in this study we examined the presence, organization, and spatial distribution of integrin β_3 in monolayers of primary embryonic aortic endothelial cells adhered to fibronectin (FN) and maintained in the presence of Ca^{2+} and in the absence of growth factors, considering that integrin $\alpha_v\beta_3$ is a receptor widely expressed on the apical surface of endothelial cells that binds proteins that are normally present in plasma, such as FN, vitronectin, fibrinogen and vWf (Bombeli et al., 1998; Soldi et al., 1999). Given that activation of c-Src, EGFR and ErbB2 may occur by association with integrins (Arias-Salgado et al., 2003; Bill et al., 2004; Cabodi et al., 2004; Desgrosellier & Cheresh, 2010; Ivaska & Heino, 2009; Huveneers & Danen, 2010; Streuli & Akhtar, 2009), we also investigated whether the activated forms of these molecules were present in these monolayers. Since some soluble growth factors can also indirectly influence integrin function by disrupting cell-to-cell contacts modulating cell-ECM interaction and facilitating cell migration and invasion events that are considered necessary in the progression of EndoMT (Arciniegas et al., 2007; Arciniegas & Candelle, 2008), we also investigated whether EGF and TGF-α as well as their activated receptors participate in the EndoMT process and if they were present in chicken embryo aortic wall during embryonic days 12-14 (days E12-E14) (stages 38 and 40) when intimal thickening is apparent and endothelial transformation occurs.

2. Materials and methods

2.1 Embryonic aortic explants

Fertilized chicken eggs (White leghorn) were obtained from local hatchery (Granja Avicola Agropollito, CA, Paracotos, Estado Miranda) and incubated at 37°C and 60% humidity for 10-11 days (stages 36 and 37 of development). Embryos were staged according to Hamburger & Hamilton (1992). Aortae were dissected in Hank`s balanced salt solution without Ca^{2+} and Mg^{2+} (Sigma-Aldrich, St. Louis, MO) at 37°C. For simplicity, this buffer is subsequently referred to as HBSS. Aortic segments, approximately 8mm² in surface area, were isolated (distal to the aortic arches) and opened along longitudinal axis. Explants were rinsed in HBSS and left in the same buffer 5-10 min before to initiate the assays.

2.1.1 Endothelial cell adhesion assays

To determine the effects of calcium (Ca^{2+}) on endothelial cell adhesion, 35mm Petri dishes (Nunclon, Delta, IL) were coated with HBSS containing plasma fibronectin (pFN) (25-50μg/ml) (Santa Cruz Biotechnology Inc., Santa Cruz, CA) and incubated at 37°C for 2 hr in a humidified atmosphere consisiting of 5% CO_2, and 95% air. The dishes were then rinsed twice with HBSS, blocked with 2% bovine serum albumin (BSA) (Sigma-Aldrich) in HBSS for 1 hr at 37°C with 5% CO_2 and finally washed three times with the same buffer. After that, 300μl of HBSS containing 0.025% BSA (Sigma-Aldrich), 100μg/ml streptomycin, and 100U/ml penicillin (GIBCO, Invitrogen, Carlsbad, CA) were added to some dishes and incubated at 37°C with 5% CO_2. Other dishes were incubated with 300μl of HBSS supplemented with either 2mM $CaCl_2$ (Ca^{2+}) (Sigma-Aldrich) or 2mM EGTA (Sigma-Aldrich) and incubated at 37°C with 5% CO_2 for 1 hr. Aortic explants were placed with the endothelial apical surface down on coated dishes and allowed to adhere for 4 hr at 37°C with 5% CO_2 . At the end of this time, 1ml of the corresponding HBSS was gently added to each dish. One hour later, the adhered explants were removed with the aid of a thin needle, leaving a monolayer of retracted endothelial cells that exhibited zones denuded of cells or wounds.

In order to emphasize the possible role of Ca^{2+} in the endothelial cell adhesion, some aortic explants were incubated on pFN-coated dishes containing either medium 199 containing 0.025% BSA (Sigma-Aldrich), 100μg/ml streptomycin, 100U/ml penicillin (GIBCO) (subsequently referred to as serum-free M199) (SFM199) or SFM199 containing 2mM EGTA (Sigma-Aldrich) and maintained as before.

Monolayers were examined with an inverted microscope (IX70 Olympus, Olympus America Inc., Melville, NY). Images were captured using an image editing capture and processing software program (Image Pro Plus, Media Cybernetics, Silver Spring, MD). Four independent experiments were performed and each one included at least 15 dishes.

2.1.2 Cell cultures

Cell cultures were initiated when the monolayers of endothelial cells adhered to the surface of the coated dishes were rinsed five times with HBSS and incubated with SFM199 for 2 hr at 37°C with 5% CO_2. Images were captured using the Image Pro Plus software program.

2.1.3 Effects of EGF and TGF-α on embryonic endothelial cells

Epidermal growth factor (EGF) and transforming growth factor-alpha (TGF-α) have been reported to stimulate cell migration, differentiation, and proliferation in presence or absence of serum (Ackland et al., 2003; Ellis et al., 2007). To determine whether EGF or TGF-α stimulates endothelial cell separation, detachment, and migration, the medium of some monolayers that had been maintained in SFM199 for 2 hr was switched to SFM199 supplemented with either recombinant human EGF (100ηg/ml) or recombinant human TGF-α (5-10ηg/ml) (R&D Systems, Inc., Minneapolis, MN) and low amount of chicken serum (ChS) (0.1%) (Sigma-Aldrich), using 10mM acetic acid as vehicle, and incubated at 37°C with 5% CO_2 for an additional 6-8 hr period. During this period the images were captured each 2 hr using the Image Pro Plus software program.

2.1.4 Immunofluorescence

Fixed and permeabilized cells were processed for immunofluorescence as previously described (Arciniegas et al., 2005) using the following antibodies: a mouse monoclonal antibody (mab) anti-human integrin $β_3$ (GPIIIa, CD61) and a mab anti-chicken integrin $β_1$

(Millipore Chemicon Corporation, Billerica, CA), a mouse mab raised against full length β-catenin of chicken origin (clone 6F9) (Santa Cruz Biotechnology), a mouse mab raised against aminoacids 8-349 of mouse p120-catenin (clone 6H11) (Santa Cruz Biotechnology), a mouse mab raised against native chick brain microtubules (clone DM1A) (Santa Cruz Biotechnology), a mouse mab raised against a phospho-peptide corresponding to amino acids 416-422 of human c-Src (clone 9A6) (Santa Cruz Biotechnology), and a rabbit polyclonal antibody (pab) phospho-FAK (Tyr397) (Sigma-Aldrich). Negative controls were performed by omitting the primary antibody incubation step or by using non immune serum in place of primary antibody. Immunofluorescence images were captured on an inverted microscope confocal laser scanning microscope (CLSM) (Eclipse TE-300 Nikon) (Nikon Instruments Inc., Melville, NY) equipped with a Nikon objective Plan-Apo BC x60, 1.2 wi coupled to a C1-LU2 unit Argon cooled air (488 ηm) laser. This laser unit was controlled by a D-eclipse C1 interface. Other immunofluorescence images were captured on a IX81 Olympus inverted microscope with the Fluo-View confocal laser scanning configuration (CLSM) (Olympus America). Fluorescence intensity was measured by using a processing software program (FV10.ASW version 02.01.01.04, Olympus America).

2.1.5 Immunoperoxidase

Fixed cells were processed for immunoperoxidase as described previously (Arciniegas et al., 2005) using a rabbit pab raised against a short amino acid sequence containing phosphorylated Tyr845 of EGFR of human origin, and a rabbit pab raised against a short amino acid sequence containing phosphorylated Tyr877 of ErbB2/Neu of human origin (Santa Cruz Biotechnology). The images were captured using the Image Pro Plus software program.

2.1.6 Flow cytometry analysis of phospho-EGFR (Tyr845) and phospho-ErbB2 (Tyr877) expression in embryonic endothelial cells

We evaluated by flow cytometry the expression of phospho-EGFR (Tyr845) and phospho-ErbB2 (Tyr877) in monolayers of endothelial cells that were maintained in SFM199 for 2 hr and monolayers whose medium was switched to SFM199 supplemented with either rhEGF (100ηg/ml) or rhTGF-α (5-10ng/ml) (R&D Systems) and low-ChS (0.1%) (Sigma-Aldrich) and incubated for an additional 6-8 period. Briefly, supernatants from cultures were removed, and the cells were harvested and incubated in permeabilizing buffer. After incubation, the cells were resuspended in PBS-0.1% BSA containing a rabbit pab anti-human phospho-EGFR (Tyr845) or a rabbit pab anti-human phospho-ErbB2 (Tyr877) (Santa Cruz Biotechnology). Negative control staining reactions were performed by incubating the cells with nonimmune rabbit Ig. After two washes with PBS, the cells were fixed with 1% paraformaldehyde in PBS. Data collection and analysis of the fluorescence intensities were carried out using a FACScalibur (Becton-Dickinson, San Jose, CA). Ten thousand events were acquired (excluding cell debris) and analyzed using the CELLQuest software program.

2.1.7 Tissue extraction

The aortae were dissected from 12-and 14-day-old embryos (stages 38 and 40 of development). The excised aortae were placed in HBSS (Sigma-Aldrich), and fixed for 20 min at room temperature with 4% formaldehyde prepared from paraformaldehyde (Sigma-Aldrich) in PBS. The aortae were dehydrated in graded ethanol and embedded in paraffin. Paraffin sections (5μm thick) were mounted on silanized slides (Dako North America, Inc., Carpinteria, CA). A total of nine aortae for each stage obtained from four different lots of fertilized chicken eggs, were processed.

2.1.8 Immunoperoxidase

For histological detection of EGF, TGF-α, EGFR and ErbB2/Neu the following antibodies were used on deparaffinized sections: a neutralizing antibody anti-human EGF and anti-TGF-α, both produced in goat (R&D Systems), a rabbit pab raised against a peptide mapping at the C-terminus of EGFR of human origin, and a rabbit pab raised against a peptide mapping at C-terminus of Neu of human origin (Santa Cruz Biotechnology). Negative controls were produced by the use of purified normal serum or PBS in place of primary antibody. The images were captured using the Image pro Plus software program.

3. Results

In order to determine the effect of Ca^{2+} on adhesion of embryonic endothelial cells to FN aortic explants from days E10 and E11 (stages 36 and 37) were placed with the endothelial apical surface down on dishes coated with pFN and containing HBSS alone or HBSS supplemented with 2mM Ca^{2+} and incubated for 5 hours.

Once the explants were removed, monolayers of endothelial cells that were transiently mechanically altered during the explant removal and therefore exhibited zones denuded of cells or wounds, were found adhered to the surface of the pFN-coated dishes that contained HBSS supplemented with Ca^{2+} (Fig. 1b), but not on the dishes that contained HBSS alone (Fig. 1a).

To emphasize the possible role of Ca^{2+} in the endothelial cell adhesion, aortic explants were incubated on pFN-coated dishes containing SFM199 or SFM199 containing 2mM EGTA to chelate extracellular Ca^{2+}. Like other culture medium, M199 is known for containing Ca^{2+} and relatively low levels of Mg^{2+}. When the explants were removed, monolayers of retracted endothelial cells exhibiting zones that were denuded of cells or wounds were found adhered to the surface of the pFN-coated dishes that contained SFM199 (Fig. 1c), but not on dishes that contained SFM199 and EGTA (Fig. 1d). When the endothelial cell monolayers were maintained in the presence SFM199 for 2-3 hr and examined, we observed that they adopted a contact inhibited cobblestone-like appearance of polygonal cells. Under this culture condition neither migrating cells from the wounded edges nor spreading, separating, detaching nor migrating cells from edges of the monolayer were observed (Figs. 2a, b). However, when, after this interval, the medium of some cultures was switched to SFM199 containing EGF or TGF-α and low-ChS and maintained for an additional 6-8 hr period, the polygonal cells from along wounds edges appeared to move toward each other extending lamellipodia into denuded area, whereas the cells located at the marginal edges of the monolayer appear to lose its cobblestone appearance, spreading, separating, detaching and migrating toward cell-free areas (Figs. 2c,d).

Integrin-Mediated Endothelial Cell Adhesion and Activation of c-Src, EGFR and ErbB2 are Required for
Endothelial-Mesenchymal Transition

49

HBSS

HBSS + 2mM Ca^{2+}

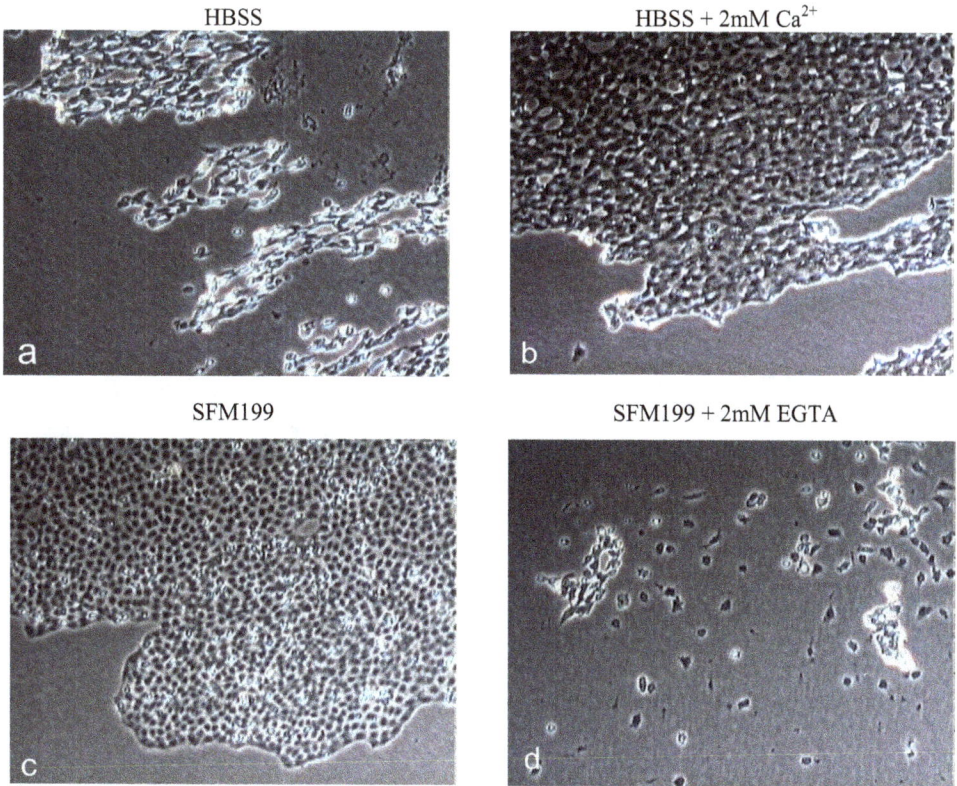

SFM199

SFM199 + 2mM EGTA

Fig. 1. Phase-contrast images captured when the aortic explants that had been incubated on pFN-coated dishes containing a) HBSS alone, b) HBSS supplemented with 2mM Ca^{2+}, c) SFM199 alone, and d) SFM199 supplemented with 2mM EGTA were removed after 5 hr. Note that only when the explants were incubated with HBSS supplemented with Ca^{2+} and with SFM199 alone monolayers of endothelial cells were found adhered to the surface of the dish after removal. Scale bar: 150µm.

Immunofluorescence analyzed by confocal microscopy determined that in the SFM199 condition in which the endothelial cells displayed a cobblestone appearance and no spreading, separating, detaching, migrating cells were observed, β-catenin and p120 catenin, proteins considered as regulators of VE-cadherin function, were localized at cell-cell contacts or AJs with MTs emanating from the microtubule organizing center (MTOC), organized radially and some of them oriented perpendicular to the cell edge probably interacting with sites of cell-cell contacts (Akhmanova et al., 2009) (Figs. 3a-c). Whereas in the EGF or TGF-α and low-ChS condition where spreading, separating, detaching and migrating cells are observed, the distribution of β-catenin and p120-catenin was disrupted at the cell-cell junctions and the organization of MTs was altered (Figs. 3d-f). Specifically, MTs were found oriented parallel to the long axis of the cell and the MTOC on the side of the cell facing the leading edge (Fig. 3f). Interestingly, β-catenin was also detected in the nucleus of some separating, detaching and migrating cells (Fig. 3d). This location indicates that translocation of β-catenin from plasma membranes to the nucleus may also occur in response to EGF or TGF-α and low-ChS. These observations indicate that the presence of Ca^{2+} in the absence of growth factors would represent an important requirement to promote the adhesion and the eventual organization of explanted embryonic endothelial cells into monolayers forming AJs, whereas the addition of EGF or TGF-α and ChS may lead to the loss of cell-cell contacts, detachment, and cell migration; in other words, to the loss of endothelial cell polarity.

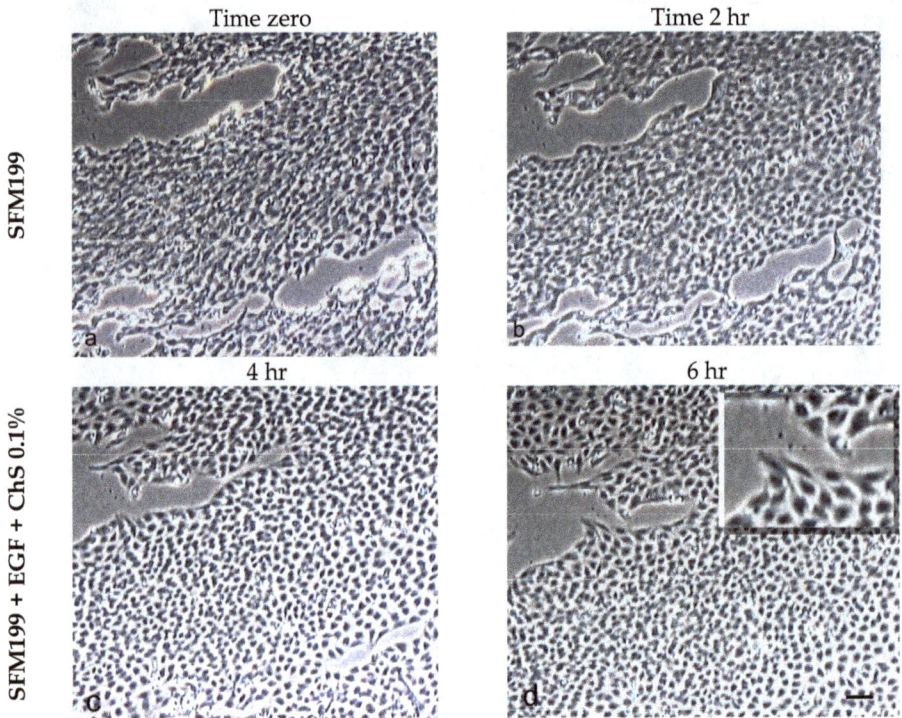

Fig. 2. Serie of phase-contrast images of a monolayer of endothelial cells adhered to the surface of the pFN-coated dish maintained in SFM199 and switched to SFM199 supplemented with EGF and low-ChS. a) time zero, shows a monolayer of retracted endothelial exhibiting zones denuded of cells or wounds after removing the explant. b) Time 2hr. Cells adopted a cobblestone appearance where neither spreading, separating, detaching nor migrating cells from the edges are observed. c) Time 4hr. cell spreading, separating detaching and migration are observed when the medium of the same culture was switched and maintained for additional 2hr (4hr). d) Time 6hr. Cells from the wound moving toward each other extending lamellipodia into denuded area. Detail of "d" showing migrating cells. Scale bar: 150µm; inset 40µm.

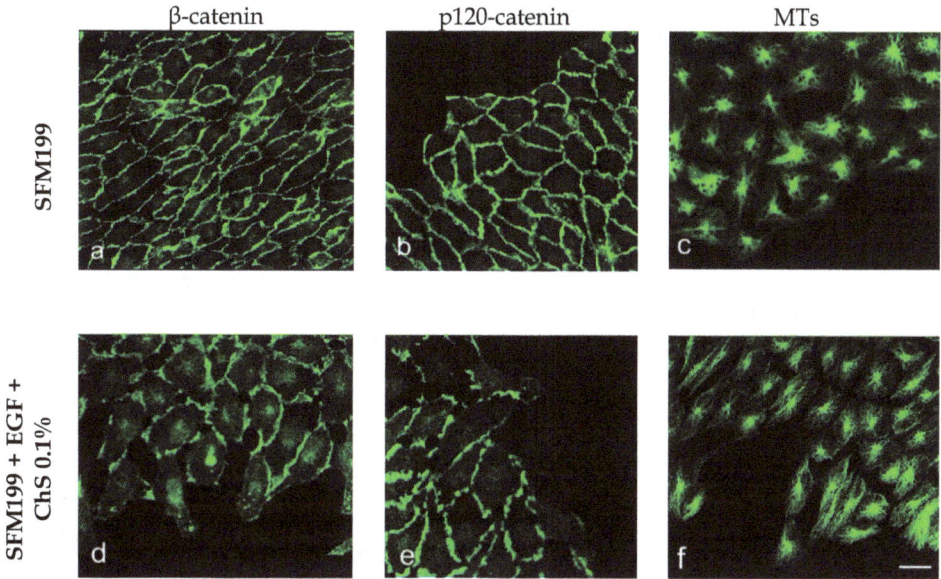

Fig. 3. Representative CLSM fluorescence images of β-catenin, p120-catenin, and MTs
localization in monolayers of endothelial cells adhered to pFN.
(a-c) Immunolocalization after 2hr in culture in SFM199. (d-f) Immunolocalization in
monolayers whose medium was switched to medium containing EGF and low-ChS and
maintained for additional 4hr (6hr). In this condition where spreading, separating,
detaching and migrating cells are observed, the distribution of β- and p120-catenins is
disrupted in the cell-cell junctions and the organization of MTs is altered. Note that
β-catenin is also detected in the nucleus and cytoplasm of some cells.
a), b), c), f) Scale bar = 30µm; d), e) scale bar = 25µm.

3.1 Endothelial cell adhesion to FN in the presence of Ca^{2+} and in the absence of serum or growth factors is mediated by integrin β_3, and addition of EGF or TGF-α produces changes in the distribution and organization of integrin β_3

As the cell-ECM adhesion in the presence of divalent cations such as Ca^{2+} and Mg^{2+} is
actually correlated with the activation, organization and spatial distribution of particular
integrins in normal and tumor cells (Cierniewska-Cieslak et al., 2002; Cluzel et al., 2005;
Leitinger et al., 2000; Luo & Springer, 2006) and as integrin $\alpha_v\beta_3$ is a receptor widely
expressed on the apical surface of endothelial cells that binds proteins that are normally
present in plasma, such as pFN, vitronectin, fibrinogen and vWf (Bombeli et al., 1998; Soldi
et al., 1999), we then examined the presence, organization and distribution of integrin β_3 by
immunofluorescence staining in monolayers of retracted endothelial cells that were found
adhered to pFN after removal of the explants and incubated with SFM199 for 2-3 hr as well
as in those whose medium was switched to medium containing EGF or TGF-α and low-ChS
and maintained for an additional 6-8 hr period.

Examination of the monolayers maintained in SFM199 revealed that integrin β_3, in addition to be localized on the apical surface, also appeared distributed delineating the margins of the cells that had adopted a cobblestone appearance (Fig. 4a). When the medium was switched to medium containing EGF or TGF-α and low-ChS the location and distribution of integrin β_3 appeared altered (Fig. 4b). Specifically, this receptor was found delineating the margin of some cells and organized into linear streaks and a punctuate pattern typical of focal adhesions in the leading edge of the cells that were spreading, separating, detaching and migrating (Fig. 4b).

These observations suggest that the adhesion to Fn and eventual organization of embryonic endothelial cells in the presence of Ca^{2+} and in the absence of serum or growth factors may be mediated by integrin β_3 and that the presence of EGF or TGF-α and low-ChS would produce changes in the spatial distribution and organization of this receptor.

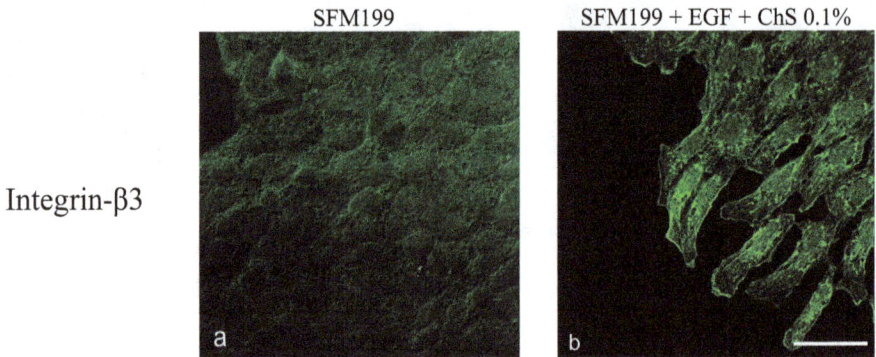

Fig. 4. a) Overlay of transmission and green fluorescence images of integrin β_3 in a monolayer of endothelial cells adhered to pFN after 2 hr in culture in the presence of SFM199. Integrin β_3 is seen on the apical surface and delineating the margin of many cells that displayed a cobblestone appearance. b) CLSM fluorescence image of integrin β_3 in a monolayer whose medium was switched to medium containing EGF and low-ChS. Integrin β_3 is seen delineating the margin of some cells and organized into linear streaks and a punctuate pattern at the leading edge of the migrating cells. Scale bar: 50µm.

3.1.1 Immunolocalization of integrin β_1 and phospho-FAK in vitro

Focal adhesions are considered not only as structural and dynamics links between the ECM and the actin cytoskeleton controlling cell shape, spreading, and migration but also as sites for signal transduction through integrins such as integrin β_1 and β_3, and adaptor proteins such as FAK and paxillin that are present in these sites (Geiger & Yamada, 2011; Gu et al., 2011; Mitra et al., 2005). We therefore examined the presence and organization and distribution of integrin β_1 and FAK when the medium was switched to medium containing EGF and low-ChS. Immunolocalization with anti-integrin β_1 and anti-phospho-FAK (Tyr397) revealed that both proteins appeared delineating the margin of some cells and organized into linear streaks typical of focal adhesions at leading edge of the cells that were separating, detaching and migrating (Figs. 5a,b).

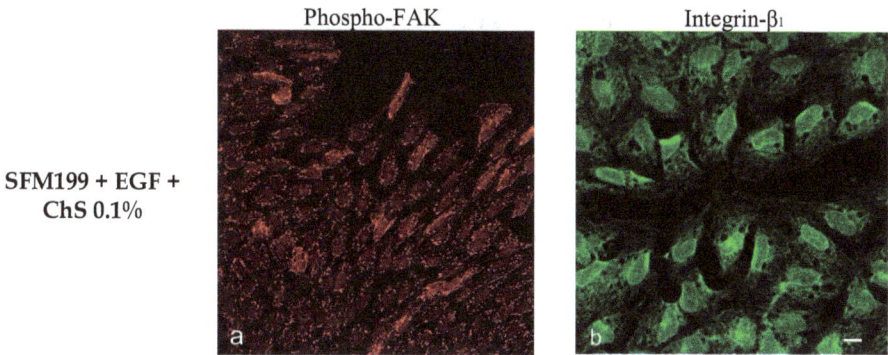

Fig. 5. Representative CLSM fluorescence images of integrin β_1 and phospho-FAK in monolayers of endothelial cells adhered to pFN after 8 hr in culture in the presence of EGF and low-ChS.
a) Integrin β_1 and b) phospho-FAK are seen delineating the margin of some cells and organized into arrays typical of focal adhesions at the leading of the migrating cells. a) Scale bar: 5µm; b) scale bar 10µm.

3.1.2 Partial activation of EGFR/ErbB1 and ErbB2/Neu mediated by integrin β_3 is increased by addition of EGF or TGF-α and low-ChS

Increasing evidence suggest that the adhesion mediated by integrins can promote the recruitment and partial activation of certain RTKs including EGFR and ErbB2/Neu in the absence of serum or growth factors after cell-matrix adhesion (Desgrosellier & Cheresh, 2010; Ivaska & Heino, 2010; Streuli & Akhtar, 2009; Yamada & Even-Ram,2002); therefore, we also investigated whether activated EGFR and ErbB2 were present in monolayers of embryonic endothelial cells adhered to pFN-coated dishes that were incubated in SFM199 for 2-3 hr and switched to SFM199 supplemented with EGF or TGF-α and low-ChS and maintained for an additional 6-8 hr period. Under these conditions the expression of both activated EGFR and ErbB2 was investigated by immunoperoxidase staining using anti-phospho-EGFR (Tyr845) and anti-phospho-ErbB2 (Tyr877). In the SFM199 condition, phospho-EGFR and phospho-ErbB2 staining was mostly localized in sites of cell-cell contacts. In addition, perinuclear and nuclear staining for these receptors suggestive of activation, internalization and nuclear translocation was observed in some cells of the monolayer that had adopted a cobblestone appearance (Figs. 6a,b). Remarkably, in the EGF or TGF-α and low-ChS condition, strong perinuclear and nuclear staining for phospho-EGFR was detected in many cells of the monolayer, as well as in many spreading, separating, detaching and migrating cells; whereas in the cell-cell contacts the staining appears disrupted (Fig. 6c). For phospho-ErbB2, less intense nuclear staining was found in many endothelial cells of the monolayer and spreading, separating, detaching and migrating cells. In this condition the staining for ErbB2 in the sites of cell-cell contacts also appeared disrupted (Fig. 6d). No immunolabeling was observed when a non immune serum was used as negative control and when the primary antibody was omitted (not shown).

Phospho-EGFR (Tyr845) and phospho-ErbB2 (Tyr877) expression was confirmed by flow cytometry in some cultures (Fig. 7). This technique revealed a relatively elevated expression of phospho-EGFR and phospho-ErbB2 in the presence of EGF or TGF-α and low-ChS, in contrast to that detected in SFM199.

Taken together, these observations would suggest that the partial phosphorylation or activation of EGFR and ErbB2 mediated by integrin $β_3$ can be increased by addition of EGF or TGF-α and low-ChS.

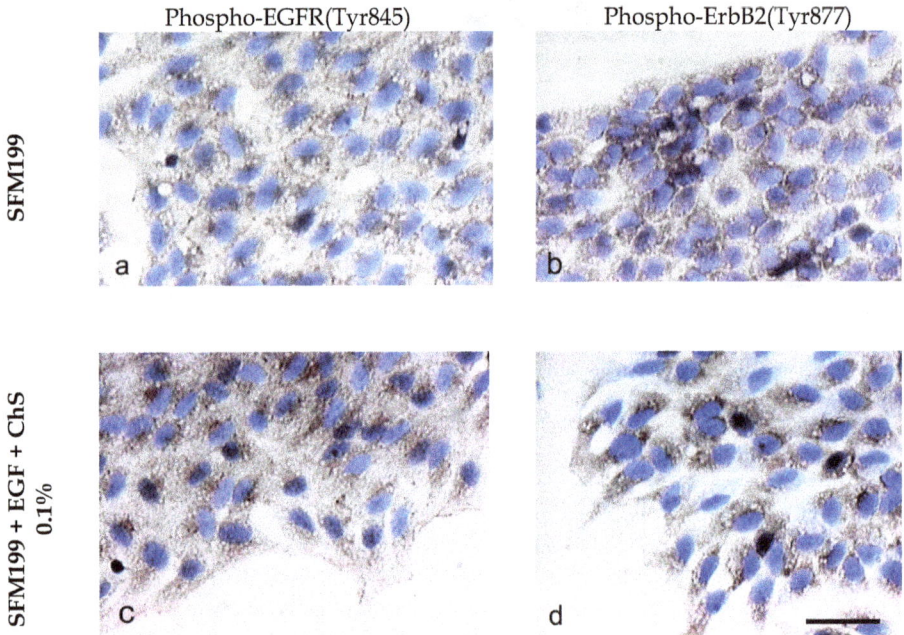

Fig. 6. (a,b) Immunolocalization of phospho-EGFR (Tyr845) and phospho-ErbB2 (Tyr877) in monolayers of endothelial cells adhered to pFN after 2hr in culture in the presence of SFM199. Staining for both receptors is detected in sites of cell-cell contacts as well as in the nucleus and perinuclear region of some cells of the monolayers. (c,d) Immunolocalization of phospho-EGFR (Tyr845) and phospho-ErbB2 (Tyr877) in monolayers whose medium were switched to medium containing EGF and low-ChS and maintained for additional 4hr (6hr). Strong nuclear and perinuclear staining for phospho-EGFR (Tyr845) is observed in many separating, detaching and migrating cells whereas in the cell-cell contacts the staining appears disrupted. For phospho-ErbB2 less intense nuclear staining is detected in many cells. Note that the staining at the sites of cell-cell contacts also appears disrupted. Scale bar: 50µm.

Integrin-Mediated Endothelial Cell Adhesion and Activation of c-Src, EGFR and ErbB2 are Required for
Endothelial-Mesenchymal Transition

55

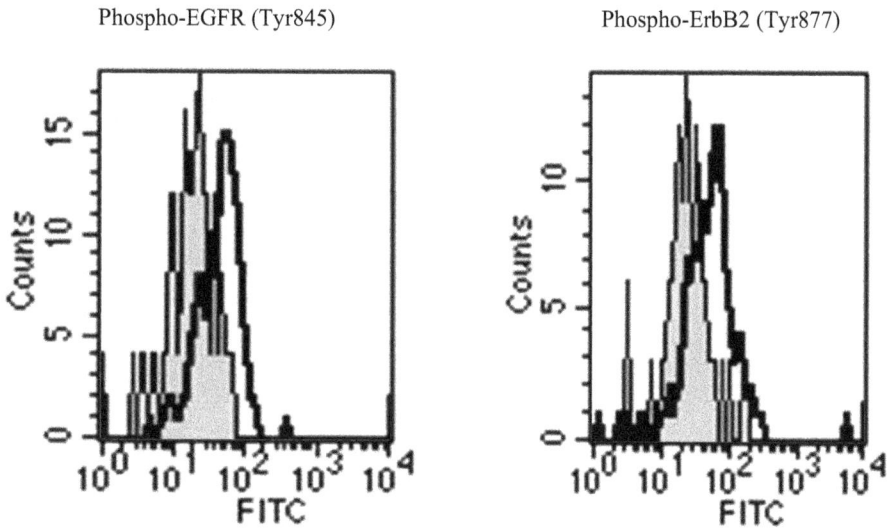

Fig. 7. Effect of TGF-α on phospho-EGFR (Tyr845) and phospho-ErbB2 (Tyr877)
expression

Expression of phospho-EGFR (Tyr845) and phospho-ErbB2 (Tyr877) analyzed by
flow cytometry in embryonic endothelial cells that were maintained for 2hr in SFM199,
and in embryonic endothelial cells where the medium was switched to SFM199
supplemented with TGF-α and low-ChS and cultured for additional 4hr (6hr). Negative
controls were stained with the respective isotype. Histograms show expression (after
substracting the background) of phospho-EGFR (Tyr845) and phospho-ErbB2 (Tyr877) by
SFM199 (black profile) or TGF-α treated (opened histograms) embryonic endothelial cells.
Results are representative of at least three independent experiments, all of which had
similar results.

3.1.3 In vitro phospho-c-Src (Tyr416) immunolocalization

Recent in vitro studies have indicated that after the adhesion of cells to the ECM, the
cytoplasmic tail of integrin β_3 can directly interact with c-Src promoting its activation and
that activated c-Src in turn phosphorylates ErbB2 at Tyr877 residue (Marcotte et al., 2009);
therefore, we also investigated whether the activated c-Src was present in monolayers of
endothelial cells when they were maintained in SFM199 and when they were switched to
medium containing EGF and low-ChS. Immunolocalization with anti-phospho-c-Src
(Tyr416 in chicken) showed that in the SFM199 condition this non-RTK was also localized at
the cell-cell contacts or AJs (Fig. 8a) whereas in the EGF and low-ChS condition, phospho-c-
Src appeared aligned with MTs and organized into linear streaks typical of focal adhesion
complexes at the leading edge as well as in the nucleus of some cells that were separating,
detaching and migrating (Fig. 8b).

SFM199   SFM199 + EGF + ChS 0.1%

Phospho-c-Src

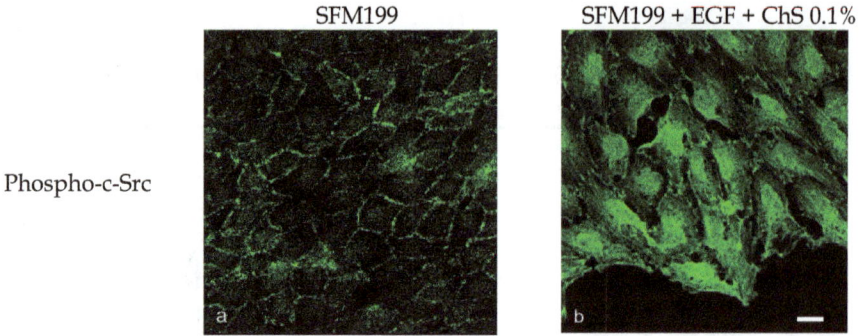

Fig. 8. a) CLSM fluorescence image of phospho-c-Src (Tyr416) in a monolayer of endothelial cells adhered to pFN after 2hr in culture in the presence of SFM199. Phospho-c-Src is seen in the cell-cell contacts. b) CLSM fluorescence image of phospho-c-Src (Tyr416) in a monolayer whose medium was switched to medium containing EGF and low-ChS. Phospho-c-Src (Tyr416) appears aligned with MTs and organized into linear streaks at the leading edge of separating, detaching and migrating cells. Note that this non-RTK is also detected in the nucleus of some cells. Scale bar: 15μm.

3.1.4 In vivo EGF, TGF-α, EGFR, and ErbB2 immunolocalization

In view of the above in vitro findings, we evaluated EGF, TGF-α, EGFR and ErbB2/Neu by immunoperoxidase staining in the aortic wall at days E12-E14 (stages 38-40) of development when intimal thickening is apparent and EndoMT occurs (Arciniegas et al., 2000).

EGF   TGF-α   EGFR   ErbB2/Neu

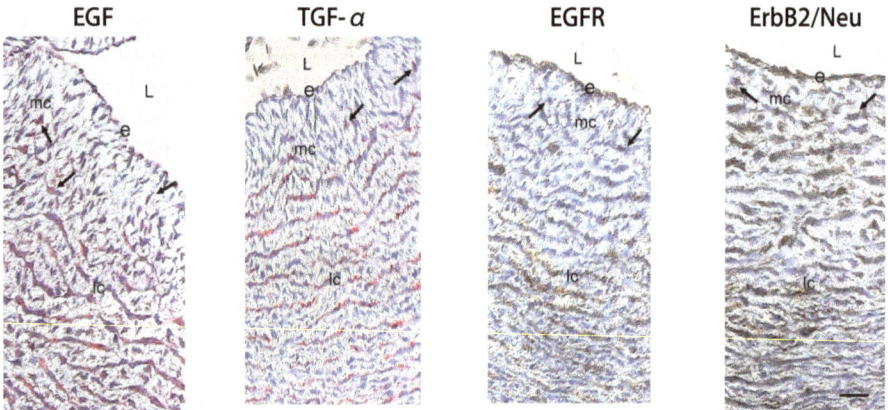

Fig. 9. Immunolocalization of EGF, TGF-α, EGFR, and ErbB2/Neu in deparaffinized sections of chicken embryo aorta at day E14 of development.
Immunoreactivity for EGF is observed in the endothelial cells (e) and some mesenchymal cells (mc) and in cells of the lamellar layers (lc). For TGF-α, a less immunoreactivity is observed in the endothelial cells (e) and some mesenchymal cells (mc) and cells of the lamellar layers (lc). Strong ErbB2/Neu and moderate EGFR immunoreactivities are detected in most endothelial cells (e) and mesenchymal cells (mc) and lamellar cells (lc). L, lumen. Scale bar = 125μm.

Integrin-Mediated Endothelial Cell Adhesion and Activation of c-Src, EGFR and ErbB2 are Required for
Endothelial-Mesenchymal Transition

57

At days E12-E14, the aortic wall is composed by the endothelium, which limits the vessel lumen, and radially oriented mesenchymal cells originating from the endothelium that constitute the intimal thickening. At these stages it is possible to distinguish cells organized in circular lamellar and interlamellar layers. The immunoreactivity observed at these stages for EGF was more intense compared to TGF-α. Even so, both immunoreactivities were detected at the endothelial cells and in some mesenchymal cells of the intimal thickening as well as in those arranged in lamellar layers (Fig. 9). Immunoperoxidase staining also revealed strong ErbB2/Neu and moderate EGFR immunoreactivities in most endothelial and mesenchymal cells and those arranged in lamellar layers (Figs. 9). No immunoreactivity was observed when the primary antibody was omitted or replaced by non immune serum in control sections (not shown).

4. Discussion

This study provides evidence that allows us to suggest that the adhesion to pFN of explanted embryonic endothelial cells is mediated by integrin β_3 and promoted by Ca^{2+} and that the organization of these cells into monolayers of polarized cells, when they were maintained in the absence of serum or growth factors, was established by adhesion to FN and by formation of endothelial cell-cell contacts or AJs.The latter involving presence of β-catenin and p120-catenin, redistribution of integrin β_3 and importantly, reorganization of MTs with the possible participation of some tyrosine phosphatases and tyrosine kinases (Dejana et al, 2009). These cellular events are considered as relevant for the maintenance of endothelial cell shape and apico-basal polarity in vitro and during embryonic development (Bryant & Mostov, 2008; Dejana et al, 2008; 2009; Iruela-Arispe & Davis, 2009). Remarkably, the adhesion to pFN and organization of the endothelial cells into monolayers of polarized cells involving formation of AJs and reorganization of MTs in the absence of serum or growth factors was accompanied by tyrosine phosphorylation in the kinase domain of EGFR and ErbB2 and the nuclear translocation of both receptors. In fact, phosphorylated EGFR and ErbB2 were detected at sites of cell-cell contacts and in the nucleus of some cells of the monolayers by using anti-phospho EGFR (Tyr845) and anti-phospho ErbB2 (Tyr877). In this respect, phosphorylated EGFR has been detected during the formation of cell-cell contacts in monolayers of epithelial cells deprived of serum and maintained in presence of Ca^{2+}, suggesting a ligand independent activation of EGFR induced by its interaction with E-cadherin or with components of the AJs (Erez et al., 2005; Pece & Gutkind, 2000; Takahashi et al., 1997). It is noteworthy that basolateral localization of EGFR and ErbB2 along with components of the AJs has been consistently reported in polarized epithelial cells (Borg et al., 2000; Feigin & Muthuswamy, 2009; Hoschuetzky et al., 1994; Shelly et al., 2003; Tanos & Rodriguez-Boulan et al., 2008). Also, studies in epithelial cancer cells have indicated that the formation of AJs mediated by E-cadherin induces activation of EGFR in the absence of ligand leading to elevation of anti-apoptotic members of Bcl-2 family of regulatory proteins to protect cells from the apoptosis (Shen & Kramer, 2004).

Activated EGFR and ErbB2 have also been observed in the nucleus of human fetal endothelial cells (Bueter et al., 2006) and in normal and tumor epithelial cells suggesting that these receptors may regulate gene activation and transcription and possibly other nuclear events (Giri et al., 2005; Wang et al., 2010). In this sense, it is known that binding of integrins to their ligands in the absence of serum or growth factors can promote cell survival by increasing Bcl-2 transcription (Matter & Ruoslahti, 2001; Zhang et al., 1995) and that clustering and occupancy of integrins in the absence of growth factors can also provoke recruitment and partial activation of several RTKs including members of the EGFR family (Desgrosellier & Cheresh, 2010; Eliceiri, 2001; Huveneers & Danen, 2010; Ivaska & Heino, 2010; ; Streuli & Akhtar, 2009; Yamada & Even-Ram, 2002). For instance, in epithelial cell lines, and human endothelial cells line ECV304, adhesion to FN mediated by integrin β_1 in the absence of serum or growth factors produces a rapid phosphorylation of EGFR at Tyr845, 1068, 1086, and 1173 residues that results critical for their survival (Bill et al., 2004; Cabodi et al., 2004; Moro et al., 2002). These levels of phosphorylation are lower than that observed with EGF. Importantly, phosphorylation of Tyr845 residue in the kinase domain of EGFR has been shown requires c-Src tyrosine kinase which is activated after integrin-mediated cell adhesion and autophosphorylated at Tyr419 residue of its kinase domain (Tyr416 in chicken) (Bill et al., 2004; Cabodi et al., 2004). Others have found that phosphorylation of Tyr877 residue in the kinase domain of ErbB2 is dependent on activated and phosphorylated c-Src (Tyr419) (Marcotte et al., 2009; Rivas et al., 2010; Xu et al., 2007). Some of them suggesting that activated and phosphorylated c-Src specifically associates with ErbB2, but not with other EGFR family members (Kim et al., 2005; Marcotte et al., 2009; Muthuswamy & Muller, 1995).

In view of above observations, we also investigated the presence and distribution of c-Src in the absence of serum or growth factors. Of note, c-Src phosphorylated at Tyr416 residue was localized at sites of cell-cell contacts or AJs displaying a pattern similar to that observed for β-catenin and p120-catenin and integrin β_3. To this respect, there is evidence showing that activated c-Src participates during the cell-ECM adhesion and formation of cell-cell adhesions where it might phosphorylate β-catenin and p120-catenin regulating certain signalling pathways that are considered as essentials for cell survival (Guarino, 2010; Schlessinger, 2000). Of interest, studies have shown that adhesion of osteoclast precursors to FN or vitronectin induces c-Src and MTs association and that this association affects the polarity of osteoclasts (Abu-Amer et al., 1997). Also, studies have revealed reciprocal interactions between c-Src and EGFR in the absence of growth factors (Donepudi & Resh, 2008). One of them, suggesting that autonomus c-Src activation may cause activation of EGFR, mimicking the effects of low concentration of EGF on EGFR activation, redistribution, and signalling (de Diesbach et al., 2010). In this context, previous studies have shown that clustering of integrin β_3 by ligands such as FN can result in the recruitment and activation of c-Src, inducing phosphorylation of Tyr416 or 419 residues in its kinase domain (Arias-Salgado et al., 2003; Desgrosellier et al., 2009; Guarino, 2010; Huveneers & Danen, 2010) and that activated and phosphorylated c-Src in turn phosphorylates ErbB2 at Tyr877 residue (Marcotte et al., 2009). Interestingly, these patterns of phosphorylation are different from those triggered by the binding of EGF.

Thus, we believe that, in the absence of serum or growth factors, the adhesion of explanted embryonic endothelial cells to pFN, mediated by activation and clustering of integrin β_3, promotes the activation of c-Src which is found associated with MTs and that activated c-Src contributes to the formation of endothelial cell-cell contacts or Ajs by phosphorylation of β-catenin and p120-catenin. This process would be accompanied by the EGFR and ErbB2 phosphorylation at the Tyr845 and Tyr877 residues respectively, leading to the partial activation and nuclear translocation of both receptors with consequent regulation of Bcl-2 proteins expression to protect cells from the apoptosis induced by serum-deprivation.

In this study, we found that the closure of the wounds (re-endothelialization) was almost complete and that endothelial cell spreading, separation, detachment and migration also took place at the marginal edges of the monolayers when the medium of some cultures was switched to medium containing EGF or TGF-α and low amount of ChS (0.1%). These observations are consistent with the possibility that EGF or TGF-α may be interacting with those EGFRs that remain exposed or accessible to ligand in the lateral cell borders after removing the explant. EGFR then would heterodimerize with ErbB2 and being internalized which results in the disruption of endothelial cell-cell contacts by remodelling of the MTs and alterations in the distribution of integrin β_3, β-catenin and p120-catenin, and therefore mediating the reparation of the wounds and the migration of the cells toward cell-free areas. This view is reinforced by previous reports suggesting that mechanical damage of monolayers of epithelial cells allows to ErbB2, which localizes on the basolateral surface, to interact with its ligand (heregulin) normally secreted to the apical surface leading to proliferation, migration and repair of the wound (Mostov & Zegers, 2003; Tanos & Rodríguez-Boulan, 2008; Vermeer et al., 2003). Notably, in this study we also found changes in the distribution and organization of phospho-c-Src (Tyr416) upon EGF or TGF-α and low-ChS addition. We believe that such changes may be associated with remodelling of MTs and alterations in the distribution of integrins β_3 and β_1 and β-catenin and p120-catenin during the disruption of endothelial cell-cell contacts. Consistent with this, studies in EGF-stimulated epithelial cells have provided evidence that MTs remodelling induces activation of c-Src which then phosphorylates β-catenin and p120-catenin, leading to the disruption of AJs, cell-ECM adhesion promoting cell migration and invasion (Guarino, 2010). Also of significance, cytoskeleton remodelling and loss of cell-cell contacts have been correlated with elevated expression of activated c-Src in tumor cells and during the EMT process (Alper & Bowden, 2005; Guarino, 2010). In relation to the nuclear localization of phospho c-Src (Tyr416) observed during EGF stimulation, emerging evidence suggest that nuclear localization of Src-family tyrosine kinases, including c-Src, upon growth factor stimulation regulates not only tyrosine phosphorylation of nuclear proteins, but also the structure of chromatin (Takahashi et al., 2009). In this study, stimulation with EGF or TGF-α also showed the localization of phospho-FAK (Tyr397), integrins β_3 and β_1 at focal adhesion when endothelial cell spreading, separation, detachment, and migration occurred. In this context, previous studies have shown that clustering of integrins β_1, β_3, and β_5 by ligands such as FN or alterations in the cytoskeleton, can result in the recruitment and autophosphorylation of FAK at Tyr397 residue and that activated FAK promotes Src binding and activation to increase FAK activity leading to the formation an activated FAK-Src signalling complex (Ilić et al., 2004; Mitra et al., 2005). Same studies propose that this activated complex affect not only the assembly and disassembly of focal adhesions, but also promotes cell migration through regulation of cytoskeleton and integrin recycling and the disruption of adherens junctions (Mitra et al., 2005). Interestingly, integrin recruitment, internalization by macropinocytosis and redistribution, have been observed during cell migration induced by growth factors (Gu et al., 2011).Thus, we believe that the endothelial cell detachment involving assembly and disassembly of focal adhesions and the migration observed upon EGF or TGF-α and low-ChS addition would be related with integrins β_3 and β_1 recruitment, internalization and redistribution, and with the activation of FAK and c-Src during EGFR and ErbB2 endocytosis. It is known that EGF or TGF-α acts by binding to EGFR leading to the receptor homo-or hetero-dimerization, activation of its receptor tyrosine kinase cytosolic domain and autophosphorylation on tyrosine residues initiating various important signal transduction pathways that could collaborate in the cell adhesion, migration, proliferation, differentiation and survival (Carpenter & Liao 2009; Olayioye et al., 2000). Upon binding of EGF, receptors clustering and endocytosis take place followed by recycling back of the ligand-complex to the cell surface or degradation. After internalization, nuclear translocation of the receptors may also occur to regulate gene expression (Giri et al., 2005; Lemmon, 2009; Roepstorff et al., 2008; Wang et al., 2010; Yarden & Sliwkowski, 2001). Of particular interest, stimulation of EGFR endocytosis accompanied by remodelling of MTs after addition of EGF has been reported in HeLa cells (Kharchenko et al., 2007).

In this study, phosphorylation, internalization, and nuclear translocation of EGFR and ErbB2 was also observed upon EGF or TGF-α and low-ChS addition. In this condition, flow cytometry analysis revealed an increased expression of phosphorylated EGFR and ErbB2, in contrast with that detected in the SFM condition or absence of growth factors. Consistent with this, previous studies have shown that treatment of endothelial ECV304 cells with EGF, increases the levels of phosphorylation of EGFR induced by adhesion to FN and mediated by integrin β_1 (Cabodi et al., 2004). Of note, a recent work by Odintsova´s laboratory has reported that the integrin-mediated epithelial cell adhesion potentiates the phosphorylation of EGFR and ErbB2 induced by EGF or TGF-α facilitating receptor homo-and hetero-dimerization of these receptors and that this process could be accompanied by actin cytoskeleton organization (Alexi et al., 2011). Accordingly, our observations suggest that the dimerization, activation and phosphorylation of EGFR and ErbB2, initiated by integrin β_3, would be increased by addition of EGF or TGF-α, and that the internalization of these receptors could be accompanied by MTs remodelling which induces the activation of c-Src and phosphorylation of β-catenin and p120-catenin to promote loss of endothelial cell polarity and disruption of cell-cell contacts, facilitating cell spreading, separation, detachment, and migration, cellular events considered as essentials in the progression of EndoMT. Interestingly, overexpression and/or activation of EGFRs have been well documented to affect epithelial polarization and cell-cell contacts and leads to EMT of normal cells (Feigin & Muthuswamy, 2009). However, the precise mechanisms by which EGFRs deregulate normal epithelial architecture to promote EMT are incompletely understood (Feigin & Muthuswamy, 2009)

In addition to these findings, this study also provides in vivo evidence that EGF, TGF-α as well as their receptors EGFR and ErbB2 were present in those stages of development (days E12-E14) where the intimal thickening are clearly evident and EndoMT is an active process. These data are interesting if we consider that in vivo expression of EGF, TGF-α as well as their respective receptors have been detected in the intimal thickening and medial smooth muscle cells of atherosclerotic lesions (Dreux et al., 2006), and that expression of activated ErbB2 and ErbB3 has been demonstrated during heart cushion development (Camenish et al., 2002), suggesting an important contribution for these receptors in the initiation of atherosclerosis and in the development of cardiac valves, respectively.

Collectively, our findings suggest that integrin-mediated endothelial cell adhesion and activation and translocation of c-Src, EGFR and ErbB2 as well as the presence of their ligands are required for EndoMT.

5. Acknowledgment

We thank Eng. Antonio Salgado (Area de informática, SAIB) for photographic assistance. This work was supported by Consejo de Desarrollo Científico y Humanístico, UCV grant PI-09-7319-2008.

6. References

Abu-Amer, Y., Ross, F., Schlesinger, P., Tondravi, M. & Teitelbaum, S. (1997). Substrate recognition by osteoclast precursors induces C-Src/microtubule association. *The Journal of Cell Biology*, 137, 1, 247-258, 0021-9525

Ackland, M., Newgreen, D., Fridman, M., Waltham, M., Arvanitis, A., Minichiello, J., Price, J. & Thompson, E. (2003). Epidermal growth factor induced epithelio mesenchymal transition in human breast carcinoma cells. *Laboratory Investigation*, 83, 3, 435-448, 0023-6837

Akhmanova, A., Stehbens, S. & Yap, A. (2009). Touch, grasp, deliver and control: functional cross-talk between microtubules and cell adhesions. *Traffic*, 10, 3, 268-274, 1398-9219

Alexi, X., Berditchevski, F. & Odintsova E. (2011). The effect of cell-ECM adhesion on signalling via the ErbB family of growth factor receptors. *Biochemical Society Transactions*, 39, 2, 568-573, 0300-5127

Alper, O. & Bowden, E. (2005). Novel insights into c-Src. *Current Pharmaceutical Design*, 11, 9, 1119-1130, 1381-6128

Arciniegas, E., Ponce, L., Hartt, Y., Graterol, A. & Carlini R. (2000). Intimal thickening involves transdifferentiation of embryonic endothelial cells. *The Anatomical Record*, 258, 1, 47-57, 1932-8494

Arciniegas, E., Neves, Y., Carrillo, L. & Zambrano, A. (2005). Endothelial – mesenchymal transition ocurrs during embryonic pulmonary artery development. *Endothelium*, 12, 4,193-200, 1062-3329

Arciniegas, E., Frid, M., Douglas, S. & Stenmark, K. (2007). Perspectives on endothelial-to-mesenchymal transition: potential contribution to vascular remodeling in chronic pulmonary hypertension. *American Journal of Physiology Lung Cellular and Molecular Physiology*, 293, 1. L1-L8, 1040-0605

Arciniegas, E. & Candelle, D. (2008). An alternate insulin-like growth factor I receptor signaling pathway for the progression of endothelial–mesenchymal transition. *Bioscience Hypotheses*, 1, 6, 312-318, 1756-2392

Arias-Salgado, E., Lizano, S., Sarkar, S., Brugge, J., Ginsberg, M. & Shattil, S. (2003). Src kinase activation by direct interaction with the integrin β cytoplasmic domain. *Proceedings of the National Academy of Sciences USA*, 100, 23, 13298-13302, 0027-8424

Baum, B., Settleman, J. & Quinlan, M. (2008). Transitions between epithelial and mesenchymal states in development and disease. *Seminars in Cell & Developmental Biology*, 19, 3, 294-308, 1084-9521

Bill, H., Knudsen, B., Moores, S., Muthuswamy, S., Rao, V., Brugge, J. & Miranti, C. (2004). Epidermal growth factor receptor-dependent regulation of integrin-mediated signaling and cell cycle entry in epithelial cells. *Molecular and Cellular Biology*, 24, 19, 8586-8599, 0270-7306

Bombeli, T., Schwartz, B. & Harlan, J. (1998). Adhesion of activated platelets to endothelial cells: evidence for a GPIIbIIIa-dependent bridging mechanism and novel roles for endothelial intercellular adhesion molecule 1 (ICAM-1), alphavbeta3 integrin, and GPIbalpha. *The Journal of Experimental Medicine*, 187, 3, 329-339, 0022-1007

Borg, J-P., Marchetto, S., Le Bivic, A., Ollendorff, V., Jaulin-Bastard, F., Saito, H., Fournier, E., Adélaïde, J., Margolis, B. & Birnbaum, D. (2000). ERBIN: a basolateral PDZ protein that interacts with the mammalian ERBB2/HER2 receptor. *Nature Cell Biology*, 2, 7, 407-414, 1476-4679

Bryant,D. & Mostov, K. (2008). From cells to organs: building polarizad tissue. *Nature Reviews Molecular Cell Biology*, 9, 9, 887-901, 1471-0072

Bueter, W., Dammann, O., Zscheppang, K., Korenbaum, E. & Dammann C. (2006). ErbB receptors in fetal endothelium – A potential linkage point for inflammation – associated neonatal disorders. *Cytokine,* 36, 5-6, 267-275, 1043-4666

Cabodi, S., Moro, L., Bergatto, E., Boeri Erba, E., Di Stefano, P., Turco, E., Tarone, E. & Defilippi P. (2004). Integrin regulation of epidermal growth factor (EGF) receptor and of EGF-dependent responses. *Biochemical Society Transactions*, 32, Pt3, 438-442, 1470-8752

Camenisch,T., Schroeder, J., Bradley, J., Klewer, S. & McDonald, J. (2002). Heart-valve mesenchyme formation is dependent on hyaluronan-augmented activation of ErbB2-ErbB3 receptors .*Nature Medicine*, 8, 8, 850-855, 1078-8956

Carpenter, G. & Liao, H. (2009). Trafficking of receptor tyrosine kinases to the nucleus. *Experimental Cell Research*, 315, 9, 1556-1566, 0014-4827

Cierniewska-Cieslak, A., Cierniewski, C., Blecka, K., Papierak, M., Michalec, L., Zhang, L., Haas, T. & Plow, E. (2002). Identification and characterization of two cation binding sites in the integrin β_3 subunit. *The Journal of Biological Chemistry*, 277, 13, 11126-11134, 0021-9258

Cluzel, C., Saltel, F., Lussi, J., Paulhe, F., Imhof, B. & Wehrle-Haller, B. (2005). The mechanisms and dynamics of $\alpha_v\beta_3$ integrin clustering in living cells. *The Journal of Cell Biology*, 171, 2, 383-392 0021-9525

de Diesbach, M., Cominelli, A., N´Kuli, F., Tyteca, D. & Courtoy, P. (2010). Acute ligand-independent Src activation mimics low EGF-induced EGFR surface signalling and redistribution into recycling endosomes. *Experimental Cell Research*, 316, 19, 3239-3253, 0014-4827

Dejana, E., Orsenigo, F. & Lampugnani, M. (2008). The role of adherens junctions and VE-cadherin in the control vascular permeability. *Journal of Cell Science*, 121, Pt13, 2115-2122, 0021-9533

Dejana, E., Tournier-Lasserve, E. & Weinstein, B. (2009). The control the vascular integrity by endothelial cell junctions: molecular basis and pathological implications. *Developmental Cell*, 16, 2, 209-221, 1534-5807

Desgrosellier, J., Barnes, L., Shields, D., Huang, M., Lau, S., Prévost, N., Tarin, D., Shattil, S. & Cheresh, D. (2009) An integrin $\alpha_v\beta_5$ c-Src oncogenic unit promotes anchorage – independence and tumor progression. *Nature Medicine*, 15, 10, 1163-1169, 1061-4036

Desgrosellier, J. & Cheresh, D. (2010). Integrins in cancer: biological implications and therapeutic opportunities. *Nature Reviews Cancer*, 10, 1, 9-22, 1474-175X

Donepudi, M. & Resh, M. (2008). c-Src trafficking and co-localization with the EGF receptor promotes EGF ligand-independent EGFR receptor activation and signaling. *Cellular Signalling*, 20, 7, 1359-1367, 0898-6568

Dreux, A., Lamb, D., Modjtahedi, H. & Ferns, G. (2006). The epidermal growth factor receptors and their family of ligands: their putative role in atherogenesis. *Atherosclerosis*, 186, 1, 38-53, 0021-9150

Eliceiri, B. (2001). Integrin and growth factor receptor crosstalk. *Circulation Research*, 89, 12, 1104-1110, 0009-7330

Ellis, I., Schor A. & Schor, S. (2007). EGF and TGF-α motogenic activities are mediated by the
    EGF receptor via distinct matrix-dependent mechanisms. *Experimental Cell Research*,
    313, 4, 732-741, 0014-4827

Erez, N., Bershadsky, A. & Geiger, B. (2005). Signaling from adherens type junctions.
    European Journal of Cell Biology, 84, 2-3, 235-244, 9335, 0171 84

Feigin, M. & Muthuswamy, S. (2009). ErbB receptors and cell polarity: new pathways and
    paradigms for understanding cell migration and invasion. *Experimental Cell
    Research*, 315, 4, 707-716, 0014-4827

Fuller, S., Sivarajah, K. & Sugden, P. (2008). ErbB receptors, their ligands, and the
    consequences of their activation and inhibition in the myocardium. *Journal of
    Molecular and Cellular Cardiology*, 44, 5, 831-854, 0022-2828

Geiger, B. & Yamada, K. (2011). Molecular architecture and function of matrix adhesions.
    Cold Spring Harbor Perspectives in Biology, 3, 5, 1-21, 1943-0264

Giri, D., Ali-Seyed, M., Li, L., Lee, D., Ling, P., Bartholomeusz, G., Wang, S. & Hung, M.
    (2005). Endosomal transport of Erbb2: mechanism for nuclear entry of the cell
    surface receptor. *Molecular and Cellular Biology*, 25, 24, 11005-11018, 0270-7306

Goumans, M., van Zonneveld, A. & ten Dijke, P. (2008). Transforming growth factor –β-
    induced endothelial to mesenchymal transition: A switch to cardiac fibrosis? *Trends
    in Cardiovascular Medicine*, 18, 8, 293-298, 1050-1738

Gu, Z., Noss, E., Hsu, V. & Brenner, M. (2011). Integrins traffic rapidly via circular dorsal
    ruffles and macropinocytosis during stimulated cell migration. *The Journal of Cell
    Biology*, 193, 1, 61-70, 0021-9525

Guarino, M. (2007). Epithelial – mesenchymal transition and tumour invasion. *The
    International Journal of Biochemistry & Cell Biology*, 39, 12, 2153-2160, 1357-2725

Guarino, M. (2010). Src signaling in cancer invasion. *Journal of Cellular Physiology*, 223, 1, 14-
    26, 0021-9541

Guo, W. & Giancotti, F. (2004). Integrin signalling during tumour progression. *Nature
    Reviews Molecular Cell Biology*, 5, 10, 816-826, 1471-0072

Guo, W., Pylayeva, Y., Pepe, A., Yoshioka, T., Muller, W., Inghirami, G. & Giancotti, F.
    (2006). β₄ integrin amplifies ErbB2 signaling to promote mammary tumorigenesis.
    Cell, 126, 3, 489-502, 0092-8674

Hamburger, V. & Hamilton, H. (1992). A series of normal stages in the development of the
    chick embryo. *Developmental Dynamics*, 195, 4, 231-272, 1097-0177.

Hoschuetzky, H., Aberle, H. & Kemler, R. (1994). Beta-catenin mediates the interaction of
    the cadherin-catenin complex with epidermal growth factor receptor. *The Journal of
    Cell Biology*, 127, 5, 1375-1380, 0021-9525

Huveneers, S. & Danen, E. (2010). The interaction of Src kinase with β₃ integrin tails: a
    potential therapeutic target in thrombosis and cancer. *The Scientific World Journal*.
    10, 1100-1106, 1537-744X

Ilić, D., Kovacic, B., Johkura, K., Schaepfer, D., Tomasević, N., Han, Q., Kim, J., Howerton,
    K., Baumbusch, C., Ogiwara, N., Streblow; D., Nelson, J., Dazin, P., Shino, Y.,
    Sasaki, K. & Damsky, C. (2004). FAK promotes organization of fibronectin matrix
    and fibrillar adhesions. *Journal of Cell Science*, 117, Pt2, 177-187, 0021-9533

Iruela-Arispe, M. & Davis, G. (2009). Cellular and molecular mechanisms of vascular lumen
    formation. *Developmental Cell*, 16, 2, 222-231, 1534-5807

Ivaska, J. & Heino, J. (2010). Interplay between cell adhesion and growth factor receptors: from the plasma membrane to the endosomes. *Cell Tissue Research*, 339, 1, 111-120, 0302-766X

Jean, C., Gravelle, P. & Laurent, G. (2011). Influence of stress on extracellular matrix and integrin biology. *Oncogene*, 30, 24, 2697-2706, 0950-9232

Kharchenko, M., Aksyonov, A., Melikova, M. & Kornilova, E. (2007). Epidermal growth factor (EGF) receptor endocytosis is accompanied by reorganization of microtubule system in HeLa cells. *Cell Biology International*, 31, 4, 349-359, 1065-6995

Kim, H., Chan, R., Dankort, D., Zuo, D., Najoukas, M., Park, M. & Muller, W. (2005). The c-Src tyrosine kinase associates with the catalytic domain of ErbB-2: implications for ErbB-2 mediated signaling and transformation. *Oncogene*, 24, 51, 7599−7607, 0950-9232

Leitinger, B., McDowall, A., Stanley, P. & Hogg N. (2000). The regulation of integrin function by Ca^{2+}. *Biochimica et Biophysica Acta*, 1498, 2-3, 91-98, 0006-3002

Lemmon, M. (2009). Ligand induced ErbB receptor dimerization. *Experimental Cell Research*, 315, 4, 638-648, 0014-4827

Li, J. & Bertram, J. (2010). Review: Endothelial-myofibroblast transition, a new player in diabetic renal fibrosis. *Nephrology*, 15, 5, 507-512, 1440-1797, 0950-9232

Luo, B. & Springer, T. (2006). Integrin structures and conformational signaling. *Current Opinion in Cell Biology*, 18, 5, 579-586, 0955-0674

Marcotte, R., Zhou, L., Kim, H., Roskelly, C. & Muller, W. (2009). c-Src associates with ErbB2 through an interaction between catalytic domains and confers enhanced transforming potential. *Molecular and Cellular Biology*, 29, 21, 5858-5871, 0270-7306

Matter, M. & Ruoslahti, E. (2001). A signaling pathway from the $\alpha_5\beta_1$ and $\alpha_v\beta_3$ integrins that elevates bcl-2 transcription. *The Journal of Biological Chemistry*, 276, 30, 27757-27763, 0021-9258

Mironov, V., Visconti, R. & Markwald, R. (2005). The role of shear stress in cardiogenesis. *Endothelium*, 12, 5-6, 259-261, 1062-3329

Mitra, S., Hanson, D. & Schlaepfer, D. (2005). Focal adhesion kinase: in command and control of cell motility. *Nature Reviews Molecular Cell Biology*, 6, 1, 1471-0072

Moro, L., Venturino, M., Bozzo, C., Silengo, L., Altruda, F., Beguinot, L., Tarone, G. & Defilippi, P. (1998). Integrins induce activation of EGF receptor: role in MAP kinase induction and adhesion-dependent cell survival. *The EMBO Journal*, 17, 22, 6622-6632, 0261-4189

Moro, L., Dolce, L., Cabodi, S., Bergatto, E., Boeri Erba, E., Smeriglio, M., Turco, E., Retta, S., Giuffrida, M., Venturino, M., Godovac-Zimmermann, J., Conti, A., Schaefer, E., Beguinot, L., Tacchetti, C., Gaggini, P., Silengo, L., Tarone, G. & Defilippi P. (2002). Integrin-induced epidermal growth factor (EGF) receptor activation requires c-Src and p130Cas and leads to phosphorylation of specific EGF receptor tyrosines. *The Journal of Biological Chemistry*. 277, 11, 9405-9414, 0021-9258

Morrell, N., Adnot, S., Archer, S., Dupuis, J., Jones, P., MacLean, R., McMurtry, I., Stenmark, K., Thistlethwaite, P, Weissmann, N, Yuan, J. & Weir, E. (2009). Cellular and molecular basis of pulmonary arterial hypertension. *Journal of the American College of Cardiology*, 54, 1, S20-S31, 0735-1097

Mostov, K. & Zegers M. (2003). Cell biology: just mix and patch. *Nature*, 422, 6929, 267-268, 0028-0836

Integrin-Mediated Endothelial Cell Adhesion and Activation of c-Src, EGFR and ErbB2 are Required for
Endothelial-Mesenchymal Transition

65

Mukherjee,S., Tessema, M. & Wandinger-Ness, A. (2006). Vesicular trafficking of tyrosine kinase receptors and associated proteins in the regulation of signaling and vascular function. *Circulation Research,* 98, 6, 743-756, 0009-7330

Muthuswamy, S. & Muller, W. (1995). Direct and specific interaction of c-Src with Neu is involved in signaling by the epidermal growth factor receptor. *Oncogene,* 11, 2, 271-279, 0950-9232

Negro, A., Brar, B. & Lee, K. (2004). Essential roles for Her2/erbB2 in cardiac development and function. *Recent Progress in Hormone Research,* 59, 1-12, 0079-9963

Olayioye, M., Neve, R., Lane, H. & Hynes, N. (2000). The ErbB signaling network: receptor heterodimerization in development and cancer. *The EMBO Journal,* 19, 13, 3159-3167, 0261-4189

Papusheva, E. & Heisenberg, C. (2010). Spatial organization of adhesion: force-dependent regulation and function in tissue morphogenesis. *The EMBO Journal,* 29, 16, 2753-2768, 0261-4189

Pece, S. & Gutkind, S. (2000). Signaling from E-cadherins to the MAPK pathway by the recruitment and activation of epidermal growth factor receptors upon cell-cell contact formation. *The Journal of Biological Chemistry,* 275, 52, 41227-41233, 0021-9258

Potenta, S., Zeisberg, E. & Kalluri, R. (2008). The endothelial -to- mesenchymal transition in cancer progression. *British Journal of Cancer,* 99, 9, 1375-1379, 0007-0920

Rivas, M., Tkach, M., Beguelin, W., Proietti, C., Rosemblit, C., Charreau, E., Elizalde, P. & Schillaci R. (2010). Transactivation of ErbB-2 induced by tumor necrosis factor α promotes NF-κB activation and breast cancer cell proliferation. *Breast Cancer Research and Treatment,* 122, 1, 111-124, 0167-6806

Roepstorff, K., Grøvdal, L., Grandal, M., Lerdrup, M. & van Deurs B. (2008). Endocytic downregulation of ErbB receptors: mechanisms and relevance in cancer. *Histochemistry and Cell Biology,* 129, 5, 563-578, 0948-6143.

Sakao, S., Tatsumi, K. & Voelkel, N. (2010). Reversible or irreversible remodeling in pulmonary arterial hypertension. *The American Journal of Respiratory Cell and Molecular Biology,* 43, 6, 629-634, 1044-1549

Schlessinger,J. (2000). New roles for Src kinases in control of cell survival and angiogenesis. *Cell,* 100, 3, 293-296, 0092-8674

Schwartz, M. (2010). Integrins and extracellular matrix in mechanotransduction. *Cold Spring Harbor Perspectives in Biology,* 2, 12, 1-13, 1943-0264

Shelly, M., Mosesson, Y., Citri, A., Lavi, S., Zwang, Y., Melamed-Book, N., Aroeti, B. & Yarden, Y. (2003). Polar expression of ErbB-2/HER2 in epithelia: Bimodal regulation by Lin-7. *Developmental Cell,* 5, 3, 475-486, 1534-5807

Shen, X. & Kramer, R. (2004). Adhesion-mediated squamous cell carcinoma survival through ligand-independent activation of epidermal growth factor receptor. *American Journal of Pathology,* 165, 4, 1315-1329, 0002-9440

Soldi, R., Mitola, S., Strasly, M., Defilippi, P., Tarone, G. & Bussolino, F. (1999). Role $α_v β_3$ integrin in the activation of vascular endothelial growth factor receptor-2. *The EMBO J,* 18, 4, 882-892, 0261-4189

Streuli, C. & Akhtar, N. (2009). Signal co-operation between integrins and other receptor systems. *Biochemical Journal,* 418, 3, 491-506, 0264-6021

Takahashi, A., Obata, Y., Fukumoto, Y., Nakayama, Y., Kasahara, K., Kuga, T., Higashiyama, Y., Saito, T., Yokoyama, K. & Yamaguchi, N. (2009). Nuclear localization of Src – family tyrosine kinases is required for growth factor induced euchromatinization. *Experimental Cell Research*, 315, 7, 1117-1141, 0014-4827

Takahashi, K., Suzuki, K. & Tsukatani, Y. (1997). Induction of tyrosine phosphorylation and association of beta-catenin with EGF receptor upon tryptic digestion of quiescent cells at confluence. *Oncogene*, 15, 1, 71-78, 0950-9232

Tanos, B. & Rodriguez-Boulan. (2008). The epithelial polarity program: machineries involved and their hijacking by cancer. *Oncogene*, 27, 55, 6939-6957, 0950-9232

Vermeer, P., Einwalter, L., Moninger, T., Rokhlina, T., Kern, J. & Weish, M. (2003). Segregation of receptor and ligand regulates activation of epithelial growth factor receptor. *Nature*, 422, 6929, 322-326, 0028-0836

Wang, Y., Yamaguchi, H., Hsu, J. & Hung, M. (2010). Nuclear trafficking of the epidermal growth factor receptor family membrane proteins. *Oncogene*, 29, 28, 3997-4006, 0950-9232

Xi-Qiao, W., Ying-Kai, L., Chun, Q. & Shu-Liang, L. (2009). Hyperactivity of fibroblasts and functional regression of endothelial cells contribute to microvessel occlusion in hypertrophic scarring. *Microsvascular Research*, 77, 2, 204-211, 0026-2862

Xu, W., Yuan, X., Beebe, K., Xiang, Z. & Neckers, L. (2007). Loss of Hsp90 association up-regulates Src – dependent ErbB2 activity. *Molecular and Cellular Biology*, 27, 1, 220-228, 0270-7306

Yamada, K. & Even-Ram, S. (2002). Integrin regulation of growth factor receptors. *Nature Cell Biology*, 4, 4, E75-E76, 1465-7392

Yarden, Y. & Sliwkowski M. (2001). Untangling the ErbB signalling network. *Nature Reviews Molecular Cell Biology*, 2, 2, 127-137, 1471-0072

Zeisberg, E., Potenta, S., Sugimoto, H., Zeisberg, M. & Kalluri, R. (2008). Fibroblasts in kidney fibrosis emerge via endothelial-to-mesenchymal transition. *Journal of the American Society of Nephrology*, 19, 12, 2282-2287, 1046-6673

Zhang, Z., Vuori, K., Reed, J. & Ruoslahti, E. (1995). The $\alpha_5\beta_1$ integrin supports survival of cells on fibronectin and up-regulates Bcl-2 expression. *Proceedings of the National Academy of Sciences USA*, 92, 13, 6161-6165, 0027-8424

ω3 and ω6 CYP450 Eicosanoid Derivatives: Key Lipid Mediators in the Regulation of Pulmonary Hypertension

Caroline Morin[1,2], Samuel Fortin[2],
Christelle Guibert[3] and Éric Rousseau[1]
[1]*Department of Physiology and Biophysics,*
Université de Sherbrooke, Sherbrooke, Québec,
[2]*SCF-Pharma, Ste-Luce, Québec,*
[3]*Centre de Recherche Cardio-Thoracique de Bordeaux,*
INSERM U1045, Université Bordeaux Segalen,
[1,2]*Canada*
[3]*France*

1. Introduction

Pulmonary arterial hypertension (PAH) is a multi-factorial, progressive disease with substantial mortality and morbidity. Despite recent improvements in treatment, mortality associated with PAH remains high, with a two-year survival rate after diagnosis of approximately 85% (Thenappan *et al.*, 2007). Although advances in the understanding of disease development and treatment have been achieved, the pathogenesis of PAH is still not clearly understood (Humbert et al., 2004). Therapeutic options remain limited despite the introduction of prostacyclin analogues, endothelin receptor antagonists and phosphodiesterase 5 inhibitors within the last 15 years. Moreover, these interventions predominantly address the endothelial and vascular dysfunction associated with the condition, and thus merely delay the progression of the disease rather than offer a cure (McLaughlin *et al.*, 2009a, McLaughlin *et al.*, 2009b).

PAH is a subset of pulmonary hypertensive syndromes, defined by a resting mean pulmonary artery pressure (PAP) >25mmHg, pulmonary vascular resistance (PVR) >3 Wood units and pulmonary wedge pressure <15mmHg, in the absence of other causes of PAH (Archer *et al.*, 1998). PAH is primarily a disease of the small pulmonary arteries, characterised by vascular proliferation, remodelling and progressive increases in PVR, ultimately leading to right ventricular failure and death (Voelkel *et al.*, 2006). These increases in PVR are attributed in part to endothelial dysfunction resulting in vasoconstriction, remodelling of the pulmonary vessel wall and thrombosis *in situ* (Budhiraja *et al.*, 2004). The role of inflammation in the development of PAH has been suggested (Voelkel et al., 1998). Inflammatory cells, including macrophages and lymphocytes, are increased in the plexiform lesions of hypertensive pulmonary vessels (Tuder et al., 1994). Elevated levels of macrophage inflammatory protein-1a, interleukin-1b and interleukin-6 are also found in patients with severe pulmonary hypertension (Humbert et al., 1995, Fartoukh et al., 1998). However, the haemodynamic aberrations represent only one aspect of PAH such that enhanced proliferation, decreased apoptosis and a shift to glycolytic metabolism in pulmonary artery smooth muscle cells, fibroblasts and endothelial cells are now recognised as central to the pathogenesis of the disease. The causes and clinical consequences of PAH have recently been reviewed by a number of international scientists and clinicians (Galie et al., 2009a). While intracellular calcium plays a pivotal role in controlling vascular tone and remodelling of the arterial wall, it became of prime interest to search for alternative biochemical or pharmacological targets in order to better understand the haemodynamic and pathophysiological shifts in the functional properties of this specific vascular bed.

Endothelial dysfunction appears to play an integral role in mediating the vasoconstriction and structural changes in pulmonary vasculature (Budhiraja *et al.*, 2004). The endothelium releases diverse growth factors, vasoactive compounds and lipidic mediators, which regulate the physical and biochemical properties of the pulmonary vessels and affect vascular contractility and cell growth, thus modifying distal pulmonary artery resistance and compliance (Budhiraja *et al.*, 2004). An altered production of various endothelial vasoactive mediators, such as NO, prostacyclin, endothelin-1 (ET-1), serotonin and thromboxane, has been increasingly recognized in patients with PAH (Giaid et al., 1993). Because most of these mediators affect the growth of smooth muscle cells, an alteration in their production may facilitate the development of pulmonary vascular hypertrophy and the structural remodelling characteristic of PAH (Galie et al., 2009a). In addition to the potential consequences of an imbalance in the endothelial production of various mediators, injury to the endothelium may expose the underlying vascular media tissue to diverse blood-borne factors that may further promote pathological changes (Galie et al., 2009a, Saouti et al., 2010). Endothelial dysfunction may also have adverse consequences on pulmonary vascular haemostasis by altering the production of anticoagulant factors. Recent reports of genetic mutations in endothelial cells of patients with PAH further underscore the role of these cells in disease pathogenesis (Galie et al., 2009a).

Several studies have demonstrated that Ca^{2+} sensitizing mechanisms of the contractile proteins may also be primed under pathophysiological conditions by various vasoactive and lipid mediators and that this Ca^{2+} sensitization process is involved in hypertension (Uehata et al., 1997, Hata et al., 2011). In vascular smooth muscle (VSM), ET-1 has been shown to enhance Ca^{2+} sensitivity through the activation of Rho-kinases and PKC-dependent phosphorylation of the 17 kDa myosin phosphatase inhibitor protein (CPI-17) pathways (Hersch et al., 2004). Contraction of VSM occurs via two related mechanisms: i) a rise in cytosolic calcium concentration ($[Ca^{2+}]_i$) which results in the formation of calcium/calmodulin complexes and activation of the myosin light chain kinase (MLCK). The activated MLCK in turn phosphorylates the 20 kDa myosin light chain (MLC) (Kimura et al., 1996), resulting in vascular smooth muscle (VSM) cell contraction; ii) a second Ca^{2+}-independent mechanism which requires the activation of Rho-kinase as well as PKC-dependent phosphorylation of myosin phosphatase inhibitor protein of 17 kDa (so called

CPI-17) to maintain tone (Somlyo et al., 2003). The calcium sensitization mechanism occurs when an agonist, which stimulates the activation of Rho-kinase or the PKC/CPI-17 pathway, results in the inhibition of MLC phosphatase (MLCP) (Uehata et al., 1997, Somlyo et al., 2003, Kitazawa et al., 2010). Rho-kinase inhibits MLCP activity by phosphorylating the myosin-binding subunit of MLCP. Alternatively, CPI-17 phosphorylation also results in an inhibition of MLCP activity, which in turn maintains steady state tension in VSM (Somlyo et al., 2003, Kitazawa et al., 2010). Hence, CPI–17 de-phosphorylation facilitates relaxation as reported previously in bronchial smooth muscle tissues (C. Morin, 2008).

Omega-6 and omega-3 poly-unsaturated fatty acids (PUFA) such as arachidonic acid (AA), eicosapentaenoic acid (EPA) and docosahexaenoic acid (DHA), respectively, can be metabolized by cytochrome P-450 (CYP450) enzymes into several classes of oxygenated and hydroxylated metabolites (Funk 2001, Fer et al., 2008). Several of these CYP450-derived eicosanoids are also known for their ability to modulate vascular (Roman 2002) and airway smooth muscle tone (Morin et al., 2009, Mouchaers et al., 2010). 20-hydroxyeicosatetraenoic acid (20-HETE) has been shown to induce relaxation of pulmonary arteries in several species including humans (Birks et al., 1997). Meanwhile, epoxyeicosatrienoic acid (EET) regioisomers have been shown to activate large conductance calcium-activated potassium channels in vascular smooth muscle cells and are considered as leading candidates for endothelium-derived hyperpolarizing factor (EDHF) in the coronary and systemic circulation (Zeldin et al., 1996, Fisslthaler et al., 1999, Node et al., 1999, Capdevila et al., 2000). Specific CYP450 epoxygenase isoforms are involved in EPA metabolism and produce 17(18)-epoxyeicosatetraenoic acid (17(18)-EpETE, see Fig.1B) (Lauterbach et al., 2002, Nguyen et al., 1999, Schwarz et al., 2004). Epoxy-docosapentaenoic acids are CYP450-dependent DHA metabolites (Fig. 1C) (Fer et al., 2004, Arnold et al., 2010, Lucas et al., 2010) and recent studies have demonstrated that these metabolites display potent vasodilatory activities on coronary arteries (Konkel et al., 2011, Wang et al., 2011). Metabolic pathways and chemical structures of CYP450-dependent AA, EPA and DHA metabolites known to modulate vascular tone are illustrated in Figure 1 A-C. Recently, pharmacological inhibitors of CYP450 epoxygenases and hydroxylases, such as N-methylsulfonyl-6-(2-propargyloxyphenyl)-hexanamide (MS-PPOH) and Dibromo-dodecenyl-methylsulfimide (DDMS), were developed to assess the specific role of these metabolites in cardiovascular circulation (Nithipatikom et al., 2006).

In this chapter, we will summarize the role and the effect of ω6 CYP-450 metabolites, such as EET regioisomers and 20-HETE, as well as their putative involvement in the control of pulmonary arterial tone. Moreover, we will review recent reports regarding the mode of action of epoxy-ω3 derivatives, such as EpETE and EpDPE, on pulmonary arteries. Although some progress has been made for the diagnosis and treatment of PAH, more effective treatments need to be developed. The omega 3 polyunsaturated fatty acids (n-3 PUFA) have recently attracted much attention in various research fields especially in cardiovascular research (McLaughlin et al., 2009a). Accordingly, we will summarize the effect of a new DHA-derivative on human pulmonary arteries. Potential involvement of this DHA derivative as a novel and prospective medicinal compound will be discussed as compared to present treatments used in the management of pulmonary arterial hypertension.

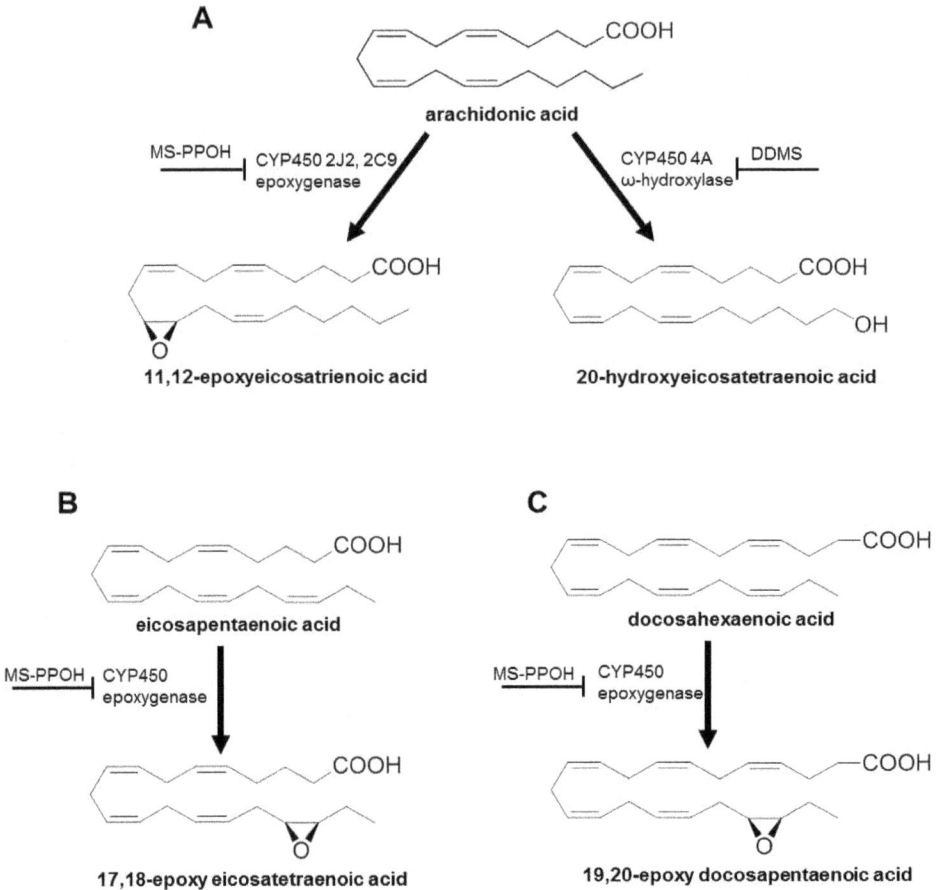

Fig. 1. Omega-3 and omega-6 metabolites produced by CYP450 enzymes in lung tissues.
A: CYP450 epoxygenase and ω-hydroxylase enzymes metabolize arachidonic acid into two
major active compounds: epoxyeicosatrienoic acid (EET) and 20-hydroxyeicosatetraenoic
acid (20-HETE), respectively. MS-PPOH and DDMS are known specific inhibitors of CYP450
enzymes. B: 17,18-epoxyeicosatetraenoic acid (17,18-EpETE) is the major active metabolite
produced by the action of CYP450 epoxygenase enzymes on eicosapentaenoic acid (EPA).
C: docosahexaenoic acid (DHA) serves as a substrate for CYP450 epoxygenase enzymes to
induce the formation of 19,20-epoxy docosapentaenoic acid (19,20-EpDPE).

2. Role of CYP450-dependent arachidonic acid metabolites in pulmonary arteries

Arachidonic acid is metabolized via cyclooxygenases, lipoxygenases, and cytochrome P-450
(CYP) enzymes to generate a range of bioactive eicosanoids. CYP enzymes, with an
important role in cardiovascular function, are epoxygenases of the CYP2C and 2J gene
families, which form four regioisomeric epoxyeicosatrienoic acids (5,6-, 8,9-, 11,12-, and

14,15-EET) and the ω-hydroxylases of the CYP4A family, which generate hydroxyeicosatetraenoic acids (19- and 20-HETE) (Roman,. 2002).

In the systemic vasculature, EETs are most commonly described as vasodilators. The mechanism of EET-induced vasodilation has been studied extensively and is dependent on the hyperpolarisation of vascular smooth muscle cells (Gebremedhin et al., 1992, Hecker et al., 1994, Campbell et al., 1996, Eckman et al., 1998, Morin et al., 2007a) resulting from EET-induced opening of smooth muscle cell potassium channels (Campbell et al., 1996, Zou et al., 1996, Eckman et al., 1998, Gebremedhin et al., 1998, Hayabuchi et al., 1998, Morin et al., 2007a). Although EETs also reduce tension in non-resistant extralobar pulmonary artery (PA) segments (Stephenson et al., 1998, Stephenson et al., 2003), all four EET regioisomers have been observed to be vasoconstrictors in small-diameter intralobar PA segments in rabbits and rats (Yaghi et al., 2001, Zhu et al., 2000). Because EETs also increase vascular resistance (and decrease compliance) in isolated perfused rabbit lungs (Stephenson et al., 2003), the predominant activity of EETs in lung vessels appears to be vasoconstriction. These data are supported by the observation that inhibition of epoxygenase activity with specific pharmacological inhibitors attenuates PA tension to phenylephrine (Zhu et al., 2000a), suggesting that endogenous EETs participate in α-adrenergic contraction of the pulmonary vasculature. Zeldin and co-workers reported that the most abundant EET regioisomer formed in the rabbit lung was 5,6-EET (Zeldin et al., 1995). Of the four EET regioisomers, 5,6-EET is also the most potent, albeit labile, constrictor of rabbit pulmonary arteries (Zhu et al., 2000b). The 5,6-EET-induced contraction of rabbit PA requires intact endothelium, cyclooxygenase activity, and activation of the thromboxane/endoperoxide (TP) receptor (Zhu et al., 2000b, Stephenson et al., 2003). Moreover data suggest that 5,6-EET induces contraction in intralobar PA by increasing Rho-kinase activity, thus phosphorylating MLC and increasing Ca^{2+} sensitivity of the contractile apparatus in rabbit lung (Losapio et al., 2005).

On the other hand, 20-hydroxyeicosatetraenoic acid (20-HETE), a CYP-450 4A metabolite of arachidonic acid, constricts renal, cerebral, coronary and mesenteric arteries via inhibitory effects on Ca^{2+}-activated K^+ channels, increased Ca^{2+} entry and modulation of Rho-kinase activity (Roman, 2002, Randriamboavonjy et al., 2003). However, 20-HETE has been shown to be an eicosanoid product of human lung tissue that acts as a potent vasodilator of isolated pressurized pulmonary arteries (Birks et al., 1997, Morin et al., 2008). Furthermore, cytochrome P-450 4A (CYP4A) protein is expressed in the pulmonary vasculature, a finding based on Western blots of PA microsomes (Zhu et al., 1998), the conversion of arachidonic acid into 20-HETE by dispersed vascular smooth muscle cells (Zhu et al., 1998), and immunohistochemistry localizing CYP4A to rabbit pulmonary capillary endothelium (Roman et al., 1993). These observations raise the possibility that products of CYP4A may contribute to the control of PA tone. However, the role of 20-HETE or other P-450 metabolites of AA in pulmonary circulation is not completely understood. In the acute hypoxic vasoconstrictive response in isolated blood-perfused rabbit lungs, 20-HETE was shown to relax rabbit PA rings, while an inhibitor of 20-HETE synthesis, DDMS, shifted the concentration response of PA rings to phenylephrine (PE) to the left, consistent with the loss of a pro-relaxing metabolite (Zhu et al., 2000b). Moreover, the inhibition of 20-HETE formation by pharmacological agents such as 17-oxydecanoic acid (17-ODYA) and DDMS enhanced the acute hypoxia-induced increase in pulmonary perfusion pressures (Zhu et al., 2000b).

In light of these findings, we postulated that, as a vasodilator, 20-HETE may counter observed increases in human pulmonary artery (HPA) tone upon serotonin (5-HT) and α-adrenergic stimulations. To perform these experiments, human lung tissues from patients undergoing surgery for lung carcinoma and distant from the malignant lesion were obtained. Pulmonary arteries of similar weight and length (inner diameter of 0.5 - 0.8 mm) were micro-dissected and placed in culture for 24 hours in a humidified incubator at 37°C under 5% CO_2 as previously reported (Guibert et al., 2005, Morin et al., 2008). Resulting data demonstrated that 20-HETE acts as a potent vasodilator on HPA pre-contracted with 5-HT and phenylephrine (PE) (Figure 2A, Morin C et al., 2008). 20-HETE displayed potent relaxing effects on HPA, with IC_{50} values in the sub-micromolar range (≈ 0.3 µM) on both resting and active tone. In HPA, the relaxing effect induced by 20-HETE was partially abolished by 30 % in the presence of iberiotoxin (IbTx) (Morin et al., 2008), suggesting that the eicosanoid activates large conducting Ca^{2+}-activated potassium (BK_{Ca}) channels which usually results in membrane hyperpolarisation. Indeed, microelectrode measurements demonstrated that 20-HETE hyperpolarizes human ASM cells, an effect abolished by 10 nM IbTx (Morin et al., 2007b). Thus, the mode of action of this compound may be related to its molecular interactions with specific ionic channels of the surface membrane, as previously demonstrated in guinea pig and human smooth muscles (Cloutier et al., 2003, Morin et al., 2007b).

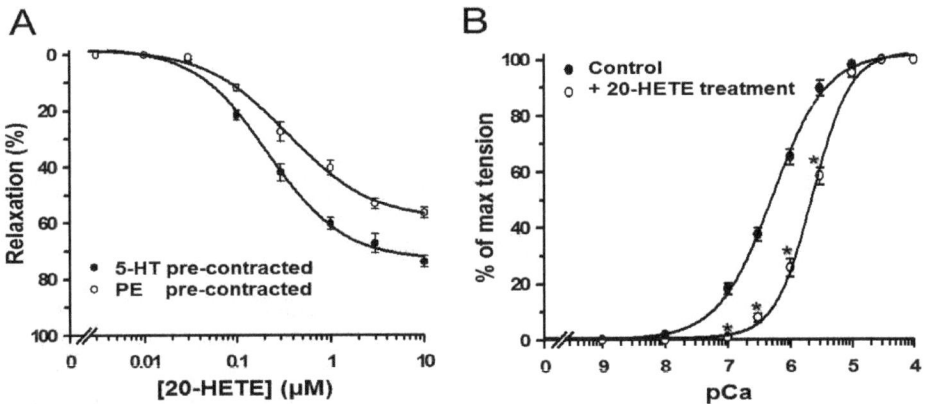

Fig. 2. Omega-6 ω-hydroxylase metabolite modulates pulmonary arterial tone.
A: Concentration-dependent relaxing responses induced by 20-HETE on distal human pulmonary arteries pre-contracted with either 1 µM 5-HT or 1 µM PE. Each point represents the mean ± S.E.M. with n=16 and n=14 for each experimental condition, respectively. B: Cumulative Concentration Response Curve (CCRC) to free [Ca^{2+}] obtained from β-escin-permeabilized pulmonary artery rings in control conditions (closed circles, n =16) and in the presence of 1 µM 20-HETE (open circles, n = 18).

The role of various ion channels in acute and chronic hypoxia in pulmonary vasculature has already been described as well (Weir et al., 2006, Guibert et al., 2007). Hence, from a physiological standpoint, it is noteworthy to emphasize the relaxing effects displayed by 20-HETE on both HPA and airway smooth muscle (Birks et al., 1997, Jacobs et al., 1999, Morin et al., 2008).

The inherent Ca^{2+} sensitivity of the myosin light chain kinase, resulting in MLC phosphorylation and contraction and subsequent de-phosphorylation by MLCP, is an important mechanism in the regulation of vascular smooth muscle tone (Somlyo et al., 2003, Koga et al., 2005). Modulation of this mechanism by 20 HETE could explain its overall effects on HPA. As shown in figure 2B, 20 HETE significantly reduces Ca^{2+} sensitivity in permeabilized preparations, suggesting that this eicosanoid modulates enzymatic systems such as Rho-Kinase and/or PKC/CPI-17 as well as down-stream MLCP activity (Morin et al., 2007a). Several studies have suggested that Ca^{2+} sensitizing mechanisms may also be primed under pathophysiological conditions and especially in PAH (Uehata et al., 1997, Somlyo et al., 2003). It was therefore of potential clinical interest to find a lipid mediator that would be able to shift the Ca^{2+} activation curve toward higher concentrations. Moreover, our group demonstrated that 20-HETE decreases CPI-17 phosphorylation levels and increase the expression of p116Rip, thus supporting the view that this eicosanoid downregulates PKC/CPI-17 and Rho kinase dependent pathways (Morin et al., 2008).

Despite the fact that CYP450 ω-hydroxylase has been identified in various lung tissues (Zeldin et al., 1995, Zhu et al., 1998, Jacob et al., 1999, Roman RJ, 2002, Miyata et al., 2005), a key issue has been to demonstrate the endogenous involvement of 20-HETE in human pulmonary arteries. Using a pharmacological ω-hydroxylase inhibitor such as DDMS, (Jacob et al., 2006, Nithipatikom et al., 2006) which minimizes the endogenous production of 20-HETE, it was now possible to amplify tonic responses to various vasoconstrictive agents. This experimental strategy enabled us to evaluate the putative role of this eicosanoid in human lung vascular tissues. Hence, it was hypothesized that 20-HETE could play the role of a paracrine mediator in the HPA wall whereby its basal production would facilitate PA dilation and help maintain low blood pressure (12-15 mm Hg) in this specific segment of the vascular apparatus. However, the difference in reactivity to 20-HETE between conduit and resistance arteries has not been addressed. In fact, 20-HETE is thought to play an important role in regulating tone in distal HPA (Diameter < 500 μm). In contrast, consistent contractions have been measured and reported in rodents such as guinea pig bronchi (Cloutier et al., 2003). Nevertheless, the relaxations induced by 20-HETE may be of pharmacological interest in pulmonary arterial hypertension, since it could be used to treat this critical clinical condition known to be refractory to classical treatments. Hence it would be relevant to analyse the expression of several genes encoding specific proteins, such as the CYP450 isoforms in the HPA wall and parenchyma. It has been reported that CYP450 4A and other isozymes represent ω-hydroxylases that are responsible for 20-HETE production in several human tissues (Gebremedhin et al., 1998), and for which their expression could be downregulated in patients diagnosed with PAH (Pierson et al., 2000). This hypothesis lends further support to the benefit of studying the functional implication of 20-HETE at both the cellular and molecular levels, despite the fact that such studies were initiated some 15 years ago in rabbit pulmonary tissues (Zeldin et al., 1995).

3. Key role of CYP450 epoxygenase-dependent metabolites derived from EPA and DHA in pulmonary hypertension

It is widely accepted that n-3 PUFA, rich in fish oils, protect against several types of cardiovascular diseases such as myocardial infarction, arrhythmia, atherosclerosis, as well as hypertension and inflammatory conditions (Abeywardena et al., 2001, Kris-Etherton et al., 2002). EPA, DHA or their derivatives may represent active biological components mediating these effects. Although the precise cellular and molecular mechanisms underlying these beneficial effects are not well understood, the protective effects of PUFA are likely related to their direct effects on VSM cells (Mizutani et al., 1997, Hirafuji et al., 2003). It has been shown that these PUFA activate K^+_{ATP} channels and inhibit specific types of Ca^{2+} channels (Ye et al., 2002). These reports suggest that modulation of VSM cell function contributes to the beneficial effects of PUFA in the systemic vascular system. EPA may also serve as an alternative substrate in CYP450-dependent epoxygenation and hydroxylation reactions as shown in rat hepatic and renal microsomes (Van Rollins et al., 1988). The CYP450-dependent EPA metabolites include the epoxyeicosatetraenoic acid regioisomers 5(6)-, 8(9)-, 11(12)-, 14(15)- and 17(18)-EpETE (Lauterbach et al., 2002). Specific CYP450 epoxygenase isoforms are involved in EPA metabolism which produce (17(18)-EpETE), and include CYP1A (Schwarz et al., 2004), CYP4A1, CYP4A3 (Nguyen et al., 1999, Lauterbach et al., 2002,) and CYP4A12A. An additional potential source for 17(18)-EpETE are endothelial CYP450 isoforms of the 2C and 2J subfamilies that otherwise produce EET from AA. Recent studies have demonstrated that EPA epoxides share and even exceed the ability of AA epoxides to stimulate large conducting Ca^{2+}-activated potassium (BK_{Ca}) channels (Lauterbach et al., 2002) and mediate vasodilatation (Zhang et al., 2001a).

However, several questions remain to be addressed as to the mode of action of EPA metabolites in human pulmonary arteries. Our group demonstrated that 17(18)-EpETE induced a relaxing effect of smooth muscle from distal human pulmonary arteries (HPA), with IC_{50} values in the sub-micromolar range on both HPA resting and active tone. To our knowledge, there are only few publications addressing the effects of 17(18) -EpETE in rodents and in cultured VSM cells (Lauterbach et al., 2002, Hercule et al., 2007). Our data showed that the relaxing effect induced by 17(18)-EpETE in HPA under normal external K^+ concentration was abolished in the presence of IbTx and glyburide (Glyb), suggesting that the eicosanoid activates BK_{Ca} and K_{ATP} channels, hence resulting in membrane hyperpolarisation. Indeed, intracellular microelectrode measurements revealed that 17(18)-EpETE induced significant hyperpolarisation of human pulmonary artery smooth muscle cells (Figure 3A). Since IbTx and Glyb prevented these hyperpolarizing effects, thereby reducing the relaxation induced by 17(18)-EpETE, BK_{Ca} and K_{ATP} channel activation thus appears to be a key determinant in the control of both HPA membrane potential and tone (Figure 3B). Moreover, it has been demonstrated that EPA epoxides share and even exceed the ability of AA epoxides to stimulate BK_{Ca} channels (Lauterbach et al., 2002) and to mediate vasodilatation in canine and porcine coronary microvessels (Zhang et al., 2001a). Using patch clamp measurements, 17(18)-EpETE has also been demonstrated to stimulate K^+ outward currents, displaying typical characteristics for BK_{Ca} channel activation in systemic VSM cells. Moreover, this effect is abolished by TEA, a BK_{Ca} channel blocker (Lauterbach et al., 2002). Recently, the $BK\alpha$ subunit, the pore-forming subunit of octameric BK_{Ca} channels, was shown to represent the main molecular target of 17(18) -EpETE in systemic VSM cells isolated from rat cerebral and mesenteric arteries (Hercule et al., 2007).

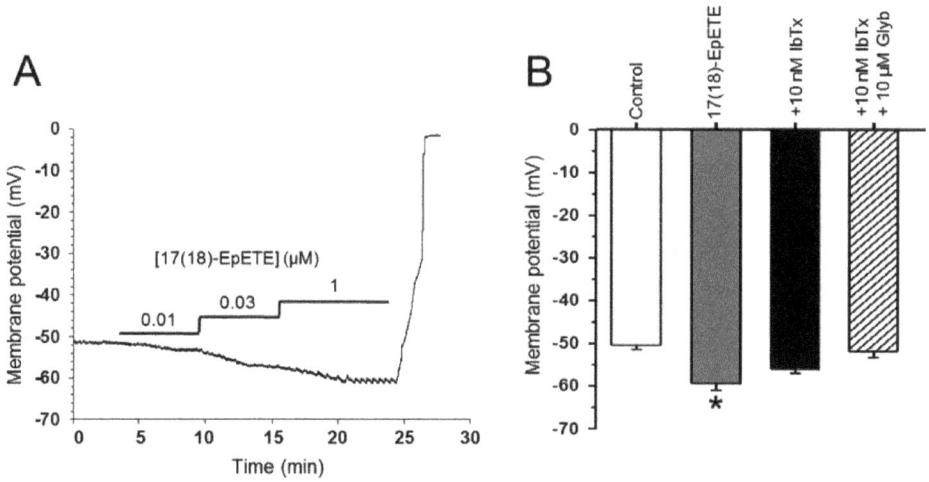

Fig. 3. EPA-derived metabolite hyperpolarisation of pulmonary arterial smooth muscles.
A: Recording of the membrane potential from pulmonary artery in control and following addition of cumulative concentrations of 17(18)-EpETE. At the end of each recording, the microelectrode was removed from the pulmonary artery smooth muscle cell to validate the electrophysiological measurements. B: Mean resting membrane potential values determined for 1 µM 17(18)-EpETE and following addition of either 10 nM IbTx or 10 nM IbTx plus 10 µM glyburide. (n = 7 for each condition).

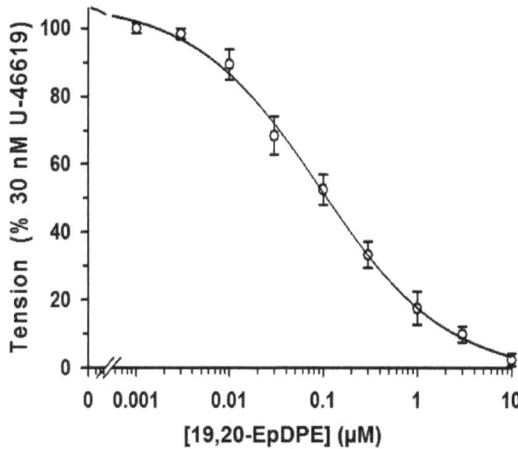

Fig. 4. DHA CYP450 epoxygenase metabolite-induced relaxation of pulmonary arterial smooth muscle.
A: Cumulative concentration response curve displaying the mean tension induced by 30 nM U46619 in control and after 24h-treatments with increasing concentrations of 19,20-EpDPE (0.001-10 µM), n=12 for each experimental condition.

CYP450-dependent DHA metabolites include the epoxy-docosapentaenoic acid regioisomers 4(5)-, 7(8)-, 10(11)-, 13(14)-, 16(17)- and 19(20)-EpDPE (Fer et al., 2008, Arnold et al., 2010, Lucas et al., 2010). Several epoxygenases have been identified in lung tissues, including 2J2, 2C8 2C9 and 1B1 (Fer et al., 2008). Recent studies have demonstrated that CYP450 epoxygenase metabolites of DHA display potent vasodilatory activities on coronary arteries. These epoxy-eicosanoids have been reported to be more potent than EET and EPA in activating BK_{Ca} channels (Konkel et al., 2011, Wang et al., 2011). In our laboratory, experiments were designed to assess the relaxing effect of 19,20-EpDPE on human pulmonary arteries pre-contracted with 30 nM U-46619, a TP receptor agonist. HPA were cultured for 24 hours in the absence or presence of increasing concentrations of 19,20-EpDPE. The tissues were then subjected to 0.6 grams of basal tone and thereafter challenged with 30 nM U-46619. The cumulative concentration response curve (CCRC) to 19,20-EpDPE (0.01-100 µM) revealed a concentration-dependent inhibitory effect on active tone, with an EC_{50} value of 0.11 µM (Figure 4).

4. Current treatments and new therapeutic strategies using omega-3 monoglyceride for PAH

Significant advances in the treatment of PAH have been made in the last 15 years. These agents target the prostacyclin pathway, the nitric oxide pathway and the endothelin pathway. A number of vasoactive substances are involved in the pathogenesis of PAH, including a major imbalance observed between prostacyclin and thromboxane. Both of these substances are by-products of arachidonic acid metabolism by endothelial cells. Prostacyclins increase intracellular cyclic AMP and reduce intracellular Ca^{2+} (Clapp et al., 2002). Transcription factors and cell cycle progression are dependent on $[Ca^{2+}]_i$. Prostacyclins also inhibit platelet activation, promote vasodilatation and inhibit smooth muscle proliferation. Thromboxane, which is also produced by endothelial cells, antagonizes the effects of prostacyclin. The imbalance between prostacyclin and thromboxane may result from a combination of genetic factors and aberrant response to certain forms of injury to endothelial cells. Intravenous prostacyclin was first introduced in the treatment of primary pulmonary arterial hypertension in the early 1980s. A cohort analysis of patients receiving intravenous prostacyclin has shown benefits in New York Heart Association (NYHA) class III and IV patients with regard to survival (McLaughlin et al., 2002b, Sitbon et al., 2002). In addition to idiopathic pulmonary arterial hypertension, epoprostenol has been successfully used in the treatment of pulmonary hypertension resulting from left to right shunt, portal hypertension and HIV infection (Rosenzweig et al., 1999, Nunes et al., 2003). While epoprostenol has shown a definite role in the treatment of primary and other forms of pulmonary hypertension, it remains expensive and very cumbersome to use. Administration of this medication requires a central line and a pump. Treatment with epoprostenol causes several side effects, with central line infection being a serious side effect (Palmer et al., 1998, Humbert et al., 1998). Other stable prostacyclins such as Treprostinil and Iloprost are also used in the treatment of PAH. However, side effects are similar to those exhibited by epoprostenol (Hoeper et al., 2000, Olschewski et al., 2002).

Endothelin-1 is produced by the vascular endothelium and serves as a vasoconstrictor and smooth muscle mitogen. While its action on endothelin-A receptors results in vasoconstriction through activation of protein kinase and an increase in $[Ca^{2+}]_i$, its effect on endothelin-B receptors results in vasodilatation secondary to prostacyclin and nitric oxide release in addition to aiding in its clearance. Endothelin receptor antagonists are also currently used in the treatment of PAH. For example, bosentan is a non-selective endothelial receptor antagonist. Endothelin A receptor stimulation results in vasoconstriction and smooth muscle proliferation, while endothelin B receptor stimulation results in endothelin clearance as well as induction of NO and prostacyclin by endothelial cells. Two randomized double-blind placebo-controlled class III and IV trials have evaluated bosentan in patients with pulmonary arterial hypertension. Study results showed a significant improvement in 6 min walk test and haemodynamics in the bosentan group. In addition, an improvement in the time to clinical worsening such as death, lung transplantation and hospitalization was also noted (Channick et al., 2001, Rubin et al., 2002). Bosentan is metabolized by the liver and an increase in transaminases has been noted during treatment with this medication. Hence, it is mandatory to perform periodic liver function tests in patients taking bosentan and ambrisentan are other examples of selective ETA receptor antagonists. Ambrisentan does not seem to have toxic effects on the liver, while bosentan induces hepatotoxicity (Barst et al., 2001, Barst et al 2006).

Often viewed as an endothelial disease, PAH has already been related i) to changes in membrane receptor and ionic channel expression (Guibert et al., 2007), ii) to a decrease in NO production, due to a lower nitric oxide synthase (NOS) activity (Guibert, 2010), and iii) to a downstream decrease in cGMP related to lower guanylate cyclase activity, which in turn activates potassium channels and hyperpolarizes VSM cells (Guibert, 2010). This process results in an inactivation of Ca^{2+} channel activity and decreases intracellular free Ca^{2+}, leading to vasodilatation. In fact, patients with PAH show impaired NO synthase activity. Impaired synthesis of endothelium-derived nitric oxide and enhanced production of vasoconstrictor endothelin have also been implicated in the pathogenesis of PAH (Giaid et al., 1993, Giaid A et al., 1995). Nitric oxide treatment is very cumbersome and is mainly used in the management of pulmonary hypertension in the neonatal intensive care unit (ICU) and occasionally in adult ICU (Giaid et al., 1993).

High-doses of Ca^{2+} channel blockers have been shown by uncontrolled studies to prolong survival in patients with PAH (Fuster et al., 1984, Rich et al., 1992), with approximately 10% of such patients belonging to this group. In a large retrospective study of 557 patients with PAH, less than 7% of patients responded to Ca^{2+}-channel blockers. Among these, patients who had a significant vasodilator response exhibited a long-term response to Ca^{2+}-channel blockers. Long-term therapy with Ca^{2+}-channel blockers is not recommended when there is no acute vasodilator response (Fuster et al., 1984).

Pulmonary vasculature contains substantial amounts of phosphodiesterase type-5 (PDE-5) enzyme and inhibition of this enzyme results in vasodilatation through the NO/cGMP pathway. Hence, the potential clinical benefit of phosphodiesterase type-5 inhibitors has been investigated in PAH (Pauvert et al., 2004). In addition, phosphodiesterase type-5 inhibitors exert anti-proliferative effects (Galie et al., 2009b). Sildenafil, a PDE-5 inhibitor, increases the levels of cyclic GMP in smooth muscle cells and causes vasodilatation. Tadalafil is a long acting PDE-5 inhibitor which has also been used in the management of PAH. The major landmark trial involving sildenafil was conducted in the pulmonary arterial hypertension (SUPER) study. Two hundred seventy-eight patients with functional class II–IV PAH were randomized to three different doses of sildenafil, namely 20, 40, or 80 mg, three times daily or to placebo. The study extended over a period of 12 weeks and, based on the convincing results, the FDA subsequently approved a thrice-daily dose of

20 mg sildenafil in the treatment of PAH (Galie et al., 2009b). The PHIRST Trial studied the efficacy and safety of the long acting phosphodiesterase-type five inhibitor (PDE 5-I) tadalafil. The study extended over a period of 16 weeks and doses of tadalafil used were 2.5, 10, 20, and 40 mg. Based on the positive responses, the FDA approved the use of tadalafil 40 mg once a day (Galie et al., 2009b). However these phosphodiesterase-5 inhibitors also induce common side effects and, in some cases, quite severe reactions such as sudden blindness, myocardial infarction, stroke and sudden cardiac death secondary to ventricular arrhythmias have been recognized.

Hence, despite the introduction of prostacyclin analogues, endothelin receptor antagonists and phosphodiesterase 5 inhibitors within the last 15 years, therapeutic options for pulmonary hypertension remain limited. To date, these interventions predominantly address the endothelial and vascular dysfunction associated with the condition, and thus merely delay the progression of the disease rather than offer a cure (McLaughlin et al., 2009). Clinical assessment of dietary supplementation of omega-3 (n-3) polyunsaturated fatty acids (PUFA) including EPA and DHA has shown their beneficial impact in a wide range of cardiovascular diseases (Connor, 2000). One explanation for these beneficial effects is that n-3 PUFA competes with arachidonic acid (AA) for enzymatic conversion by COX, LOX and CYP450 enzymes. This competition can lead to reduced formation of vasoactive AA metabolites while alternative PUFA-metabolites originating from DHA and EPA are increased. In a recent study, the DHA metabolite 16,17-EpDPE was shown to mediate vasodilatation of coronary arteries by the activation of BK channels (Wang et al., 2011). These n-3 PUFA effects are also mediated by a variety of mechanisms that involve both indirect (by eicosanoids and hormones) and direct genomic effects. In addition, EPA and DHA have been reported to reduce the expression of genes for interleukins, vascular cell adhesion molecule-1, intracellular adhesion molecule-1, endothelial adhesion molecule and E-selectin (Clarke et al., 1993, De Caterina et al., 1994, Tagawa et al., 1999). Recently our group has synthesized a new DHA monoglyceride derivative (Figure 5A, Fortin, 2008) in order to assess the effect of n-3 PUFA on pulmonary arterial tone and their involvement in key components of PAH pathogenesis. Fatty acids in monoglyceride form are generally recognized as safe and are widely used as emulsifying agents in the food industry. Pharmacokinetic experiments were thus performed on rats treated with an oral dose of 309 mg/kg of either DHA monoglyceride (MAG-DHA), DHA triglycerides (DHA-TG) or DHA ethyl ester (DHA-EE), based on the recommended daily dose of DHA for humans following dose translation from human to rat by the equation described by Reagan-Shaw et al., 2008. Blood samples from different groups were taken at 0, 0.5, 4, 8 and 24 h post-drug administration and DHA concentration (%) in plasma was determined by high performance liquid chromatography (HPLC). Figure 5B demonstrates that DHA monoacylglyceride increases the oral bioavailability of DHA compared to commercially available marine oil (Fortin, 2008).

The Rho-kinase pathway participates in vasoconstriction elicited by numerous agents involved in PAH, including TXA_2, ET-1 and 5-HT (Rodat-Despoix et al., 2009; Rodat-Despoix et al., 2008; Connolly & Aaronson, 2011). Rho is a small monomeric GTPase which activates Rho-associated kinase (ROCK) which in turn phosphorylates and inhibits myosin light chain phosphatase, leading to prolonged, refractory vasoconstriction. Rho kinase is considered to be a major determinant of arterial tone, through its essential role in the regulation of Ca^{2+} sensitivity of the contractile machinery in smooth muscle cells (Somlyo et al., 2003). Moreover, Rho kinase regulates a variety of cellular functions including motility, proliferation, apoptosis, contraction and gene expression. Amongst promising targets recently identified is the Rho-kinase pathway (Loirand et al., 2006). Recent pharmacological studies suggest that activation of the small G protein RhoA and its target Rho kinase is a critical shared mechanism in the pathogenesis of PAH (Loirand et al., 2006). *In vivo*, potent effects of treatment with Rho-kinase inhibitors (Y-27632 or fasudil) have been demonstrated in several animal models of PAH (Abe et al., 2004, Fagan et al., 2004, Nagaoka et al., 2006). Furthermore, acute intravenous administration of low dose fasudil has been shown to reduce PVR and Ppa in patients with PAH (Fukumoto et al., 2005, Ishikura et al., 2006, Fujita et al., 2010).

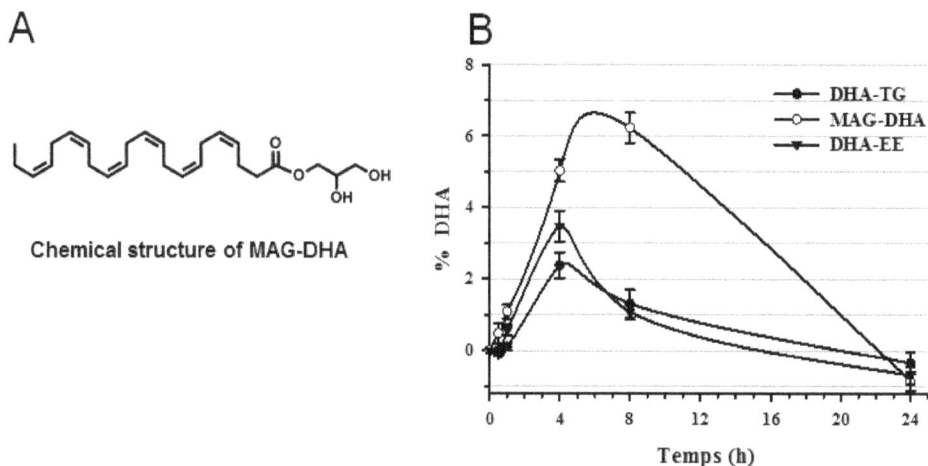

Fig. 5. Chemical structure and oral absorption of DHA monoacylglyceride (MAG-DHA). A: MAG-DHA was synthesized from highly purified DHA attached to a monoglycerol in sn-1 position. B: Pharmacokinetic experiments showing DHA concentration (%) in plasma derived from rats treated with an oral dose (309 mg/kg) of either DHA triglycerides (TG-DHA), DHA monoglyceride (MAG-DHA) or DHA ethyl ester (DHA-EE). Blood samples were taken at 0, 0.5, 4, 8 and 24 h post-drug administration, (n=6 for each experimental condition).

To investigate the potential usefulness of MAG-DHA, complementary approaches were used in our laboratory to assess putative changes in Ca^{2+} sensitivity and to determine the activation of RhoA in human pulmonary arteries. Comparative analyses were performed on β-escin-permeabilized human pulmonary arterial rings to assess the effect of MAG-DHA pre-treatments on Ca^{2+} sensitivity. Figure 6A illustrates CCRC to free Ca^{2+} concentrations on permeabilized HPA rings obtained from control and treated tissues. When compared to control (untreated) condition (Fig. 6A, dashed line), addition of the TP receptor agonist U-46619 to the organ bath enhanced Ca^{2+} sensitivity to pre-calibrated Ca^{2+} step increases in HPA explants (Fig. 6A, open circles). However, MAG-DHA pretreatment resulted in a marked inhibitory effect on Ca^{2+}-sensitivity (right shift) developed by U-46619-treated explants. Data analysis demonstrated that MAG-DHA treatment induced a shift in EC_{50} values (0.94 µM) toward higher Ca^{2+} concentrations when compared to untreated tissues challenged with U-46619 (0.13 µM) (Fig. 6A). However, the difference in Ca^{2+} sensitivity between control HPA and tissues pre-treated with 3 µM MAG-DHA was not significant, with EC_{50} values of 0.65 µM and 0.51 µM, respectively (Figure 6A). Furthermore, the involvement of the Rho-kinase pathway was examined using a RhoA pull down assay to evaluate RhoA activity following MAG-DHA treatment in HPA-derived homogenates. Thus, in order to investigate whether these observations were correlated with a modulation status of contractile proteins, RhoA activity level was assessed in HPA following MAG-DHA treatment in the absence or presence of MSPPOH, a CYP450 epoxygenase inhibitor and in 19,20-EpDPE-treated tissues alone. Western blot and quantitative analyses of GTP-RhoA/RhoA ratio revealed that MAG-DHA treatment reduced the activity of RhoA induced by U-46619, while an increased RhoA activity level was observed in the presence of MS-PPOH. Hence, 19,20-EpDPE pre-treatment resulted in a reduction in RhoA activity level when compared to the activity level detected upon U-46619 treatment (Figure 6B). These data suggest that MAG-DHA can be metabolized by CYP450 epoxygenase enzymes, leading to the sequential production of 19,20-EpDPE. This CYP450 metabolite in turn decreases RhoA activity level leading to an inhibition of Rho-kinase activation, thus resulting in a lower Ca^{2+}-sensitivity of HPA.

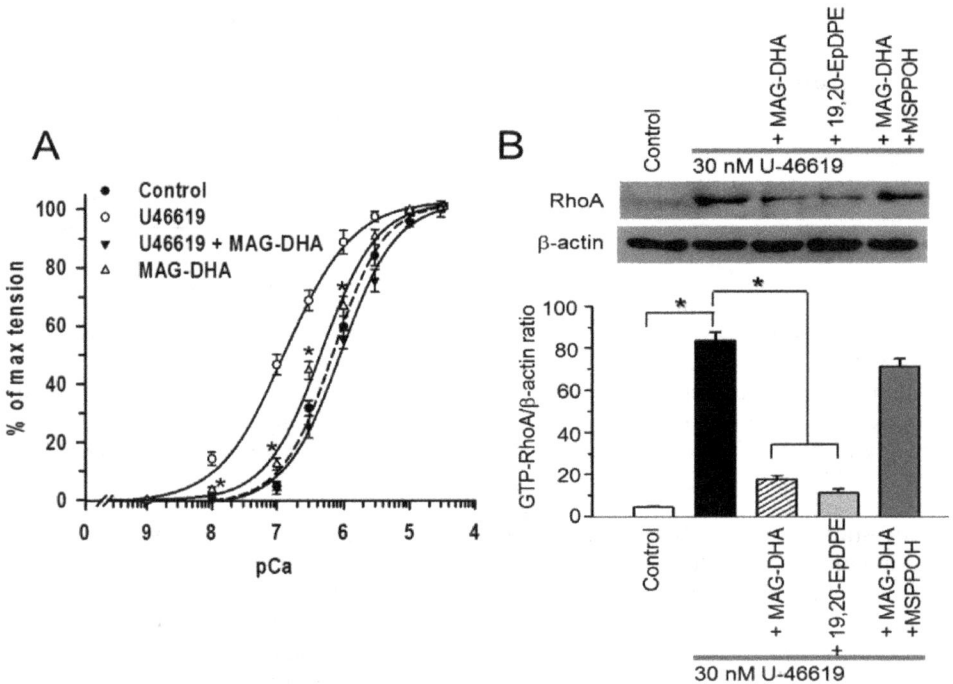

Fig. 6. MAG-DHA modulates Ca^{2+} sensitivity and Rho A activity in human pulmonary arteries.
A: Cumulative Concentration Response Curve to free $[Ca^{2+}]$ obtained in control (untreated HPA) and after short term (20 min) stimulation with 30 nM U-46619; as well as on 3 μM MAG-DHA-treated HPA alone and after 30 nM U46619 challenge. Each point represents the mean ± s.e.m., n= 12 for each experimental condition, * p < 0.05. B: RhoA activity was quantified in human pulmonary artery homogenates by measurement of RhoA-GTP using a Rhotekin pull-down assay, (n=8 for each experimental condition, * p < 0.05).

Several studies have demonstrated that the use of Rho-kinase inhibitors reduces PAH in many animal models (Oka et al., 2007, Mouchaers et al., 2010). Y-27632 inhaled at 10 – 100 mM was shown to reduce mean pulmonary arterial pressure without altering systemic arterial pressure in a hypoxic rat model of hypertension (Nagaoka et al., 2004). In the monocrotaline model, fasudil 30 or 100 mg/kg/day per os improved survival, pulmonary hypertension, right ventricular hypertrophy as well as pulmonary vascular lesions (Abe et al., 2004). In Fawn-hooded rats exhibiting a raised pulmonary arterial pressure (PAP), inhaled fasudil reduced PAP to 55 mmHg without altering mean systemic arterial pressure (Nagaoka et al., 2006). In humans, Rho-kinase inhibition with fasudil has also been shown to bring about an immediate, albeit modest, reduction in PVR, although this Rho kinase inhibitor must be administered by nebulisation to avoid systemic hypotension (Fujita et al., 2010, Ishikura et al., 2006). Our data attest that MAG-DHA, a newly synthesized DHA derivative, targets the Rho-kinase pathway to reduce U-46619-induced tension in HPA. Moreover, we were able to demonstrate that MAG-DHA treatment reduced RhoA activation which in turn inactivated the Rho-kinase pathway resulting in a reduction in U-46619-induced Ca^{2+} sensitivity of human pulmonary arterial smooth muscle cells. Finally, our data with the newly synthesized DHA derivative, MAG-DHA, could represent a new pharmacological agent of clinical interest in the management of PAH. Further investigations using *in vivo* models, such as a hypoxic rat model or a monocrotaline model of hypertension would however be required to determine the efficacy of MAG-DHA *per os* treatments in reversing pulmonary hypertension. Furthermore, the identification of CYP450 epoxygenase metabolites using high performance liquid chromatography coupled to tandem mass spectrometry (HPLC/MS/MS) may prove useful to explain the effect of MAG-DHA in these *in vivo* hypertension models.

5. Conclusion

Long-chain PUFAs are metabolized by CYP450 epoxygenase and ω-hydroxylase enzymes in the lung which induce the production of several bioactive eicosanoids, such as the EET regioisomers, 20-HETE, 17,18-EpETE and docosanoids, such as 19,20-EpDPE. These epoxy- and hydroxyl-derivatives are able to modulate the electrophysiological and mechanical properties of human pulmonary arterial smooth muscle. In addition, these vasoactive metabolites induce the activation of K^+ channels and reduce the Ca^{2+} sensitivity of the contractile apparatus in preparations derived from human pulmonary arteries. The main limitation of these compounds is their relative instability, further justifying the use of biochemical precursors or stable analogues (Roman, 2002). Thus we propose that PUFA derivatives, possessing selective pulmonary vasodilation capabilities, may provide an interesting new approach for various forms of PAH. Moreover, we have evaluated and summarized the effects of DHA monoacylglycerol on the reactivity of pulmonary arterial smooth muscle. Data revealed that MAG-DHA is likely metabolized into 19,20-EpDPE by the action of CYP450 epoxygenases in human lung. This epoxy-metabolite prevents U-46619-induced vasoconstriction through a decrease in RhoA activation thus leading to a reduction in Ca^{2+} sensitivity of smooth muscle cells. Since the activated RhoA/Rho kinase pathway is associated with both acute pulmonary vasoconstriction and chronic pulmonary artery remodelling, it is of potential clinical interest to find a lipid mediator able to reduce the activation of Rho-kinase. Moreover, animal and clinical studies have demonstrated that Rho-kinase inhibitors could inhibit signal transductions initiated by many vasoactive drugs;

hence it is possible that MAG-DHA may exert broader beneficial effects as compared to single receptor antagonists due to its mode of action on intracellular targets. In this respect, it is postulated that DHA-monoacylglyceride leads to the production of bioactive metabolites which represent new and prospective pharmacological compounds of low toxicity and medicinal interest in modulating pulmonary vasoconstriction. Collectively, the present review provides new insight regarding the mode of actions of specific epoxy and hydroxy eicosanoids and docosanoids, which represent biochemical compounds of putative clinical relevance in pulmonary hypertension.

6. Acknowledgment

The authors thank Drs Marco Sirois and Chantal Sirois for their help in patient recruitment. The authors thank Dr Roula Albadine and Edmond Riscallah, the pulmonary pathologists, and the technicians of the pathology laboratory for their technical support. We wish to thank Mr. Pierre Pothier for critical review of the manuscript and the members of the pathology laboratory for their technical support. This work was supported by a transition grant from the FMSS and CRC E-LeBel CHUS. ER is a member of the Respiratory Health Network of the FRSQ.

7. References

Abe, K., Shimokawa, H., Morikawa, K., Uwatoku, T., Oi, K., Matsumoto, Y., Hattori, T., Nakashima, Y., Kaibuchi, K., Sueishi, K. & Takeshit, A. (2004), Long-term treatment with a Rho-kinase inhibitor improves monocrotaline-induced fatal pulmonary hypertension in rats. *Circulation research*, Vol.94, No.3, pp.385-393, 1524-4571; 0009-7330

Abeywardena, M. Y. & Head, R. J. (2001), Longchain n-3 polyunsaturated fatty acids and blood vessel function. *Cardiovascular research*, Vol.52, No.3, pp.361-371, 0008-6363; 0008-6363

Archer, S. L., Djaballah, K., Humbert, M., Weir, K. E., Fartoukh, M., Dall'ava-Santucci, J., Mercier, J. C., Simonneau, G. & Dinh-Xuan, A. T. (1998), Nitric oxide deficiency in fenfluramine- and dexfenfluramine-induced pulmonary hypertension. *American journal of respiratory and critical care medicine*, Vol.158, No.4, pp.1061-1067, 1073-449X; 1073-449X

Arnold, C., Markovic, M., Blossey, K., Wallukat, G., Fischer, R., Dechend, R., Konkel, A., von Schacky, C., Luft, F. C., Muller, D. N., Rothe, M. & Schunck, W. H. (2010), Arachidonic acid-metabolizing cytochrome P450 enzymes are targets of {omega}-3 fatty acids. *The Journal of biological chemistry*, Vol.285, No.43, pp.32720-32733, 1083-351X; 0021-9258

Barst R. J. (2001), Medical therapy of pulmonary hypertension. An overview of treatment and goals. *Clinics in chest medicine*, Vol.22, No.3, pp.509-15, ix, 0272-5231; 0272-5231

Barst, R. J., Langleben, D., Badesch, D., Frost, A., Lawrence, E. C., Shapiro, S., Naeije, R. & Galie, N. STRIDE-2 Study Group. (2006), Treatment of pulmonary arterial hypertension with the selective endothelin-A receptor antagonist sitaxsentan. *Journal of the American College of Cardiology*, Vol.47, No.10, pp.2049-2056, 1558-3597; 0735-1097

Birks, E. K., Bousamra, M., Presberg, K., Marsh, J. A., Effros, R. M.& Jacobs, E. R.. (1997), Human pulmonary arteries dilate to 20-HETE, an endogenous eicosanoid of lung tissue. *The American Journal of Physiology*, Vol.272, No.5 Pt 1, pp.L823-9, 0002-9513; 0002-9513

Budhiraja, R., Tuder, R. M. & Hassoun, P. M. (2004), Endothelial dysfunction in pulmonary hypertension. *Circulation*, Vol.109, No.2, pp.159-165, 1524-4539; 0009-7322

Campbell, W. B., Gebremedhin, D., Pratt, P. F. & Harder, D. R. (1996), Identification of epoxyeicosatrienoic acids as endothelium-derived hyperpolarizing factors. *Circulation research*, Vol.78, No.3, pp.415-423, 0009-7330; 0009-7330

Capdevila, J. H., Falck, J. R. & Harris, R. C. (2000), Cytochrome P450 and arachidonic acid bioactivation. Molecular and functional properties of the arachidonate monooxygenase. *Journal of lipid research*, Vol.41, No.2, pp.163-181, 0022-2275; 0022-2275

Channick, R. N., Simonneau, G., Sitbon, O., Robbins, I. M., Frost, A., Tapson, V. F., Badesch, D. B., Roux, S., Rainisio, M., Bodin, F. & Rubin, L. J. (2001), Effects of the dual endothelin-receptor antagonist bosentan in patients with pulmonary hypertension: a randomised placebo-controlled study. *Lancet*, Vol.358, No.9288, pp.1119-1123, 0140-6736; 0140-6736

Clapp, L. H., Finney, P., Turcato, S., Tran, S., Rubin, L. J. & Tinker, A. (2002), Differential effects of stable prostacyclin analogs on smooth muscle proliferation and cyclic AMP generation in human pulmonary artery. *American journal of respiratory cell and molecular biology*, Vol.26, No.2, pp.194-201, 1044-1549; 1044-1549

Clarke, S. D. & Jump, D. B. (1993), Regulation of gene transcription by polyunsaturated fatty acids. *Progress in lipid research*, Vol.32, No.2, pp.139-149, 0163-7827; 0163-7827

Cloutier, M., Campbell, S., Basora, N., Proteau, S., Payet, M. D. & Rousseau, E. (2003), 20-HETE inotropic effects involve the activation of a nonselective cationic current in airway smooth muscle. *American journal of physiology.Lung cellular and molecular physiology*, Vol.285, No.3, pp.L560-8, 1040-0605; 1040-0605

Connolly, M. J. & Aaronson, P. I. (2011), Key role of the RhoA/Rho kinase system in pulmonary hypertension. *Pulmonary pharmacology & therapeutics*, Vol.24, No.1, pp.1-14, 1522-9629; 1094-5539

Connor, W. E. (2000), Importance of n-3 fatty acids in health and disease. *The American Journal of Clinical Nutrition*, Vol.71, No.1 Suppl, pp.171S-5S, 0002-9165; 0002-9165

De Caterina, R., Cybulsky, M. I., Clinton, S. K., Gimbrone Jr, M. A. & Libby, P. (1994), The omega-3 fatty acid docosahexaenoate reduces cytokine-induced expression of proatherogenic and proinflammatory proteins in human endothelial cells. *Arteriosclerosis and Thrombosis : A Journal of Vascular Biology / American Heart Association*, Vol.14, No.11, pp.1829-1836, 1049-8834; 1049-8834

Eckman, D. M., Hopkins, N., McBride, C. & Keef, K. D. (1998), Endothelium-dependent relaxation and hyperpolarization in guinea-pig coronary artery: role of epoxyeicosatrienoic acid. *British journal of pharmacology*, Vol.124, No.1, pp.181-189, 0007-1188; 0007-1188

Fagan, K. A., Oka, M., Bauer, N. R., Gebb, S. A., Ivy, D. D., Morris, K. G. & McMurtry, I. F. (2004), Attenuation of acute hypoxic pulmonary vasoconstriction and hypoxic pulmonary hypertension in mice by inhibition of Rho-kinase. *American journal of physiology.Lung cellular and molecular physiology,* Vol.287, No.4, pp.L656-64, 1040-0605; 1040-0605

Fartoukh, M., Emilie, D., Le Gall, C., Monti, G., Simonneau, G. & Humbert, M. (1998), Chemokine macrophage inflammatory protein-1alpha mRNA expression in lung biopsy specimens of primary pulmonary hypertension. *Chest,* Vol.114, No.1 Suppl, pp.50S-51S, 0012-3692; 0012-3692

Fer, M., Dreano, Y., Lucas, D., Corcos, L., Salaun, J. P., Berthou, F. & Amet, Y. (2008), Metabolism of eicosapentaenoic and docosahexaenoic acids by recombinant human cytochromes P450. *Archives of Biochemistry and Biophysics,* Vol.471, No.2, pp.116-125, 1096-0384; 0003-9861

Fisslthaler, B., Popp, R., Kiss, L., Potente, M., Harder, D. R., Fleming, I. & Busse, R. (1999), Cytochrome P450 2C is an EDHF synthase in coronary arteries. *Nature,* Vol.401, No.6752, pp.493-497, 0028-0836; 0028-0836

Fortin, S. Polyunsaturated fatty acid monoglycerides, derivatives, and uses thereof. No.Can. Patent 2 672 513,

Fujita, H., Fukumoto, Y., Saji, K., Sugimura, K., Demachi, J., Nawata, J. & Shimokawa, H. (2010), Acute vasodilator effects of inhaled fasudil, a specific Rho-kinase inhibitor, in patients with pulmonary arterial hypertension. *Heart and vessels,* Vol.25, No.2, pp.144-149, 1615-2573; 0910-8327

Fukumoto, Y., Matoba, T., Ito, A., Tanaka, H., Kishi, T., Hayashidani, S., Abe, K., Takeshita, A. & Shimokawa, H. (2005), Acute vasodilator effects of a Rho-kinase inhibitor, fasudil, in patients with severe pulmonary hypertension. *Heart (British Cardiac Society),* Vol.91, No.3, pp.391-392, 1468-201X; 1355-6037

Funk, C. D. (2001), Prostaglandins and leukotrienes: advances in eicosanoid biology. *Science (New York, N.Y.),* Vol.294, No.5548, pp.1871-1875, 0036-8075; 0036-8075

Fuster, V., Steele, P. M., Edwards, W. D., Gersh, B. J., McGoon, M. D. & Frye, R. L.. (1984), Primary pulmonary hypertension: natural history and the importance of thrombosis. *Circulation,* Vol.70, No.4, pp.580-587, 0009-7322; 0009-7322

Galie, N., Brundage, B. H., Ghofrani, H. A., Oudiz, R. J., Simonneau, G., Safdar, Z., Shapiro, S., White, R. J., Chan, M., Beardsworth, A., Frumkin, L. & Barst, R. J. Pulmonary Arterial Hypertension and Response to Tadalafil (PHIRST) Study Group. (2009), Tadalafil therapy for pulmonary arterial hypertension. *Circulation,* Vol.119, No.22, pp.2894-2903, 1524-4539; 0009-7322 (b)

Galie, N., Hoeper, M. M., Humbert, M., Torbicki, A., Vachiery, J. L., Barbera, J. A., Beghetti, M., Corris, P., Gaine, S., Gibbs, J. S., Gomez-Sanchez, M. A., Jondeau, G., Klepetko, W., Opitz, C., Peacock, A., Rubin, L., Zellweger, M. & Simonneau, G. (2009), Guidelines for the diagnosis and treatment of pulmonary hypertension. *The European respiratory journal : official journal of the European Society for Clinical Respiratory Physiology,* Vol.34, No.6, pp.1219-1263, 1399-3003; 0903-1936 (a)

Gebremedhin, D., Lange, A. R., Narayanan, J., Aebly, M. R., Jacobs, E. R. & Harder, D. R. (1998), Cat cerebral arterial smooth muscle cells express cytochrome P450 4A2 enzyme and produce the vasoconstrictor 20-HETE which enhances L-type Ca2+

current. *The Journal of physiology,* Vol.507 (Pt 3), No.Pt 3, pp.771-781, 0022-3751; 0022-3751

Gebremedhin, D., Ma, Y. H., Falck, J. R., Roman, R. J., VanRollins, M. & Harder, D. R. (1992), Mechanism of action of cerebral epoxyeicosatrienoic acids on cerebral arterial smooth muscle. *The American Journal of Physiology,* Vol.263, No.2 Pt 2, pp.H519-25, 0002-9513; 0002-9513

Giaid, A. & Saleh, D. (1995), Reduced expression of endothelial nitric oxide synthase in the lungs of patients with pulmonary hypertension. *The New England journal of medicine,* Vol.333, No.4, pp.214-221, 0028-4793; 0028-4793

Giaid, A., Yanagisawa, M., Langleben, D., Michel, R. P., Levy, R., Shennib, H., Kimura, S., Masaki, T., Duguid, W. P. & Stewart, D. J. (1993), Expression of endothelin-1 in the lungs of patients with pulmonary hypertension. *The New England journal of medicine,* Vol.328, No.24, pp.1732-1739, 0028-4793; 0028-4793

Guibert, C. (2010), Plasma membrane Ca2+-ATPase equals no NO. *Cardiovascular research,* Vol.87, No.3, pp.401-402, 1755-3245; 0008-6363

Guibert, C., Marthan, R. & Savineau, J. P. (2007), Modulation of ion channels in pulmonary arterial hypertension. *Current pharmaceutical design,* Vol.13, No.24, pp.2443-2455, 1873-4286; 1381-6128

Guibert, C., Savineau, J. P., Crevel, H., Marthan, R. & Rousseau, E. (2005), Effect of short-term organoid culture on the pharmaco-mechanical properties of rat extra- and intrapulmonary arteries. *British journal of pharmacology,* Vol.146, No.5, pp.692-701, 0007-1188; 0007-1188

Hata, T., Soga, J., Hidaka, T., Idei, N., Fujii, Y., Fujimura, N., Mikami, S., Maruhashi, T., Kihara, Y., Chayama, K., Kato, H., Noma, K., JLiao, K. & Higashi, Y. ROCK Study Group. (2011), Calcium channel blocker and Rho-associated kinase activity in patients with hypertension. *Journal of hypertension,* Vol.29, No.2, pp.373-379, 1473-5598; 0263-6352

Hayabuchi, Y., Nakaya, Y., Matsuoka, S. & Kuroda, Y. (1998), Endothelium-derived hyperpolarizing factor activates Ca2+-activated K+ channels in porcine coronary artery smooth muscle cells. *Journal of cardiovascular pharmacology,* Vol.32, No.4, pp.642-649, 0160-2446; 0160-2446

Hecker, M., Bara, A. T., Bauersachs, J. & Busse, R. (1994), Characterization of endothelium-derived hyperpolarizing factor as a cytochrome P450-derived arachidonic acid metabolite in mammals. *The Journal of physiology,* Vol.481 (Pt 2), No.Pt 2, pp.407-414, 0022-3751; 0022-3751

Hercule, H. C., Salanova, B., Essin, K., Honeck, H., Falck, J. R., Sausbier, M., Ruth, P., Schunck, W. H., Luft, F. C. & Gollasch, M. (2007), The vasodilator 17,18-epoxyeicosatetraenoic acid targets the pore-forming BK alpha channel subunit in rodents. *Experimental physiology,* Vol.92, No.6, pp.1067-1076, 0958-0670; 0958-0670

Hersch, E., Huang, J., Grider, J. R. & Murthy, K. S. (2004), Gq/G13 signaling by ET-1 in smooth muscle: MYPT1 phosphorylation via ETA and CPI-17 dephosphorylation via ETB. *American journal of physiology.Cell physiology,* Vol.287, No.5, pp.C1209-18, 0363-6143; 0363-6143

Hirafuji, M., Machida, T., Hamaue, N. & Minami, M. (2003), Cardiovascular protective effects of n-3 polyunsaturated fatty acids with special emphasis on docosahexaenoic acid. *Journal of pharmacological sciences,* Vol.92, No.4, pp.308-316, 1347-8613; 1347-8613

Hoeper, M. M., Schwarze, M., Ehlerding, S., Adler-Schuermeyer, A., Spiekerkoetter, E., Niedermeyer, J., Hamm, M. & Fabel, H. (2000), Long-term treatment of primary pulmonary hypertension with aerosolized iloprost, a prostacyclin analogue. *The New England journal of medicine,* Vol.342, No.25, pp.1866-1870, 0028-4793; 0028-4793

Humbert, M., Maitre, S., Capron, F., Rain, B., Musset, D. & Simonneau, G. (1998), Pulmonary edema complicating continuous intravenous prostacyclin in pulmonary capillary hemangiomatosis. *American journal of respiratory and critical care medicine,* Vol.157, No.5 Pt 1, pp.1681-1685, 1073-449X; 1073-449X

Humbert, M., Monti, G., Brenot, F., Sitbon, O., Portier, A., Grangeot-Keros, L., Duroux, P., Galanaud, P., Simonneau, G. & Emilie, D. (1995), Increased interleukin-1 and interleukin-6 serum concentrations in severe primary pulmonary hypertension. *American journal of respiratory and critical care medicine,* Vol.151, No.5, pp.1628-1631, 1073-449X; 1073-449X

Humbert, M., Yaici, A., Sztrymf, B. & Montani, D. (2004), Pulmonary hypertension: from genetics to treatments. *Revue de pneumologie clinique,* Vol.60, No.4, pp.196-201, 0761-8417; 0761-8417

Ishikura, K., Yamada, N., Ito, M., Ota, S., Nakamura, M., Isaka, N. & Nakano, T. (2006), Beneficial acute effects of rho-kinase inhibitor in patients with pulmonary arterial hypertension. *Circulation journal : official journal of the Japanese Circulation Society,* Vol.70, No.2, pp.174-178, 1346-9843; 1346-9843

J. L. Losapio, R. S. Sprague, A. J. Lonigro and A. H. Stephenson. (2005), 5,6-EET-induced contraction of intralobar pulmonary arteries depends on the activation of Rho-kinase. *Journal of applied physiology (Bethesda, Md.: 1985),* Vol.99, No.4, pp.1391-1396, 8750-7587; 0161-7567

Jacobs, E. R., Effros, R. M., Falck, J. R., Reddy, K. M., Campbell, W. B. & Zhu, D. (1999), Airway synthesis of 20-hydroxyeicosatetraenoic acid: metabolism by cyclooxygenase to a bronchodilator. *The American Journal of Physiology,* Vol.276, No.2 Pt 1, pp.L280-8, 0002-9513; 0002-9513

Jacobs, E. R., Zhu, D., Gruenloh, S., Lopez, B. & Medhora, M. (2006), VEGF-induced relaxation of pulmonary arteries is mediated by endothelial cytochrome P-450 hydroxylase. *American journal of physiology.Lung cellular and molecular physiology,* Vol.291, No.3, pp.L369-77, 1040-0605; 1040-0605

Kimura, K., Ito, M., Amano, M., Chihara, K., Fukata, Y., Nakafuku, M., Yamamori, B., Feng, J., Nakano, T., Okawa, K., Iwamatsu, A. & Kaibuchi, K. (1996), Regulation of myosin phosphatase by Rho and Rho-associated kinase (Rho-kinase). *Science (New York, N.Y.),* Vol.273, No.5272, pp.245-248, 0036-8075; 0036-8075

Kitazawa, T. (2010), G protein-mediated Ca(2)+-sensitization of CPI-17 phosphorylation in arterial smooth muscle. *Biochemical and biophysical research communications,* Vol.401, No.1, pp.75-78, 1090-2104; 0006-291X

Koga, Y. & Ikebe, M. (2005), p116Rip decreases myosin II phosphorylation by activating myosin light chain phosphatase and by inactivating RhoA. *The Journal of biological chemistry*, Vol.280, No.6, pp.4983-4991, 0021-9258; 0021-9258

Konkel, A. & Schunck, W. H. (2011), Role of cytochrome P450 enzymes in the bioactivation of polyunsaturated fatty acids. *Biochimica et biophysica acta*, Vol.1814, No.1, pp.210-222, 0006-3002; 0006-3002

Kris-Etherton, P. M., Etherton, T. D., Carlson, J. & Gardner, C. (2002), Recent discoveries in inclusive food-based approaches and dietary patterns for reduction in risk for cardiovascular disease. *Current opinion in lipidology*, Vol.13, No.4, pp.397-407, 0957-9672; 0957-9672

Kris-Etherton, P. M., Harris, W. S. & Appel, L. J. American Heart Association. Nutrition Committee. (2002), Fish consumption, fish oil, omega-3 fatty acids, and cardiovascular disease. *Circulation*, Vol.106, No.21, pp.2747-2757, 1524-4539; 0009-7322

Lauterbach, B., Barbosa-Sicard, E., Wang, M. H., Honeck, H., Kargel, E., Theuer, J., Schwartzman, M. L., Haller, H., Luft, F. C., Gollasch, M. & Schunck, W. H. (2002), Cytochrome P450-dependent eicosapentaenoic acid metabolites are novel BK channel activators. *Hypertension*, Vol.39, No.2 Pt 2, pp.609-613, 1524-4563; 0194-911X

Loirand, G., Guilluy, C. & Pacaud, P. (2006), Regulation of Rho proteins by phosphorylation in the cardiovascular system. *Trends in cardiovascular medicine*, Vol.16, No.6, pp.199-204, 1050-1738; 1050-1738

Lucas, D., Goulitquer, S., Marienhagen, J., Fer, M., Dreano, Y., Schwaneberg, U., Amet, Y. & Corcos, L. (2010), Stereoselective epoxidation of the last double bond of polyunsaturated fatty acids by human cytochromes P450. *Journal of lipid research*, Vol.51, No.5, pp.1125-1133, 0022-2275; 0022-2275

McLaughlin, V. V., Badesch, D. B., Delcroix, M., Fleming, T. R., Gaine, S. P., Galie, N., Gibbs, J. S., Kim, N. H., Oudiz, R. J., Peacock, A., Provencher, S., Sitbon, O., Tapson, V. F. & Seeger, W. (2009), End points and clinical trial design in pulmonary arterial hypertension. *Journal of the American College of Cardiology*, Vol.54, No.1 Suppl, pp.S97-107, 1558-3597; 0735-1097 (a)

McLaughlin, V. V., Shillington, A. & Rich, S. (2002), Survival in primary pulmonary hypertension: the impact of epoprostenol therapy. *Circulation*, Vol.106, No.12, pp.1477-1482, 1524-4539; 0009-7322 (b)

Miyata, N. & Roman, R. J.. (2005), Role of 20-hydroxyeicosatetraenoic acid (20-HETE) in vascular system. *Journal of smooth muscle research* = *Nihon Heikatsukin Gakkai kikanshi*, Vol.41, No.4, pp.175-193, 0916-8737; 0916-8737

Mizutani, M., Asano, M., Roy, S., Nakajima, T., Soma, M., Yamashita, K. & Okuda, Y. (1997), Omega-3 polyunsaturated fatty acids inhibit migration of human vascular smooth muscle cells in vitro. *Life Sciences*, Vol.61, No.19, pp.PL269-74, 0024-3205; 0024-3205

Morin, C., Guibert C., Sirois, M., Echave, V., Gomes, M. M. & Rousseau, E. (2008), Effects of omega-hydroxylase product on distal human pulmonary arteries. *American journal of physiology.Heart and circulatory physiology*, Vol.294, No.3, pp.H1435-43, 0363-6135; 0363-6135

Morin, C., Sirois, M., Echave, V., Gomes, M. M. & Rousseau, E. (2007), Epoxyeicosatrienoic acid relaxing effects involve Ca2+-activated K+ channel activation and CPI-17 dephosphorylation in human bronchi. *American journal of respiratory cell and molecular biology*, Vol.36, No.5, pp.633-641, 1044-1549; 1044-1549 (a)

Morin, C., Sirois, M., Echave, V., Gomes, M. M. & Rousseau, E. (2007), Functional effects of 20-HETE on human bronchi: hyperpolarization and relaxation due to BKCa channel activation. *American journal of physiology.Lung cellular and molecular physiology*, Vol.293, No.4, pp.L1037-44, 1040-0605; 1040-0605 (b)

Morin, C., Sirois, M., Echave, V., Rizcallah, E. & Rousseau, E. (2009), Relaxing effects of 17(18)-EpETE on arterial and airway smooth muscles in human lung. *American journal of physiology.Lung cellular and molecular physiology*, Vol.296, No.1, pp.L130-9, 1040-0605; 1040-0605

Mouchaers, K. T., Schalij, I., de Boer, M. A., Postmus, P. E., van Hinsbergh, V. W., van Nieuw Amerongen, G. P., Vonk Noordegraaf, A. & van der Laarse, W. J. (2010), Fasudil reduces monocrotaline-induced pulmonary arterial hypertension: comparison with bosentan and sildenafil. *The European respiratory journal : official journal of the European Society for Clinical Respiratory Physiology*, Vol.36, No.4, pp.800-807, 1399-3003; 0903-1936

Nagaoka, T. Morio, Y., Casanova, N., Bauer, N., Gebb, S., McMurtry, I. & Oka, M. (2004), Rho/Rho kinase signaling mediates increased basal pulmonary vascular tone in chronically hypoxic rats. *American journal of physiology.Lung cellular and molecular physiology*, Vol.287, No.4, pp.L665-72, 1040-0605; 1040-0605

Nagaoka, T., Gebb, S. A., Karoor, V., Homma, N., Morris, K. G., McMurtry, I. F. & Oka, M.. (2006), Involvement of RhoA/Rho kinase signaling in pulmonary hypertension of the fawn-hooded rat. *Journal of applied physiology (Bethesda, Md.: 1985)*, Vol.100, No.3, pp.996-1002, 8750-7587; 0161-7567

Nguyen, X., Wang, M. H., Reddy, K. M., Falck, J. R. & Schwartzman, M. L. (1999), Kinetic profile of the rat CYP4A isoforms: arachidonic acid metabolism and isoform-specific inhibitors. *The American Journal of Physiology*, Vol.276, No.6 Pt 2, pp.R1691-700, 0002-9513; 0002-9513

Nithipatikom, K., Endsley, M. P., Moore, J. M., Isbell, M. A., Falck, J. R., Campbell, W. B. & Gross, G. J.. (2006), Effects of selective inhibition of cytochrome P-450 omega-hydroxylases and ischemic preconditioning in myocardial protection. *American journal of physiology.Heart and circulatory physiology*, Vol.290, No.2, pp.H500-5, 0363-6135; 0363-6135

Node, K., Huo Y., Ruan X., Yang, B., Spiecker, M., Ley, K., Zeldin, D. C. & Liao, J. K.. (1999), Anti-inflammatory properties of cytochrome P450 epoxygenase-derived eicosanoids. *Science (New York, N.Y.)*, Vol.285, No.5431, pp.1276-1279, 0036-8075; 0036-8075

Nunes, H., Humbert, M., Sitbon, O., Morse, J. H., Deng, Z., Knowles, J. A., Le Gall, C., Parent, F., Garcia, G., Herve, P., Barst, R. J. & Simonneau, G. (2003), Prognostic factors for survival in human immunodeficiency virus-associated pulmonary arterial hypertension. *American journal of respiratory and critical care medicine*, Vol.167, No.10, pp.1433-1439, 1073-449X; 1073-449X

Oka, M., Homma, N., Taraseviciene-Stewart, L., Morris, K. G., Kraskauskas, D., Burns, N., Voelkel, N. F. & McMurtry, I. F. (2007), Rho kinase-mediated vasoconstriction is important in severe occlusive pulmonary arterial hypertension in rats. *Circulation research,* Vol.100, No.6, pp.923-929, 1524-4571; 0009-7330

Olschewski, H., Simonneau, G., Galie, N., Higenbottam, T., Naeije, R., Rubin, L. J., Nikkho, S., Speich, R., Hoeper, M. M., Behr, J., Winkler, J., Sitbon, O., Popov, W., Ghofrani, H. A., Manes, A., Kiely, D. G., Ewert, R., Meyer, A., Corris, P. A., Delcroix, M., Gomez-Sanchez, M., Siedentop, H. & Seeger, W. Aerosolized Iloprost Randomized Study Group. (2002), Inhaled iloprost for severe pulmonary hypertension. *The New England journal of medicine,* Vol.347, No.5, pp.322-329, 1533-4406; 0028-4793

Palmer, S. M., Robinson, L. J., Wang, A., Gossage, J. R., Bashore, T. & Tapson, V. F. (1998), Massive pulmonary edema and death after prostacyclin infusion in a patient with pulmonary veno-occlusive disease. *Chest,* Vol.113, No.1, pp.237-240, 0012-3692; 0012-3692

Pauvert, O., Bonnet, S., Rousseau, E., Marthan, R. & Savineau, J. P. (2004), Sildenafil alters calcium signaling and vascular tone in pulmonary arteries from chronically hypoxic rats. *American journal of physiology. Lung cellular and molecular physiology,* Vol.287, No.3, pp.L577-83, 1040-0605; 1040-0605

Pierson, D. J. (2000), Pathophysiology and clinical effects of chronic hypoxia. *Respiratory care,* Vol.45, No.1, pp.39-51; discussion 51-3, 0020-1324; 0020-1324

Randriamboavonjy, V., Busse, R. & Fleming, I. (2003), 20-HETE-induced contraction of small coronary arteries depends on the activation of Rho-kinase. *Hypertension,* Vol.41, No.3 Pt 2, pp.801-806, 1524-4563; 0194-911X

Reagan-Shaw, S., Nihal, M. & Ahmad, N. (2008), Dose translation from animal to human studies revisited. *The FASEB journal : official publication of the Federation of American Societies for Experimental Biology,* Vol.22, No.3, pp.659-661, 1530-6860; 0892-6638

Rich, S., Kaufmann, E. & Levy, P. S. (1992), The effect of high doses of calcium-channel blockers on survival in primary pulmonary hypertension. *The New England journal of medicine,* Vol.327, No.2, pp.76-81, 0028-4793; 0028-4793

Rodat-Despoix, L., Aires, V., Ducret, T., Marthan, R., Savineau, J. P., Rousseau, E. & Guibert, C. (2009), Signalling pathways involved in the contractile response to 5-HT in the human pulmonary artery. *The European respiratory journal : official journal of the European Society for Clinical Respiratory Physiology,* Vol.34, No.6, pp.1338-1347, 1399-3003; 0903-1936

Rodat-Despoix, L., Crevel, H., Marthan, R., Savineau, J. P. & Guibert, C. (2008), Heterogeneity in 5-HT-induced contractile and proliferative responses in rat pulmonary arterial bed. *Journal of vascular research,* Vol.45, No.3, pp.181-192, 1423-0135; 1018-1172

Roman, L. J., Palmer, C. N., Clark, J. E., Muerhoff, A. S., Griffin, K. J., Johnson, E. F. & Masters, B. S. (1993), Expression of rabbit cytochromes P4504A which catalyze the omega-hydroxylation of arachidonic acid, fatty acids, and prostaglandins. *Archives of Biochemistry and Biophysics,* Vol.307, No.1, pp.57-65, 0003-9861; 0003-9861

Roman, R. J. (2002), P-450 metabolites of arachidonic acid in the control of cardiovascular function. *Physiological reviews,* Vol.82, No.1, pp.131-185, 0031-9333; 0031-9333

Rosenzweig, E. B., Kerstein, D. & Barst, R. J. (1999), Long-term prostacyclin for pulmonary hypertension with associated congenital heart defects. *Circulation,* Vol.99, No.14, pp.1858-1865, 1524-4539; 0009-7322

Rubin, L. J., Badesch, D. B., Barst, R. J., Galie, N., Black, C. M., Keogh, A., Pulido, T., Frost, A., Roux, S., Leconte, I., Landzberg, M. & Simonneau, G. (2002), Bosentan therapy for pulmonary arterial hypertension. *The New England journal of medicine,* Vol.346, No.12, pp.896-903, 1533-4406; 0028-4793

Saouti, N., Westerhof, N., Postmus, P. E. & Vonk-Noordegraaf, A. (2010), The arterial load in pulmonary hypertension. *European respiratory review : an official journal of the European Respiratory Society,* Vol.19, No.117, pp.197-203, 1600-0617; 0905-9180

Schwarz, D., Kisselev, P., Ericksen, S. S., Szklarz, G. D., Chernogolov, A., Honeck, H., Schunck, W. H. & Roots, I. (2004), Arachidonic and eicosapentaenoic acid metabolism by human CYP1A1: highly stereoselective formation of 17(R),18(S)-epoxyeicosatetraenoic acid. *Biochemical pharmacology,* Vol.67, No.8, pp.1445-1457, 0006-2952; 0006-2952

Sitbon, O., Humbert, M., Nunes, H., Parent, F., Garcia, G., Herve, P., Rainisio, M. & Simonneau, G. (2002), Long-term intravenous epoprostenol infusion in primary pulmonary hypertension: prognostic factors and survival. *Journal of the American College of Cardiology,* Vol.40, No.4, pp.780-788, 0735-1097; 0735-1097

Somlyo, A. P. & Somlyo, A. V. (2003), Ca2+ sensitivity of smooth muscle and nonmuscle myosin II: modulated by G proteins, kinases, and myosin phosphatase. *Physiological reviews,* Vol.83, No.4, pp.1325-1358, 0031-9333; 0031-9333

Stephenson, A. H., Sprague, R. S. & Lonigro, A. J. (1998), 5,6-Epoxyeicosatrienoic acid reduces increases in pulmonary vascular resistance in the dog. *The American Journal of Physiology,* Vol.275, No.1 Pt 2, pp.H100-9, 0002-9513; 0002-9513

Stephenson, A. H., Sprague, R. S., Losapio, J. L. & Lonigro, A. J. (2003), Differential effects of 5,6-EET on segmental pulmonary vasoactivity in the rabbit. *American journal of physiology.Heart and circulatory physiology,* Vol.284, No.6, pp.H2153-61, 0363-6135; 0363-6135

Tagawa H., Shimokawa, H., Tagawa, T., Kuroiwa-Matsumoto, M., Hirooka, Y. & Takeshita, A. (1999), Long-term treatment with eicosapentaenoic acid augments both nitric oxide-mediated and non-nitric oxide-mediated endothelium-dependent forearm vasodilatation in patients with coronary artery disease. *Journal of cardiovascular pharmacology,* Vol.33, No.4, pp.633-640, 0160-2446; 0160-2446

Thenappan, T., Shah, S. J., Rich, S. & Gomberg-Maitland, M. (2007), A USA-based registry for pulmonary arterial hypertension: 1982-2006. *The European respiratory journal : official journal of the European Society for Clinical Respiratory Physiology,* Vol.30, No.6, pp.1103-1110, 0903-1936; 0903-1936

Tuder, R. M., Groves, B., Badesch, D. B. & Voelkel, N. F. (1994), Exuberant endothelial cell growth and elements of inflammation are present in plexiform lesions of pulmonary hypertension. *The American journal of pathology,* Vol.144, No.2, pp.275-285, 0002-9440; 0002-9440

Uehata, M., Ishizaki, T., Satoh, H., Ono, T., Kawahara, T., Morishita, T., Tamakawa, H., Yamagami, K., Inui, J., Maekawa, M. & Narumiya, S. (1997), Calcium sensitization of smooth muscle mediated by a Rho-associated protein kinase in hypertension. *Nature,* Vol.389, No.6654, pp.990-994, 0028-0836; 0028-0836

Van Rollins, M., Frade, P. D. & Carretero, O. A.. (1988), Oxidation of 5,8,11,14,17-eicosapentaenoic acid by hepatic and renal microsomes. *Biochimica et biophysica acta,* Vol.966, No.1, pp.133-149, 0006-3002; 0006-3002

Voelkel, N. F., Quaife, R. A., Leinwand, L. A., Barst, R. J., McGoon, M. D., Meldrum, D. R., Dupuis, J., Long, C. S., Rubin, L. J., Smart, F. W., Suzuki, Y. J., Gladwin, M., Denholm, E. M. & Gail, D. B. National Heart, Lung, and Blood Institute Working Group on Cellular and Molecular Mechanisms of Right Heart Failure. (2006), Right ventricular function and failure: report of a National Heart, Lung, and Blood Institute working group on cellular and molecular mechanisms of right heart failure. *Circulation,* Vol.114, No.17, pp.1883-1891, 1524-4539; 0009-7322

Wang, R. X., Chai, Q., Lu, T. & Lee, H. C. (2011), Activation of vascular BK channels by docosahexaenoic acid is dependent on cytochrome P450 epoxygenase activity. *Cardiovascular research,* Vol.90, No.2, pp.344-352, 1755-3245; 0008-6363

Weir, E. K. & Olschewski, A. (2006), Role of ion channels in acute and chronic responses of the pulmonary vasculature to hypoxia. *Cardiovascular research,* Vol.71, No.4, pp.630-641, 0008-6363; 0008-6363

Yaghi, A., Webb, C. D., Scott, J. A., Mehta, S., Bend, J. R. & McCormack, D. G. (2001), Cytochrome P450 metabolites of arachidonic acid but not cyclooxygenase-2 metabolites contribute to the pulmonary vascular hyporeactivity in rats with acute Pseudomonas pneumonia. *The Journal of pharmacology and experimental therapeutics,* Vol.297, No.2, pp.479-488, 0022-3565; 0022-3565

Ye, D., Zhang, D., Oltman, C., Dellsperger, K., Lee, H. C. & VanRollins, M. (2002), Cytochrome p-450 epoxygenase metabolites of docosahexaenoate potently dilate coronary arterioles by activating large-conductance calcium-activated potassium channels. *The Journal of pharmacology and experimental therapeutics,* Vol.303, No.2, pp.768-776, 0022-3565; 0022-3565

Zeldin, D. C., Foley, J., Ma, J., Boyle, J. E., Pascual, J. M., Moomaw, C. R., Tomer, K. B., Steenbergen, C. & Wu, S. (1996), CYP2J subfamily P450s in the lung: expression, localization, and potential functional significance. *Molecular pharmacology,* Vol.50, No.5, pp.1111-1117, 0026-895X; 0026-895X

Zeldin, D. C., Plitman, J. D., Kobayashi, J., Miller, R. F., Snapper, J. R., Falck, J. R., Szarek, J. L., Philpot, R. M. & Capdevila, J. H. (1995), The rabbit pulmonary cytochrome P450 arachidonic acid metabolic pathway: characterization and significance. *The Journal of clinical investigation,* Vol.95, No.5, pp.2150-2160, 0021-9738; 0021-9738

Zhang, Y., Oltman, C. L., Lu, T., Lee, H. C., Dellsperger, K. C. & VanRollins, M. (2001), EET homologs potently dilate coronary microvessels and activate BK(Ca) channels. *American journal of physiology.Heart and circulatory physiology,* Vol.280, No.6, pp.H2430-40, 0363-6135; 0363-6135

Zhu, D., Birks, E. K., Dawson, C. A., Patel, M., Falck, J. R., Presberg, K., Roman, R. J. & Jacobs, E. R.. (2000), Hypoxic pulmonary vasoconstriction is modified by P-450 metabolites. *American journal of physiology.Heart and circulatory physiology,* Vol.279, No.4, pp.H1526-33, 0363-6135; 0363-6135 (a)

Zhu, D., Bousamra 2nd, M., Zeldin, D. C., Falck, J. R., Townsley, M., Harder, D. R., Roman, R. J. & Jacobs, E. R. (2000), Epoxyeicosatrienoic acids constrict isolated pressurized rabbit pulmonary arteries. *American journal of physiology.Lung cellular and molecular physiology,* Vol.278, No.2, pp.L335-43, 1040-0605; 1040-0605 (b)

Zhu, D., Effros, R. M., Harder, D. R., Roman, R. J. & Jacobs, E. R. (1998), Tissue sources of cytochrome P450 4A and 20-HETE synthesis in rabbit lungs. *American journal of respiratory cell and molecular biology,* Vol.19, No.1, pp.121-128, 1044-1549; 1044-1549

Zou, A. P., Fleming, J. T., Falck, J. R., Jacobs, E. R., Gebremedhin, D., Harder, D. R. & Roman, R. J. (1996), Stereospecific effects of epoxyeicosatrienoic acids on renal vascular tone and K(+)-channel activity. *The American Journal of Physiology,* Vol.270, No.5 Pt 2, pp.F822-32, 0002-9513; 0002-9513

5

Deregulation of BMP Signaling in the Pathogenesis of Pulmonary Hypertension

Miriam de Boeck and Peter ten Dijke
Department of Molecular Cell Biology and Centre for Biomedical Genetics,
Leiden University Medical Center
The Netherlands

1. Introduction

Idiopathic pulmonary arterial hypertension (IPAH) is a rare disease that is defined by a sustained pulmonary arterial pressure of >25 mmHg at rest and a pulmonary capillary wedge pressure (PCWP) or left ventricular end-diastolic pressure (LVEDP) of no more than 15 mmHg. The disease is characterized by a constriction of the precapillary pulmonary arteries due to vascular remodeling. The excessive proliferation of endothelial cells and vascular smooth muscle cells gives rise to medial hypertrophy, plexiform lesions and narrowing of the vascular lumina due to the formation of a neointima (Figure 1) (Cool et al., 1999; Humbert et al., 2004). Patients develop right ventricular hypertrophy due to increased vascular resistance and are prone to heart failure (Farber & Loscalzo, 2004; Sastry, 2006).

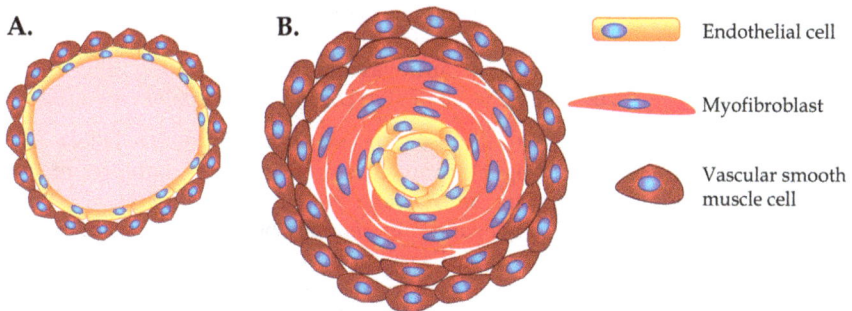

Fig. 1. Vascular remodeling in pulmonary arterial hypertension (PAH). A.) A healthy small pulmonary artery is lined by a single layer of endothelial cells (ECs) supported by vascular smooth muscle cells (VSMCs). B.) In PAH, excessive proliferation of ECs, myofibroblasts and VSMCs leads to a narrowing of the vascular lumen. (Adapted from ten Dijke & Arthur, 2007)

Most cases of idiopathic pulmonary arterial hypertension are sporadic, but in 6-10% of cases one or more family members are also affected thereby marking it as heritable pulmonary arterial hypertension (HPAH). The sporadic and heritable cases of PAH present with identical symptoms, yet HPAH occurs at a younger age and prognosis is worse (Sztrymf et al., 2008). Interestingly, females have an increased risk of developing IPAH compared to males and the disease occurs mostly at 30-40 years of age, yet it can present at any age (Gaine & Rubin, 1998; Rich et al., 1987).

HPAH is inherited in an autosomal-dominant pattern, yet only 10-20% of family members develop overt pulmonary hypertension. This incomplete penetrance highlights the role of environmental factors and currently unknown genetic factors in the pathogenesis of PAH. However, in 70-80% of heritable cases heterozygous germ line mutations in the bone morphogenetic protein (BMP) receptor II gene (BMPRII) have been found. These mutations were also found to be the underlying cause of about 20% of IPAH cases (Machado et al., 2009). Also in patients suffering from non-hereditary forms of PAH a deregulation of BMP signaling has been observed in vascular beds of the lungs (Atkinson et al., 2002). These findings have driven researchers to investigate the role of BMPs and its family members in the pathogenesis of PAH.

In this chapter we will discuss the basic molecular biology and regulation of BMP signaling and the role of subverted BMP responses in vascular disease. In particular, we will focus on the pathogenesis of PAH and the effects of mutations in the BMP pathway in both murine models and PAH patients.

2. Transforming growth factor-β and bone morphogenetic protein signaling

BMPs are members of the transforming growth factor-β (TGF-β) superfamily of cytokines (Miyazono et al., 2010). Although the name BMP originates from its discovery as an inducer of bone formation (Wozney et al., 1988), it is currently well known to be important for many processes including the development (Wu & Hill, 2009) and homeostasis of the vascular system (David et al., 2009; Lowery & de Caestecker, 2010). The members of the TGF-β superfamily of signal transduction molecules are indispensible during both embryonic development and throughout adult life and are therefore well conserved through evolution. Disruptions in the various TGF-β family signaling pathways give rise to developmental disorders, fibrotic diseases, cancer and cardiovascular diseases among others (Bertolino et al., 2005; Goumans et al., 2009; Meulmeester & ten Dijke, 2011; Pardali et al., 2010) .

TGF-β family ligands are subject to intracellular cleavage by proteases before secretion as biologically active dimers. They signal through heterotetrameric complexes of type II and type I serine/threonine kinase transmembrane receptors (Heldin et al., 1997; Shi & Massague, 2003). Each TGF-β family ligand preferentially binds to a subset of the five type II receptors and seven type I receptors. BMPs signal via the type I receptors activin receptor-like kinase (ALK) 1/2/3/6 and the type II receptors BMPRII, activin receptor type IIA (ActIIA) and ActIIB. The signal can be enhanced by co-receptors such as betaglycan and endoglin. Type II receptors are constitutively active kinases that phosphorylate serine and threonine residues of type I receptors after ligand-induced oligomerization. This results in an activation of the kinase domain of the type I receptor and the recruitment of receptor-regulated Smads (R-Smads) to the receptor. R-Smads are subsequently phosphorylated and thereby activated. Type I TGF-β/Activin receptors activate Smad2 and Smad3, while type I BMP receptors activate Smad1, Smad5 and Smad8. These activated R-Smads form heteromeric complexes with the common Smad (co-Smad), Smad4. After translocation to the nucleus these complexes participate in the transcriptional control of target genes (Figure 2) (Feng & Derynck, 2005; Schmierer & Hill, 2007).

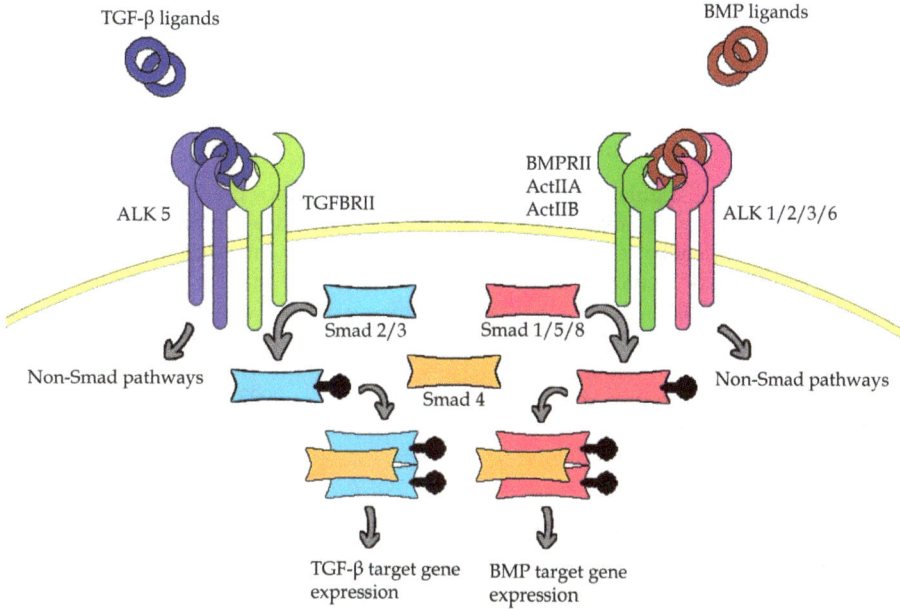

Fig. 2. Schematic overview of the TGF-β and BMP signaling pathways. Binding of ligand induces complex formation of type I and type II receptors. After activation by type II receptors, the type I receptors phosphorylate R-Smads. R-Smads form complexes with Smad4 and translocate to the nucleus to regulate target gene expression. Besides Smad-dependent signaling, also non-Smad pathways are involved.

TGF-β family members can also exert their effect via non-Smad pathways such as mitogen-activated protein kinase (MAPK) pathways, phosphatidylinositol-3-kinase/AKT pathways and Rho-like GTPase signaling pathways (Moustakas & Heldin, 2005; Zhang, 2009). TGF-β receptors directly activate components of these pathways. The cellular responses depend on the cell type and context and include proliferation, apoptosis, cytoskeletal rearrangements and modulation of Smad-dependent signaling. A well studied example of Smad-independent signaling is the activation of c-Jun N-terminal kinase (JNK) and p38 MAPK by TGF-β/BMPs. This pathway is mediated by TGF-β activated kinase 1 (TAK1), which is activated via BMP receptors (Shibuya et al., 1998). TAK1 not only activates MAP kinase pathways, but it also induces the phosphorylation of Smad1, Smad5 and Smad8, the BMP Smads, thereby linking the Smad-dependent and –independent pathways (Shim et al., 2009).

Because of the diverse effects BMPs have on cells, both the intensity and the duration of the signal are tightly regulated. First, the expression and maturation of ligands is a complex multi-step process that allows strict regulation prior to secretion (Saremba et al., 2008; von Einem et al., 2011). After secretion, BMPs are subjected to various extracellular regulatory mechanisms (ten Dijke & Arthur, 2007; Zakin & De Robertis, 2010). They can be sequestered by extracellular matrix molecules from which they can be released at the appropriate time (Nistala et al., 2010). They can also be bound by BMP antagonists such as chordin, noggin, twisted gastrulation, gremlin, DAN and cerberus, which inhibit the interaction of BMPs with their receptors (Yanagita, 2005). Once BMPs reach the membrane of the target cell, they first interact with auxiliary receptors, such as those of the Dragon family (Corradini et al., 2009), which are expressed at higher levels but have lower BMP affinity than signaling BMP type I and type II receptors. Auxiliary receptors present BMP ligands to signaling receptors. Inhibitory decoy-receptors that inhibit BMP interaction with BMP type II/I receptor complexes have also been identified (Onichtchouk et al., 1999).

The BMP signal can be regulated intracellularly as well. Besides the R-Smads and Smad4, there are also inhibitory (I)-Smads, Smad6 and Smad7, which are induced by TGF-β and BMPs as a negative feedback mechanism. Smad6 acts as an inhibitor of BMP signaling, while Smad7 can inhibit signals of many members of the TGF-β family (Hariharan & Pillai, 2008; Itoh & ten Dijke, 2007). These I-Smads can compete with R-Smads for binding to type I receptors and can induce the dephosphorylation of the receptor by phosphatases. Smad6 has been found to compete with Smad1 for complex formation with Smad4, but it can also recruit transcriptional co-repressors in the nucleus (Lin et al., 2003). I-Smads can recruit E3 ubiquitin ligases such as Smurf1 to the receptors and thereby mediate ubiquitination and subsequent proteasomal degradation of the receptor complexes (Kavsak et al., 2000; Murakami et al., 2003).

Smurf1 also targets other components of BMP signaling for degradation, most importantly Smad1 (Zhu et al., 1999). Interestingly, activation of BMPRII leads to degradation of Smurf1, thereby stabilizing Smad1. BMPRII accomplishes this via the release of Tribbles-like protein 3 (Trb3) from its long carboxyl terminal tail domain upon activation by BMP. Trb3 subsequently induces the degradation of Smurf1 (Chan et al., 2007). Besides Trb3, the tail domain of BMPRII has been shown to interact with proteins such as c-Src, cGMP-dependent protein kinase I (Schwappacher et al., 2009), Tctex1 and LIM domain kinase 1 (LIMK1). The latter is a cofilin kinase and plays a role in the regulation of cell polarity and migration. LIMK1 is released from BMPRII and activated upon stimulation with BMP4 (Foletta et al., 2003). The importance of the tail domain of BMPRII is highlighted by the finding that mutations in it lead to PAH.

3. The role of BMP signaling in vascular homeostasis

BMP signaling plays an important role in the development of the vascular system, demonstrated by the embryonic lethality caused by the loss of any one of several components of this pathway in mice (Goumans & Mummery, 2000). Also in several human vascular diseases the underlying causal mutations were identified to affect BMP signaling. BMP signaling is thought to be involved in the maintenance of homeostasis in adult vasculature (David et al., 2009; Lowery & de Caestecker, 2010). Disruptions of homeostasis by vascular injury, hypertension or atherosclerosis have been shown to affect the expression of BMPs, thereby suggesting a role of BMPs in vascular responses.

The role of BMPs in the pathogenesis of vascular diseases is complex. First, different BMPs may exert very different effects. BMP2 and BMP4 have partly overlapping effects, but can also oppose each other depending on the spatial and temporal context. Second, the cellular response to a specific BMP can vary enormously with changing concentrations of the ligand. Another consideration worth taking is the presence of antagonists that preferentially inhibit one BMP over the other. Finally, BMPs can be produced locally by neighbouring cells in the tissue or be released into the circulation.

Regarding the pathogenesis of pulmonary vascular disease, it is important to note that while much research has been done on BMPs and the systemic vasculature, the pulmonary vasculature responds very differently. BMP4 exerts pro-inflammatory and prohypertensive effects in the systemic circulation, whereas the pulmonary circulation responds differently in an *in vitro* setting (Csiszar et al., 2008). This could explain why a systemic loss of one functional BMPRII allele results in a pulmonary phenotype.

The main cell types involved in vascular homeostasis are endothelial cells (ECs) and vascular smooth muscle cells (VSMCs). Each cell type has its own expression pattern of BMP ligands, receptors, antagonists and intracellular signaling components. The response to BMPs also depends on temporal and spatial factors, for instance, there are differences between ECs in capillaries compared to the ECs of small arteries (Kiyono & Shibuya, 2006). *In vitro* studies in vascular cells have proven to be difficult to interpret, since contradicting results have been reported in for instance early versus late passage VSMCs (Frank et al., 2005). *In vitro* data also does not always match the *in vivo* observations (David et al., 2009; Lowery & de Caestecker, 2010).

In ECs, BMP2 was found to promote pulmonary arterial endothelial cell (PAEC) survival and proliferation *in vitro* (Teichert-Kuliszewska et al., 2006). BMP2 also induces the expression of endothelial nitric oxide synthase (eNOS), which is important for proper vascular function and vasodilation. Heterozygous null BMP2 mice show an increased susceptibility for hypoxic PAH. Conversely, heterozygous null BMP4 mice are protected from hypoxia-induced PAH (Anderson et al., 2010). BMP4 is expressed in lung epithelium and ECs and is upregulated by hypoxia. BMP2 and BMP4 are considered to be regulators of EC and VSMC proliferation and migration, therefore their deregulation may lead to vascular pathologies (Southwood et al., 2008; Yu et al., 2008).

BMP9 has been reported to be a circulating factor that inhibits angiogenesis (David et al., 2007). It is a ligand for ALK1, an endothelial specific type I receptor, and the type II receptors BMPRII and ActRII. BMP9 signaling via BMPRII induces transcription of target genes by activating Smad1 and Smad5 (David et al., 2007; Scharpfenecker et al., 2007). Signaling via ActRII also activates Smad2 (Upton et al., 2009). Interestingly, BMP9 stimulates the transcription of BMPRII and endoglin in pulmonary endothelial cells, thereby maintaining their expression (David et al., 2007). BMP9 was also shown to stimulate the production of endothelin-1 (ET-1) by ECs *in vitro* (Star et al., 2010). ET-1 is a vasoconstrictor and mitogen, which is possibly involved in the pathogenesis of PAH. BMP9 exerts its effects on endothelial cells while circulating in the blood. It is regarded as an important regulator of vascular quiescence (David et al., 2008), yet its precise role remains to be elucidated.

4. Deregulation of BMP signaling in pulmonary arterial hypertension

In the majority of HPAH cases and a subset of IPAH cases a mutation in the BMPRII gene is the likely cause of disease (Morrell, 2010). Over a hundred different mutations have been identified in HPAH families occurring in different regions of the gene (Cogan et al., 2005; Lane et al., 2000; Machado et al., 2006; Moller et al., 2010). Some mutations occur in the extracellular domain or the kinase domain of the receptor, yet others are present in the tail domain. Since the various mutations lead to the same phenotype it is generally believed that they cause a loss of function of the receptor leading to haploinsufficiency (Jiang et al., 2011; Machado et al., 2001). The expression of BMPRII by ECs and VSMCs is significantly reduced in HPAH cases with a BMPRII mutation, but also in patients with secondary PAH the expression level of BMPRII is reduced (Atkinson et al., 2002; Du et al., 2003; Menon et al., 2011).

In PAH, excessive proliferation of ECs and VSMCs is an important part of the pathogenic process. Previously, and quite simplistically, it was thought that the reduction in BMP signaling through the BMPRII results in a loss of growth inhibitory signals. Yet the pathogenesis of PAH is more complex. It involves excessive proliferation, vascular inflammation, increased vasoconstriction and reduced dilation. The reduction in BMPRII was shown to not simply lead to a reduction in BMP signaling. As stated before, there are multiple BMP ligands and multiple type I and type II receptors. Yu et.al. have shown that the disruption of BMPRII in pulmonary arterial smooth muscle cells (PASMCs) leads to reduced signaling by BMP2 and BMP4, yet conversely signaling by BMP6 and BMP7 is enhanced (Yu et al., 2005). Also, a loss of BMP Smad signaling is accompanied by an activation of the p38 MAPK pathway causing aberrant PASMC proliferation (Dewachter et al., 2009; Rudarakanchana et al., 2002; Yang et al., 2005). PAEC dysfunction is also caused by a loss of BMP-induced eNOS expression and thereby increases pulmonary vasoconstriction (Anderson et al., 2010; Frank et al., 2008). Alterations in BMP signaling thereby lead to EC dysfunction and apoptosis, increased vasoconstriction, increased inflammation, excessive VSMC proliferation and the formation of plexiform lesions by apoptosis-resistant EC clones (Morrell, 2006).

Much attention is being paid to loss of BMP2 and BMP4 signaling through BMPRII, yet a mutation in ALK1 has also been found in PAH patients (Harrison et al., 2003). These patients suffer from hereditary hemorrhagic telangiectasia (HHT), a severe vascular disorder in which mucocutaneous telangiectasias and arteriovenous malformations develop in multiple organs (Shovlin, 2010). A subset of patients carrying an ALK1 mutation also develops PAH (Fujiwara et al., 2008; Harrison et al., 2003). ALK1 mediates both TGF-β and BMP9 signaling in endothelial cells. As described earlier, BMP9 induces the expression of BMPRII, therefore a loss of ALK1 signaling might result in a reduced expression of BMPRII (Upton et al., 2009). Also, a reduction of BMP9 signaling leads to reduced vascular quiescence, which may have pathogenic effects as well.

The role of TGF-β in PAH is also being investigated. BMP signaling through Smad1/5/8 is connected to TGF-β signaling through Smad2/3. Multiple mechanisms of crosstalk exist between the two pathways and it is thereby not surprising that TGF-β is involved in PAH next to BMPs. Abnormal TGF-β signaling has been observed in the pulmonary vasculature of PAH patients (Arcot et al., 1993; Morrell et al., 2001). TGF-β has various effects on vascular cells depending on context. The mechanisms by which TGF-β and BMP exert their pleiotropic effects in the adult vasculature are not yet understood. However, it is clear that they are interconnected and crucial for vascular homeostasis, making them both interesting therapeutic targets.

5. Evidence from animal models of PAH

In order to study the pathogenesis of PAH and to test potential treatments, we need reliable animal models of PAH. Since a heterozygous germ line mutation in the BMPRII is found in a large percentage of HPAH cases, various transgenic and knockout mouse models have been developed trying to mimic the pathogenesis seen in patients. A homozygous null mutation in BMPRII is lethal early during embryogenesis (Beppu et al., 2000). A RNAi germline 90% knockdown of BMPRII gives rise to a severe vascular phenotype including mucosal hemorrhage, vascular dysmorphogenesis and dysplasia (Liu et al., 2007). Heterozygous null mice initially show no phenotype, yet after challenge with serotonin (Long et al., 2006), chronic hypoxia (Frank et al., 2008), or inflammatory stress (Song et al., 2005) they are more susceptible to PAH. These findings support the idea that the development of PAH requires a second insult besides BMPRII mutation. The phenotype does not show the vascular remodeling seen in patients, which is a limitation to the use of this model.

An inducible transgenic mouse model that overexpresses a dominant-negative BMPRII specifically in smooth muscle cells develops PAH spontaneously (West et al., 2004). These mice show muscularization of small pulmonary arteries and an increase in medial thickness due to SMC proliferation. The loss of BMPRII signaling in VSMCs was sufficient to induce PAH, yet it does not reconstitute the complexity of human PAH (West et al., 2004). Mice with an inducible SMC specific expression of BMPRII with a truncating mutation in the tail domain (R899X) also show vascular abnormalities. About one third of the animals develop PAH. Interestingly this mutation does not lead to a loss of Smad signaling, yet it increases MAPK signaling (West et al., 2008).

Heterozygous or homozygous deletion of BMPRII in pulmonary ECs predisposes mice to PAH. A subset of animals develop PAH spontaneously, including right ventricular hypertrophy, vascular inflammation and histopathological changes (Hong et al., 2008; Majka et al., 2011). Disruptions in BMPRII signaling in either ECs or VSMCs lead to phenotypes resembling aspects of human PAH. Therefore, in patients both cell types most likely play a role in the complex pathogenesis of this disease.

A mutation in Smad8 has been identified as the cause in one IPAH case (Shintani et al., 2009). Smad8 is highly expressed in the pulmonary vasculature. Loss of Smad8 function in mice does not cause developmental problems. These mice do however show abnormal vascular remodeling, increased vascular inflammation and pulmonary tumors (Huang et al., 2009). Since other mouse models of PAH often do not present with the excessive vascular remodeling seen in patients, this Smad8 mutant is interesting in the way it recapitulates an important aspect of PAH.

Two commonly used rat models are the chronic hypoxia model and the monocrotaline (MCT)-induced PAH model (Altiere et al., 1986). Both models develop PAH and right ventricular hypertrophy within only a few weeks. A disruption of BMP signaling via the BMPRII has been documented in the pulmonary arteries of these animals (Long et al., 2009; Morty et al., 2007; Ramos et al., 2008). Murakami et al. have shown an increase in Smurf1 and I-Smad expression in the arteries of rats after MCT treatment or chronic hypoxia. The BMPRII is downregulated and BMP-Smad signaling is inhibited. This potentiates MAPK pathways and could be responsible for the observed proliferation and remodeling of the pulmonary vasculature (Murakami et al., 2010).

6. Implications for the treatment of PAH

This review has focussed on the pathogenesis of primary forms of PAH, IPAH and HPAH. PAH can arise as a secondary disease, which means the underlying medical condition should be taken into account when deciding on the course of treatment. Since right heart failure develops as a consequence of PAH, patients are treated with anticoagulants, diuretics and oxygen. Furthermore, patients can be treated with calcium channel blockers, prostanoids, endothelin antagonists or phosphodiesterase inhibitors (Badesch et al., 2007; Sastry, 2006). In severe cases, patients need a lung or heart/lung transplant.

Because of the role of BMPs in the pathogenesis of PAH and the crosstalk between BMP and TGF-β signaling, both pathways are regarded as potential drug targets. However, it is crucial to realize that the TGF-β family signaling pathways are tightly regulated and important for all tissues. Inhibition of TGF-β signaling as a potential treatment for PAH is currently under investigation. In rats with monocrotaline-induced PAH, anti-TGF-β treatment has prevented the development of PAH, right ventricular hypertrophy, vascular remodeling and reduced the loss in exercise capacity (Long et al., 2009; Megalou et al., 2010; Zaiman et al., 2008). Specific BMP agonists or TGF-β antagonists might prove to be valuable in fighting both BMPRII mutation positive and negative PAH. However, it is uncertain whether a reversal of the pathogenic processes is possible. It remains crucial to diagnose and start treatment early.

7. Conclusion

Transforming growth factor (TGF)-β family members are cytokines which are crucial for embryonic development and adult tissue homeostasis. This large family includes TGF-β isoforms, activins and bone morphogenetic proteins (BMPs), which act on cells via their type I and II serine/threonine kinase receptors and a specific subset of Smad transcription factors.

BMP signaling has been shown to be involved in vascular development and angiogenesis and deregulation gives rise to vascular disease. Mutations in the BMP receptor II gene are responsible for 80% of heritable pulmonary arterial hypertension cases, yet also in non-hereditary forms of PAH deregulation of BMP signaling occurs. PAH is characterised by an increase in blood pressure due to the constriction of small pulmonary arteries. Aberrant BMP signaling has been shown to be involved in the proliferation and dysfunction of ECs and VSMCs and vascular remodeling leading to PAH. In rat models of PAH, induced by hypoxia or monocrotaline, a disruption in BMP signaling has been found. Additionally, mouse models in which BMP signaling is disturbed in either ECs or VSMCs show a predisposition to develop PAH.

It is clear that BMP and TGF-β signaling play an important role in the pathogenesis of PAH. However, the exact roles of various signaling components and cell types remain unclear due to the complexity of these pathways. By studying different animal models of PAH we have learned much about the underlying processes and we can use these models to test whether BMP and TGF-β signaling can be targeted for treatment.

8. Acknowledgement

We thank José Maring, Anton Vonk Noordegraaf, Nick Morrell, Paul Upton, Valeria Orlova and Gonzalo Sánchez-Duffhues for critical reading of our chapter. Studies on TGF-β family members in vascular diseases in our laboratory are supported by the Le Ducq foundation,

Netherlands Organization of Scientific Research, Dutch Cancer Society, and the Centre for Biomedical Genetics. Miriam de Boeck is supported by the LUMC grant for excellent students in Biomedical Sciences.

9. List of abbreviations

ActIIA/B	Activin receptor type IIA/B
ALK	Activin receptor-like kinase
BMP	Bone morphogenetic protein
BMPRII	Bone morphogenetic protein receptor II
EC	Endothelial cell
eNOS	Endothelial nitric oxide synthase
ET-1	Endothelin-1
HHT	Hereditary hemorrhagic telangiectasia
HPAH	Heritable pulmonary arterial hypertension
IPAH	Idiopathic pulmonary arterial hypertension
I-Smad	Inhibitory Smad
JNK	c-Jun N-terminal kinase
LIMK	LIM domain kinase 1
MAPK	Mitogen-activated protein kinase
MCT	Monocrotaline
PAEC	Pulmonary arterial endothelial cell
PAH	Pulmonary arterial hypertension
PASMC	Pulmonary arterial smooth muscle cell
R-Smad	Receptor-regulated Smad
Smad	Sma and Mad related protein
TAK1	TGF-β activated kinase 1
TGF-β	Transforming growth factor-β
Trb3	Tribbles-like protein 3
VSMC	Vascular smooth muscle cell

10. References

Altiere, R.J., Olson, J.W. & Gillespie, M.N.(1986). Altered pulmonary vascular smooth muscle responsiveness in monocrotaline-induced pulmonary hypertension. *J.Pharmacol.Exp.Ther.*, Vol. 236, No. 2, pp. (390-395)

Anderson, L., Lowery, J.W., Frank, D.B., Novitskaya, T., Jones, M., Mortlock, D.P., Chandler, R.L. & de Caestecker, M.P.(2010). Bmp2 and Bmp4 exert opposing effects in hypoxic pulmonary hypertension. *Am.J.Physiol Regul.Integr.Comp Physiol*, Vol. 298, No. 3, pp. (R833-R842)

Arcot, S.S., Lipke, D.W., Gillespie, M.N. & Olson, J.W.(1993). Alterations of growth factor transcripts in rat lungs during development of monocrotaline-induced pulmonary hypertension. *Biochem.Pharmacol.*, Vol. 46, No. 6, pp. (1086-1091)

Atkinson, C., Stewart, S., Upton, P.D., Machado, R., Thomson, J.R., Trembath, R.C. & Morrell, N.W.(2002). Primary pulmonary hypertension is associated with reduced pulmonary vascular expression of type II bone morphogenetic protein receptor. *Circulation*, Vol. 105, No. 14, pp. (1672-1678)

Badesch, D.B., Abman, S.H., Simonneau, G., Rubin, L.J. & McLaughlin, V.V.(2007). Medical therapy for pulmonary arterial hypertension: updated ACCP evidence-based clinical practice guidelines. *Chest*, Vol. 131, No. 6, pp. (1917-1928)

Beppu, H., Kawabata, M., Hamamoto, T., Chytil, A., Minowa, O., Noda, T. & Miyazono, K.(2000). BMP type II receptor is required for gastrulation and early development of mouse embryos. *Dev.Biol.*, Vol. 221, No. 1, pp. (249-258)

Bertolino, P., Deckers, M., Lebrin, F. & ten Dijke, P.(2005). Transforming growth factor-β signal transduction in angiogenesis and vascular disorders. *Chest*, Vol. 128, No. 6 Suppl, pp. (585S-590S)

Chan, M.C., Nguyen, P.H., Davis, B.N., Ohoka, N., Hayashi, H., Du, K., Lagna, G. & Hata, A.(2007). A novel regulatory mechanism of the bone morphogenetic protein (BMP) signaling pathway involving the carboxyl-terminal tail domain of BMP type II receptor. *Mol.Cell Biol.*, Vol. 27, No. 16, pp. (5776-5789)

Cogan, J.D., Vnencak-Jones, C.L., Phillips, J.A., III, Lane, K.B., Wheeler, L.A., Robbins, I.M., Garrison, G., Hedges, L.K. & Loyd, J.E.(2005). Gross BMPR2 gene rearrangements constitute a new cause for primary pulmonary hypertension. *Genet.Med.*, Vol. 7, No. 3, pp. (169-174)

Cool, C.D., Stewart, J.S., Werahera, P., Miller, G.J., Williams, R.L., Voelkel, N.F. & Tuder, R.M.(1999). Three-dimensional reconstruction of pulmonary arteries in plexiform pulmonary hypertension using cell-specific markers. Evidence for a dynamic and heterogeneous process of pulmonary endothelial cell growth. *Am.J.Pathol.*, Vol. 155, No. 2, pp. (411-419)

Corradini, E., Babitt, J.L. & Lin, H.Y.(2009). The RGM/DRAGON family of BMP co-receptors. *Cytokine Growth Factor Rev.*, Vol. 20, No. 5-6, pp. (389-398)

Csiszar, A., Labinskyy, N., Jo, H., Ballabh, P. & Ungvari, Z.(2008). Differential proinflammatory and prooxidant effects of bone morphogenetic protein-4 in coronary and pulmonary arterial endothelial cells. *Am.J.Physiol Heart Circ.Physiol*, Vol. 295, No. 2, pp. (H569-H577)

David, L., Feige, J.J. & Bailly, S.(2009). Emerging role of bone morphogenetic proteins in angiogenesis. *Cytokine Growth Factor Rev.*, Vol. 20, No. 3, pp. (203-212)

David, L., Mallet, C., Keramidas, M., Lamande, N., Gasc, J.M., Dupuis-Girod, S., Plauchu, H., Feige, J.J. & Bailly, S.(2008). Bone morphogenetic protein-9 is a circulating vascular quiescence factor. *Circ.Res.*, Vol. 102, No. 8, pp. (914-922)

David, L., Mallet, C., Mazerbourg, S., Feige, J.J. & Bailly, S.(2007). Identification of BMP9 and BMP10 as functional activators of the orphan activin receptor-like kinase 1 (ALK1) in endothelial cells. *Blood*, Vol. 109, No. 5, pp. (1953-1961)

Dewachter, L., Adnot, S., Guignabert, C., Tu, L., Marcos, E., Fadel, E., Humbert, M., Dartevelle, P., Simonneau, G., Naeije, R. & Eddahibi, S.(2009). Bone morphogenetic protein signalling in heritable versus idiopathic pulmonary hypertension. *Eur.Respir.J.*, Vol. 34, No. 5, pp. (1100-1110)

Du, L., Sullivan, C.C., Chu, D., Cho, A.J., Kido, M., Wolf, P.L., Yuan, J.X., Deutsch, R., Jamieson, S.W. & Thistlethwaite, P.A.(2003). Signaling molecules in nonfamilial pulmonary hypertension. *N.Engl.J.Med.*, Vol. 348, No. 6, pp. (500-509)

Farber, H.W. and Loscalzo, J.(2004). Pulmonary arterial hypertension. *N.Engl.J.Med.*, Vol. 351, No. 16, pp. (1655-1665)

Feng, X.H. and Derynck, R.(2005). Specificity and versatility in TGF-β signaling through Smads. *Annu.Rev.Cell Dev.Biol.*, Vol. 21, pp. (659-693)

Foletta, V.C., Lim, M.A., Soosairajah, J., Kelly, A.P., Stanley, E.G., Shannon, M., He, W., Das, S., Massague, J. & Bernard, O.(2003). Direct signaling by the BMP type II receptor via the cytoskeletal regulator LIMK1. *J.Cell Biol.*, Vol. 162, No. 6, pp. (1089-1098)

Frank, D., Johnson, J. & de, C.M.(2005). Bone morphogenetic protein 4 promotes vascular remodeling in hypoxic pulmonary hypertension. *Chest*, Vol. 128, No. 6 Suppl, pp. (590S-591S)

Frank, D.B., Lowery, J., Anderson, L., Brink, M., Reese, J. & de Caestecker, M.(2008). Increased susceptibility to hypoxic pulmonary hypertension in Bmpr2 mutant mice is associated with endothelial dysfunction in the pulmonary vasculature. *Am.J.Physiol Lung Cell Mol.Physiol*, Vol. 294, No. 1, pp. (L98-109)

Fujiwara, M., Yagi, H., Matsuoka, R., Akimoto, K., Furutani, M., Imamura, S., Uehara, R., Nakayama, T., Takao, A., Nakazawa, M. & Saji, T.(2008). Implications of mutations of activin receptor-like kinase 1 gene (ALK1) in addition to bone morphogenetic protein receptor II gene (BMPR2) in children with pulmonary arterial hypertension. *Circ.J.*, Vol. 72, No. 1, pp. (127-133)

Gaine, S.P. and Rubin, L.J.(1998). Primary pulmonary hypertension. *Lancet*, Vol. 352, No. 9129, pp. (719-725)

Goumans, M.J., Liu, Z. & ten Dijke, P.(2009). TGF-β signaling in vascular biology and dysfunction. *Cell Res.*, Vol. 19, No. 1, pp. (116-127)

Goumans, M.J. and Mummery, C.(2000). Functional analysis of the TGF-β receptor/Smad pathway through gene ablation in mice. *Int.J.Dev.Biol.*, Vol. 44, No. 3, pp. (253-265)

Hariharan, R. and Pillai, M.R.(2008). Structure-function relationship of inhibitory Smads: Structural flexibility contributes to functional divergence. *Proteins*, Vol. 71, No. 4, pp. (1853-1862)

Harrison, R.E., Flanagan, J.A., Sankelo, M., Abdalla, S.A., Rowell, J., Machado, R.D., Elliott, C.G., Robbins, I.M., Olschewski, H., McLaughlin, V., Gruenig, E., Kermeen, F., Halme, M., Raisanen-Sokolowski, A., Laitinen, T., Morrell, N.W. & Trembath, R.C.(2003). Molecular and functional analysis identifies ALK-1 as the predominant cause of pulmonary hypertension related to hereditary haemorrhagic telangiectasia. *J.Med.Genet.*, Vol. 40, No. 12, pp. (865-871)

Heldin, C.H., Miyazono, K. & ten Dijke, P.(1997). TGF-β signalling from cell membrane to nucleus through SMAD proteins. *Nature*, Vol. 390, No. 6659, pp. (465-471)

Hong, K.H., Lee, Y.J., Lee, E., Park, S.O., Han, C., Beppu, H., Li, E., Raizada, M.K., Bloch, K.D. & Oh, S.P.(2008). Genetic ablation of the BMPR2 gene in pulmonary endothelium is sufficient to predispose to pulmonary arterial hypertension. *Circulation*, Vol. 118, No. 7, pp. (722-730)

Huang, Z., Wang, D., Ihida-Stansbury, K., Jones, P.L. & Martin, J.F.(2009). Defective pulmonary vascular remodeling in Smad8 mutant mice. *Hum.Mol.Genet.*, Vol. 18, No. 15, pp. (2791-2801)

Humbert, M., Morrell, N.W., Archer, S.L., Stenmark, K.R., MacLean, M.R., Lang, I.M., Christman, B.W., Weir, E.K., Eickelberg, O., Voelkel, N.F. & Rabinovitch, M.(2004). Cellular and molecular pathobiology of pulmonary arterial hypertension. *J.Am.Coll.Cardiol.*, Vol. 43, No. 12 Suppl S, pp. (13S-24S)

Itoh, S. and ten Dijke, P.(2007). Negative regulation of TGF-β receptor/Smad signal transduction. *Curr.Opin.Cell Biol.*, Vol. 19, No. 2, pp. (176-184)

Jiang, Y., Nohe, A., Bragdon, B., Tian, C., Rudarakanchana, N., Morrell, N.W. & Petersen, N.O.(2011). Trapping of BMP receptors in distinct membrane domains inhibits their function in pulmonary arterial hypertension. *Am.J.Physiol Lung Cell Mol.Physiol,*

Kavsak, P., Rasmussen, R.K., Causing, C.G., Bonni, S., Zhu, H., Thomsen, G.H. & Wrana, J.L.(2000). Smad7 binds to Smurf2 to form an E3 ubiquitin ligase that targets the TGF β receptor for degradation. *Mol.Cell*, Vol. 6, No. 6, pp. (1365-1375)

Kiyono, M. and Shibuya, M.(2006). Inhibitory Smad transcription factors protect arterial endothelial cells from apoptosis induced by BMP4. *Oncogene*, Vol. 25, No. 54, pp. (7131-7137)

Lane, K.B., Machado, R.D., Pauciulo, M.W., Thomson, J.R., Phillips, J.A., III, Loyd, J.E., Nichols, W.C. & Trembath, R.C.(2000). Heterozygous germline mutations in BMPR2, encoding a TGF-β receptor, cause familial primary pulmonary hypertension. *Nat.Genet.*, Vol. 26, No. 1, pp. (81-84)

Lin, X., Liang, Y.Y., Sun, B., Liang, M., Shi, Y., Brunicardi, F.C., Shi, Y. & Feng, X.H.(2003). Smad6 recruits transcription corepressor CtBP to repress bone morphogenetic protein-induced transcription. *Mol.Cell Biol.*, Vol. 23, No. 24, pp. (9081-9093)

Liu, D., Wang, J., Kinzel, B., Mueller, M., Mao, X., Valdez, R., Liu, Y. & Li, E.(2007). Dosage-dependent requirement of BMP type II receptor for maintenance of vascular integrity. *Blood*, Vol. 110, No. 5, pp. (1502-1510)

Long, L., Crosby, A., Yang, X., Southwood, M., Upton, P.D., Kim, D.K. & Morrell, N.W.(2009). Altered bone morphogenetic protein and transforming growth factor-β signaling in rat models of pulmonary hypertension: potential for activin receptor-like kinase-5 inhibition in prevention and progression of disease. *Circulation*, Vol. 119, No. 4, pp. (566-576)

Long, L., MacLean, M.R., Jeffery, T.K., Morecroft, I., Yang, X., Rudarakanchana, N., Southwood, M., James, V., Trembath, R.C. & Morrell, N.W.(2006). Serotonin increases susceptibility to pulmonary hypertension in BMPR2-deficient mice. *Circ.Res.*, Vol. 98, No. 6, pp. (818-827)

Lowery, J.W. and de Caestecker, M.P.(2010). BMP signaling in vascular development and disease. *Cytokine Growth Factor Rev.*, Vol. 21, No. 4, pp. (287-298)

Machado, R.D., Aldred, M.A., James, V., Harrison, R.E., Patel, B., Schwalbe, E.C., Gruenig, E., Janssen, B., Koehler, R., Seeger, W., Eickelberg, O., Olschewski, H., Elliott, C.G., Glissmeyer, E., Carlquist, J., Kim, M., Torbicki, A., Fijalkowska, A., Szewczyk, G., Parma, J., Abramowicz, M.J., Galie, N., Morisaki, H., Kyotani, S., Nakanishi, N., Morisaki, T., Humbert, M., Simonneau, G., Sitbon, O., Soubrier, F., Coulet, F., Morrell, N.W. & Trembath, R.C.(2006). Mutations of the TGF-β type II receptor BMPR2 in pulmonary arterial hypertension. *Hum.Mutat.*, Vol. 27, No. 2, pp. (121-132)

Machado, R.D., Eickelberg, O., Elliott, C.G., Geraci, M.W., Hanaoka, M., Loyd, J.E., Newman, J.H., Phillips, J.A., III, Soubrier, F., Trembath, R.C. & Chung, W.K.(2009). Genetics and genomics of pulmonary arterial hypertension. *J.Am.Coll.Cardiol.*, Vol. 54, No. 1 Suppl, pp. (S32-S42)

Machado, R.D., Pauciulo, M.W., Thomson, J.R., Lane, K.B., Morgan, N.V., Wheeler, L., Phillips, J.A., III, Newman, J., Williams, D., Galie, N., Manes, A., McNeil, K.,

Yacoub, M., Mikhail, G., Rogers, P., Corris, P., Humbert, M., Donnai, D., Martensson, G., Tranebjaerg, L., Loyd, J.E., Trembath, R.C. & Nichols, W.C.(2001). BMPR2 haploinsufficiency as the inherited molecular mechanism for primary pulmonary hypertension. *Am.J.Hum.Genet.*, Vol. 68, No. 1, pp. (92-102)

Majka, S., Hagen, M., Blackwell, T., Harral, J., Johnson, J.A., Gendron, R., Paradis, H., Crona, D., Loyd, J.E., Nozik-Grayck, E., Stenmark, K.R. & West, J.(2011). Physiologic and Molecular Consequences of Endothelial Bmpr2 Mutation. *Respir.Res.*, Vol. 12, No. 1, pp. (84-

Megalou, A.J., Glava, C., Oikonomidis, D.L., Vilaeti, A., Agelaki, M.G., Baltogiannis, G.G., Papalois, A., Vlahos, A.P. & Kolettis, T.M.(2010). Transforming growth factor-β inhibition attenuates pulmonary arterial hypertension in rats. *Int.J.Clin.Exp.Med.*, Vol. 3, No. 4, pp. (332-340)

Menon, S., Fessel, J. & West, J.(2011). Microarray studies in pulmonary arterial hypertension. *Int.J.Clin.Pract.Suppl*, No. 169, pp. (19-28)

Meulmeester, E. and ten Dijke, P.(2011). The dynamic roles of TGF-β in cancer. *J.Pathol.*, Vol. 223, No. 2, pp. (205-218)

Miyazono, K., Kamiya, Y. & Morikawa, M.(2010). Bone morphogenetic protein receptors and signal transduction. *J.Biochem.*, Vol. 147, No. 1, pp. (35-51)

Moller, T., Leren, T.P., Eiklid, K.L., Holmstrom, H., Fredriksen, P.M. & Thaulow, E.(2010). A novel BMPR2 gene mutation associated with exercise-induced pulmonary hypertension in septal defects. *Scand.Cardiovasc.J.*, Vol. 44, No. 6, pp. (331-336)

Morrell, N.W.(2006). Pulmonary hypertension due to BMPR2 mutation: a new paradigm for tissue remodeling? *Proc.Am.Thorac.Soc.*, Vol. 3, No. 8, pp. (680-686)

Morrell, N.W.(2010). Role of bone morphogenetic protein receptors in the development of pulmonary arterial hypertension. *Adv.Exp.Med.Biol.*, Vol. 661, pp. (251-264)

Morrell, N.W., Yang, X., Upton, P.D., Jourdan, K.B., Morgan, N., Sheares, K.K. & Trembath, R.C.(2001). Altered growth responses of pulmonary artery smooth muscle cells from patients with primary pulmonary hypertension to transforming growth factor-β(1) and bone morphogenetic proteins. *Circulation*, Vol. 104, No. 7, pp. (790-795)

Morty, R.E., Nejman, B., Kwapiszewska, G., Hecker, M., Zakrzewicz, A., Kouri, F.M., Peters, D.M., Dumitrascu, R., Seeger, W., Knaus, P., Schermuly, R.T. & Eickelberg, O.(2007). Dysregulated bone morphogenetic protein signaling in monocrotaline-induced pulmonary arterial hypertension. *Arterioscler.Thromb.Vasc.Biol.*, Vol. 27, No. 5, pp. (1072-1078)

Moustakas, A. and Heldin, C.H.(2005). Non-Smad TGF-β signals. *J.Cell Sci.*, Vol. 118, No. Pt 16, pp. (3573-3584)

Murakami, G., Watabe, T., Takaoka, K., Miyazono, K. & Imamura, T.(2003). Cooperative inhibition of bone morphogenetic protein signaling by Smurf1 and inhibitory Smads. *Mol.Biol.Cell*, Vol. 14, No. 7, pp. (2809-2817)

Murakami, K., Mathew, R., Huang, J., Farahani, R., Peng, H., Olson, S.C. & Etlinger, J.D.(2010). Smurf1 ubiquitin ligase causes downregulation of BMP receptors and is induced in monocrotaline and hypoxia models of pulmonary arterial hypertension. *Exp.Biol.Med.(Maywood.)*, Vol. 235, No. 7, pp. (805-813)

Nistala, H., Lee-Arteaga, S., Smaldone, S., Siciliano, G., Carta, L., Ono, R.N., Sengle, G., Arteaga-Solis, E., Levasseur, R., Ducy, P., Sakai, L.Y., Karsenty, G. & Ramirez,

F.(2010). Fibrillin-1 and -2 differentially modulate endogenous TGF-β and BMP bioavailability during bone formation. *J.Cell Biol.*, Vol. 190, No. 6, pp. (1107-1121)

Onichtchouk, D., Chen, Y.G., Dosch, R., Gawantka, V., Delius, H., Massague, J. & Niehrs, C.(1999). Silencing of TGF-β signalling by the pseudoreceptor BAMBI. *Nature*, Vol. 401, No. 6752, pp. (480-485)

Pardali, E., Goumans, M.J. & ten Dijke, P.(2010). Signaling by members of the TGF-β family in vascular morphogenesis and disease. *Trends Cell Biol.*, Vol. 20, No. 9, pp. (556-567)

Ramos, M.F., Lame, M.W., Segall, H.J. & Wilson, D.W.(2008). Smad signaling in the rat model of monocrotaline pulmonary hypertension. *Toxicol.Pathol.*, Vol. 36, No. 2, pp. (311-320)

Rich, S., Dantzker, D.R., Ayres, S.M., Bergofsky, E.H., Brundage, B.H., Detre, K.M., Fishman, A.P., Goldring, R.M., Groves, B.M., Koerner, S.K. & .(1987). Primary pulmonary hypertension. A national prospective study. *Ann.Intern.Med.*, Vol. 107, No. 2, pp. (216-223)

Rudarakanchana, N., Flanagan, J.A., Chen, H., Upton, P.D., Machado, R., Patel, D., Trembath, R.C. & Morrell, N.W.(2002). Functional analysis of bone morphogenetic protein type II receptor mutations underlying primary pulmonary hypertension. *Hum.Mol.Genet.*, Vol. 11, No. 13, pp. (1517-1525)

Saremba, S., Nickel, J., Seher, A., Kotzsch, A., Sebald, W. & Mueller, T.D.(2008). Type I receptor binding of bone morphogenetic protein 6 is dependent on N-glycosylation of the ligand. *FEBS J.*, Vol. 275, No. 1, pp. (172-183)

Sastry, B.K.(2006). Pharmacologic treatment for pulmonary arterial hypertension. *Curr.Opin.Cardiol.*, Vol. 21, No. 6, pp. (561-568)

Scharpfenecker, M., van Dinther, M., Liu, Z., van Bezooijen, R.L., Zhao, Q., Pukac, L., Lowik, C.W. & ten Dijke, P.(2007). BMP-9 signals via ALK1 and inhibits bFGF-induced endothelial cell proliferation and VEGF-stimulated angiogenesis. *J.Cell Sci.*, Vol. 120, No. Pt 6, pp. (964-972)

Schmierer, B. and Hill, C.S.(2007). TGF-β-SMAD signal transduction: molecular specificity and functional flexibility. *Nat.Rev.Mol.Cell Biol.*, Vol. 8, No. 12, pp. (970-982)

Schwappacher, R., Weiske, J., Heining, E., Ezerski, V., Marom, B., Henis, Y.I., Huber, O. & Knaus, P.(2009). Novel crosstalk to BMP signalling: cGMP-dependent kinase I modulates BMP receptor and Smad activity. *EMBO J.*, Vol. 28, No. 11, pp. (1537-1550)

Shi, Y. and Massague, J.(2003). Mechanisms of TGF-β signaling from cell membrane to the nucleus. *Cell*, Vol. 113, No. 6, pp. (685-700)

Shibuya, H., Iwata, H., Masuyama, N., Gotoh, Y., Yamaguchi, K., Irie, K., Matsumoto, K., Nishida, E. & Ueno, N.(1998). Role of TAK1 and TAB1 in BMP signaling in early Xenopus development. *EMBO J.*, Vol. 17, No. 4, pp. (1019-1028)

Shim, J.H., Greenblatt, M.B., Xie, M., Schneider, M.D., Zou, W., Zhai, B., Gygi, S. & Glimcher, L.H.(2009). TAK1 is an essential regulator of BMP signalling in cartilage. *EMBO J.*, Vol. 28, No. 14, pp. (2028-2041)

Shintani, M., Yagi, H., Nakayama, T., Saji, T. & Matsuoka, R.(2009). A new nonsense mutation of SMAD8 associated with pulmonary arterial hypertension. *J.Med.Genet.*, Vol. 46, No. 5, pp. (331-337)

Shovlin, C.L.(2010). Hereditary haemorrhagic telangiectasia: pathophysiology, diagnosis and treatment. *Blood Rev.*, Vol. 24, No. 6, pp. (203-219)

Song, Y., Jones, J.E., Beppu, H., Keaney, J.F., Jr., Loscalzo, J. & Zhang, Y.Y.(2005). Increased susceptibility to pulmonary hypertension in heterozygous BMPR2-mutant mice. *Circulation*, Vol. 112, No. 4, pp. (553-562)

Southwood, M., Jeffery, T.K., Yang, X., Upton, P.D., Hall, S.M., Atkinson, C., Haworth, S.G., Stewart, S., Reynolds, P.N., Long, L., Trembath, R.C. & Morrell, N.W.(2008). Regulation of bone morphogenetic protein signalling in human pulmonary vascular development. *J.Pathol.*, Vol. 214, No. 1, pp. (85-95)

Star, G.P., Giovinazzo, M. & Langleben, D.(2010). Bone morphogenic protein-9 stimulates endothelin-1 release from human pulmonary microvascular endothelial cells: a potential mechanism for elevated ET-1 levels in pulmonary arterial hypertension. *Microvasc.Res.*, Vol. 80, No. 3, pp. (349-354)

Sztrymf, B., Coulet, F., Girerd, B., Yaici, A., Jais, X., Sitbon, O., Montani, D., Souza, R., Simonneau, G., Soubrier, F. & Humbert, M.(2008). Clinical outcomes of pulmonary arterial hypertension in carriers of BMPR2 mutation. *Am.J.Respir.Crit Care Med.*, Vol. 177, No. 12, pp. (1377-1383)

Teichert-Kuliszewska, K., Kutryk, M.J., Kuliszewski, M.A., Karoubi, G., Courtman, D.W., Zucco, L., Granton, J. & Stewart, D.J.(2006). Bone morphogenetic protein receptor-2 signaling promotes pulmonary arterial endothelial cell survival: implications for loss-of-function mutations in the pathogenesis of pulmonary hypertension. *Circ.Res.*, Vol. 98, No. 2, pp. (209-217)

ten Dijke, P. and Arthur, H.M.(2007). Extracellular control of TGF-β signalling in vascular development and disease. *Nat.Rev.Mol.Cell Biol.*, Vol. 8, No. 11, pp. (857-869)

Upton, P.D., Davies, R.J., Trembath, R.C. & Morrell, N.W.(2009). Bone morphogenetic protein (BMP) and activin type II receptors balance BMP9 signals mediated by activin receptor-like kinase-1 in human pulmonary artery endothelial cells. *J.Biol.Chem.*, Vol. 284, No. 23, pp. (15794-15804)

von Einem, S., Erler, S., Bigl, K., Frerich, B. & Schwarz, E.(2011). The pro-form of BMP-2 exhibits a delayed and reduced activity when compared to mature BMP-2. *Growth Factors*, Vol. 29, No. 2-3, pp. (63-71)

West, J., Fagan, K., Steudel, W., Fouty, B., Lane, K., Harral, J., Hoedt-Miller, M., Tada, Y., Ozimek, J., Tuder, R. & Rodman, D.M.(2004). Pulmonary hypertension in transgenic mice expressing a dominant-negative BMPRII gene in smooth muscle. *Circ.Res.*, Vol. 94, No. 8, pp. (1109-1114)

West, J., Harral, J., Lane, K., Deng, Y., Ickes, B., Crona, D., Albu, S., Stewart, D. & Fagan, K.(2008). Mice expressing BMPR2R899X transgene in smooth muscle develop pulmonary vascular lesions. *Am.J.Physiol Lung Cell Mol.Physiol*, Vol. 295, No. 5, pp. (L744-L755)

Wozney, J.M., Rosen, V., Celeste, A.J., Mitsock, L.M., Whitters, M.J., Kriz, R.W., Hewick, R.M. & Wang, E.A.(1988). Novel regulators of bone formation: molecular clones and activities. *Science*, Vol. 242, No. 4885, pp. (1528-1534)

Wu, M.Y. and Hill, C.S.(2009). TGF-β superfamily signaling in embryonic development and homeostasis. *Dev.Cell*, Vol. 16, No. 3, pp. (329-343)

Yanagita, M.(2005). BMP antagonists: their roles in development and involvement in pathophysiology. *Cytokine Growth Factor Rev.*, Vol. 16, No. 3, pp. (309-317)

Yang, X., Long, L., Southwood, M., Rudarakanchana, N., Upton, P.D., Jeffery, T.K., Atkinson, C., Chen, H., Trembath, R.C. & Morrell, N.W.(2005). Dysfunctional Smad signaling contributes to abnormal smooth muscle cell proliferation in familial pulmonary arterial hypertension. *Circ.Res.*, Vol. 96, No. 10, pp. (1053-1063)

Yu, P.B., Beppu, H., Kawai, N., Li, E. & Bloch, K.D.(2005). Bone morphogenetic protein (BMP) type II receptor deletion reveals BMP ligand-specific gain of signaling in pulmonary artery smooth muscle cells. *J.Biol.Chem.*, Vol. 280, No. 26, pp. (24443-24450)

Yu, P.B., Deng, D.Y., Beppu, H., Hong, C.C., Lai, C., Hoyng, S.A., Kawai, N. & Bloch, K.D.(2008). Bone morphogenetic protein (BMP) type II receptor is required for BMP-mediated growth arrest and differentiation in pulmonary artery smooth muscle cells. *J.Biol.Chem.*, Vol. 283, No. 7, pp. (3877-3888)

Zaiman, A.L., Podowski, M., Medicherla, S., Gordy, K., Xu, F., Zhen, L., Shimoda, L.A., Neptune, E., Higgins, L., Murphy, A., Chakravarty, S., Protter, A., Sehgal, P.B., Champion, H.C. & Tuder, R.M.(2008). Role of the TGF-β/Alk5 signaling pathway in monocrotaline-induced pulmonary hypertension. *Am.J.Respir.Crit Care Med.*, Vol. 177, No. 8, pp. (896-905)

Zakin, L. and De Robertis, E.M.(2010). Extracellular regulation of BMP signaling. *Curr.Biol.*, Vol. 20, No. 3, pp. (R89-R92)

Zhang, Y.E.(2009). Non-Smad pathways in TGF-β signaling. *Cell Res.*, Vol. 19, No. 1, pp. (128-139)

Zhu, H., Kavsak, P., Abdollah, S., Wrana, J.L. & Thomsen, G.H.(1999). A SMAD ubiquitin ligase targets the BMP pathway and affects embryonic pattern formation. *Nature*, Vol. 400, No. 6745, pp. (687-693)

Part 2

Hypoxia and Its Effects on Pulmonary Vasculature and Heart

6

Hypoxic Pulmonary Arterial Hypertension in the Chicken Model

Aureliano Hernández and Martha de Sandino

Universidad Nacional de Colombia,
Facultad de Medicina Veterinaria y de Zootecnia, Bogotá
Colombia

1. Introduction

Pulmonary hypertension (PH) in modern genetic strains of chicken broilers is a world wide distributed entity, which has a recognized economical impact (Maxwell et al., 1997; Pavlidis et al., 2007). Also, the commercial chicken has been a model to study PH in man, because encountered pathological changes in that animal closely resemble the human condition.

Under natural atmospheric conditions, two determining causes for PH are known: hypobaric hypoxia and low temperatures exposure (i.e. birds exposure to temperatures below 16° C (Pakdel et al., 2005; Pan et al., 2005).

The incidence and clinical evolution of PH in various strains of commercial chickens maintained under a natural hypoxic tropical environment in the Bogotá plane at 2638 m above sea level (masl) have been evaluated over several years, using direct observation of animals, electrocardiography, morphometric studies, hematocrit and hemoglobin changes, histochemical, immunohistochemical and molecular procedures.

Morphometric cardiac and pulmonary changes allowed in post-mortem studies to define mass cardiac index values (CI) to differentiate non-pulmonary hypertensive chickens (NPHC) from the pulmonary hypertensive ones (PHC) (Hernández, 1982, 1987; Cárdenas et al., 1985; Areiza, 2010, Vásquez, 2010). CI is defined as the right ventricular muscle mass weight expressed as a percentage of the total ventricular muscle weight (Alexander and Jensen, 1959). It is now clear that PHC have a CI value of 25 and higher and, below 22, birds can be safely allocated in the NPHC group (Gómez et al., 2007; Areiza, 2010; Vásquez, 2010). The remodeling process of pulmonary arterioles has been studied by morphometric analysis of smooth muscle and adventitia layers in PHC (Useche et al., 1981 Sandino and Hernández, 2005).

Electrocardiography was found to have a predictive value to define which animals would develop PH. Also, it determined that there is not a defined time course in the evolution of PH in chickens. The latter has been corroborated with daily field observations (Pulido, 1996).

Several studies showed that low temperatures and pulmonary diseases have an enhancing effect in the occurrence of PH (Mejía, 1982; Hernández, 1984).

Hypobaric hypoxia and low temperature are determinants of PH occurrence in the pulmonary vasculature of broilers. Sensitivity is species dependent and the domestic chicken appears to be most prone to develop that condition, whereas South American camelids and the bovine yak are highly resistant, among studied species. Man is believed to occupy a low place in this context (Grover et al., 1983; Monge and León-Velarde, 1991). However, there is a genetic component within species, which is responsible for susceptibility or resistance, as seen in human native Tibetans and the bovine yak (Durmowicz et al., 1993; Moore et al., 1998). The bar-headed goose and the Himalayan domestic chicken are well adapted avian species to altitudes above 3000 masl. The bar-headed goose can reach altitudes of 9000 masl (Graham and Milsom, 2007). The modern broiler chicken´s strains also differ in their susceptibility (Hernández, 1982; Huchzermeyer et al, 1988).

There is a large amount of scientific data which give capital importance to the energy density of feed as causative of PH, but, at least under low altitude and respiratory healthy conditions, commercial chickens do not develop PH (Useche et al., 1981, Cárdenas et al, 1985; Gómez et al, 2007; Vásquez, 2010). Nevertheless, the energy content is in fact an undeniable adjuvant factor to increase incidence of PH when low temperatures and/or hypobaric hypoxia are present, although its mechanism has not been clearly elucidated (Tarquino et al., 1990). Interesting theories and well carried studies have been advanced, which include thyroid hormones metabolism (hypothyroidism) and hypoxemia (Camacho-Fernández et al, 2002; Hassanzadeh et al., 2005), but they do not focus on the principal issue which is pulmonary vasoconstriction due to low temperature and/or hypobaric hypoxia. In fact, they attribute PH to a metabolic disarrangement which results in hypoxemia. Another element to enhance or probably cause PH, most likely through hypoxia, is the presence of pulmonary obstructive diseases (Huchzermeyer et al., 1987; Guzmán et al., 2001), which are common entities in the broiler´s industry nowadays.

It is important to note that when both temperature and energy density of feed are controlled, hypobaric hypoxia *per se* is sufficient to cause PH (Tarquino et al, 1990; Vásquez, 2010).

2. Compensatory mechanisms and development of PH

Elevation of pulmonary artery pressure is an immediate response to hypobaric hypoxia. If the level of this increment is maintained above physiological limits, that is, in susceptible (non- adapted) individuals, PH ensues (Cueva et al., 1974). From there on, cardiac output is maintained due to ventricular adaptation to high pulmonary vascular resistance. There is right ventricular mass increment through hypertrophy and hyperplasia (Bernal et al., 1984) and the II Q wave in electrocardiographic readings becomes progressively more negative, until ventricular dilatation determines cardiac failure (table 2). This process does not have a defined time pattern and may begin as early as 10 days post-hatching, ranging from 4 to 20 days (Pulido, 1996).

Another compensatory mechanism is augmentation of hematocrit (Ht) and hemoglobin (Hb) content (Table 2; Cárdenas et al, 1985; Colmenares et al, 1990). Hypoxia induces the expression of the hypoxia inducible factor 2α (HIF-2α) which stimulates renal secretion of erythropoietin by cortical fibroblasts in the kidney, a molecule responsible for hematocrit increment, by diminishing apoptosis in erythrocyte progenitor cells (Paliege et al., 2010). As a consequence, blood viscosity is augmented, a change believed to increase resistance in the pulmonary vasculature, which can be considered as an aggravating factor in the development of PH. One compensatory mechanism is increased hemoglobin affinity for oxygen, as exhibited by well adapted avian species such as the bar headed and Andean geese as well as the Tibetan chicken (Weber et al. 1993, Zhang et al, 2007).

Hypoxemia results from low pO2 in the air spaces in the lung (alveoli in mammals and respiratory capillaries in avian species). Oxygen and carbon dioxide low blood pressure sensing structures such as the carotid cell bodies (Lahiri et al., 2006), intrapulmonary and peripheral neural receptors elicit a rise in respiratory rate through vagal neural efferent inputs originated in neural respiratory centers (Glogowska et al., 1972).

3. Gross and light microscopic changes in pulmonary hypertension

The lungs appear congested, but no signs of edema are evident as known to occur in mammals. Microscopically, the most prominent finding relates to the engrossment of the medial muscle layer in arterioles (figures 9 and 10). This subjective appreciation has been thoroughly corroborated by morphometric methods in several studies (Sillau and Montalvo, 1982; Useche et al., 1981, Moreno de Sandino and Hernández, 2006). Cartilage and/or bone neo-formations can be seen in variable amounts within the pulmonary parenchyma (figure 3), together with fibrosis of the adventitial layer of arterioles. The degree of fibrosis varies (figure 2). Muscle hypertrophy is also found in peribronchial walls (Dalmau, 1997). Atelectasia can be encountered in many areas of the lung.

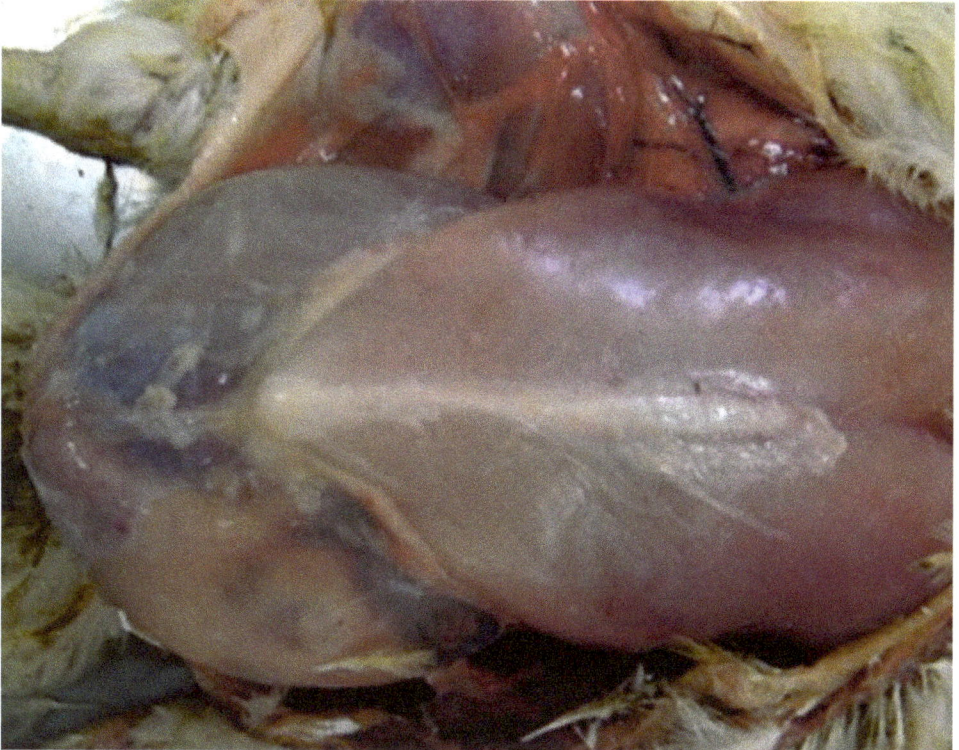

Fig. 1. Pulmonary hypertensive chicken. Ascites

In the heart, different degrees of right ventricular dilatation are present, which are presumably connected to the severity of PH. The increase in ventricular mass weight is due to both hyperplasia and hypertrophy (Bernal et al, 1984). No signs of vascular changes in the heart are detected, as seen with the light microscope.

As a result of right ventricular insufficiency secondary to increased pulmonary vascular resistance, detention of returning venous blood becomes increasingly difficult. Hence, generalized passive congestion is evident, which includes portal congestion. Ascites results from plasma leaking from the congested liver (Figure 1). Liver hypertrophy is a common finding in necropsies. Microscopically, some degree of fibrosis and sinusoidal dilatation can be seen.

In most cases of PH, hydropericardium is encountered. Some individuals may die with this lesion, and absence of ascites. Furthermore, a few animals die with none of the abovementioned lesions. The latter cases probably correspond to more susceptible individuals.

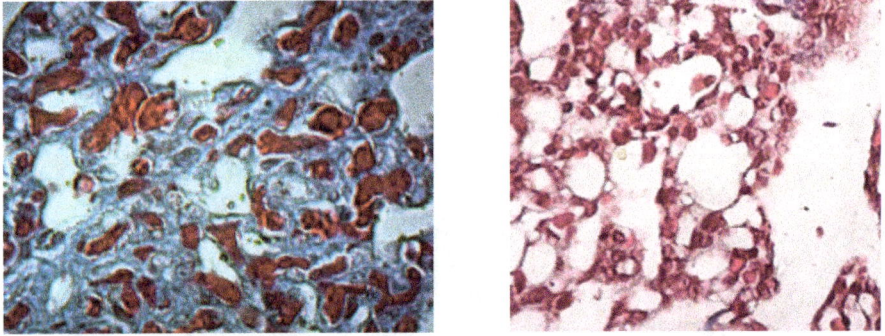

Fig. 2. Lung fibrosis (left). Pulmonary hypertensive chicken. Lung from a non-pulmonary hypertensive chicken (right). Masson´s trichromic stain

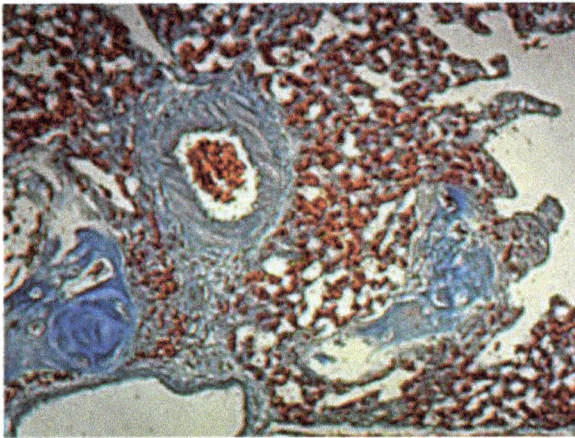

Fig. 3. Fibrosis and bone neo-formation. Pulmonary hipertensive chicken Masson's trichromic stain

Altitude m above sea level	Hemoglobine g/100 mm		Hematocrit % PVC		Red blood cells millions/cc *	
	Mean	SD	Mean	SD	Mean	SD
225	8.54	1.26	27.30	2.88	4.72	0.97
2638 NPHC	10.82	1.36	33.91	3.15	4.40	0.71
2638 PHC	13.15	2.30	40.10	8.30	2.43	1.31

SD: standard deviation. NPHC and PHC: non-pulmonary and pulmonary hypertensive chickens
* Red blood cells values should be multiplied by 10000
Cárdenas et al., 1985.

Table 1. Hemoglobine, hematocrit and red blood cells counts in healthy and pulmonary hypertensive broilers maintained under normoxia and hypobaric hypoxia

L(II) s (- mV) values at different age ranges (in days)

8-10	15-17	22-24	29-31	36-41 days	CI	D
0.20	0.40				35.2	15
0.35					42.9	17
0.40	0.40				38.5	22
0.10	0.30				37.5	22
0.30	0.20				33.3	22
0.05	0.15	0.30			38.7	22
0.35	0.60	0.65			41.7	23
0.30	0.60	0.65			36.4	23
0.15	0.40				37.5	24
0.25	0.25	0.50			34.8	29
0.15	0.25	0.60	0.80		37.0	30
0.35	0.60	0.75			40.0	30
0.10	0.10	0.20	0.50		36.2	30
0.25	0.15	0.45	0.65		37.5	31
0.30	0.10	0.50	1.00		48.9	31
0.20	0.20	0.30	0.50	0.90	40.5	37
0.30	0.40	0.30	0.35		35.4	37
0.20	0.10	0.20	0.25	0.30	41.3	41

CI= cardiac mass index. D= age-day of spontaneous animal's death. Data taken and modified from Pulido, 1996

Table 2. Electrocardiographic wave 2. derivative II [L (II)s] (mV) and cardiac mass index in pulmonary hypertensive chickens

4. Pathogenesis

As already stated, chronic exposure to hypoxia leads to PH due to pulmonary vasoconstriction, structural remodeling of pulmonary vessels and increased blood viscosity in mammals and chickens (Bartsch et al., 2005; Burton and Smith, 1967; Burton et al., 1967; Cueva et al., 1974; Currie, 1999; Cogo et al., 2004; Huchzermeyer, 1988; Kanazawa et al., 2005; Meyrick and Reid, 1978; Remillard and Yuan, 2005; Reeves and Grover, 2005; Rhodes, 2005). Pulmonary vascular resistance is enhanced by constriction of pulmonary vascular smooth muscle and structural remodeling of the vascular bed (Reid, 1979; Stenmark and Mecham, 1997).

The pathogenesis of PH involves a complex and multifactorial process. Vasoconstriction and remodeling of the pulmonary vessel wall contribute to increased pulmonary vascular resistance in PH (Voelkel et al., 1997). Hypoxic pulmonary vasoconstriction (HPV) is an important physiological property of the pulmonary circulation and can optimize the ventilation: perfusion ratio by diverting blood away from poorly ventilated areas of the lung. However, in global hypoxia, which is found in high altitude environments, HPV results in a rise in pulmonary vascular resistance (PVR) and concomitant PH. This severely increases the afterload on the right heart and, in combination with associated pulmonary vascular remodelling, leads to a right ventricular dilatation and heart failure. Sustained vasoconstriction in response to moderate hypoxia is unique to the pulmonary vasculature. In despite of the progress made from many studies, the precise mechanisms involved are elusive. Recent advances in the field have opened up new areas of investigation, particularly in regard to the role of the vascular endothelium.

The first modern observation of HPV was made in 1894 when Bradford and Dean (1894) described increases in pulmonary arterial pressure (PAP) in response to asphyxia. Half a century later, HPV was recognized as an adaptive phenomenon by von Euler and Liljestrand (1946). They ventilated anesthetized cats with either hypoxic (10% O_2) or hypercapnic gas mixtures and found that PAP increased, with minimal change in left atrial pressure, predominantly with the hypoxic challenge. They concluded that HPV might "increase the blood flow to better aerated lung areas, which leads to improved conditions for the utilization of alveolar air". HPV shunts blood from poorly oxygenated areas to better ventilated lung segments, thereby optimizing ventilation-perfusion matching, reducing shunt fraction and optimizing systemic O_2 delivery in conditions such as atelectasis and pneumonia (Brimioulle et al, 1996). HPV onsets within seconds of moderate hypoxia and reverses quickly on restoration of normoxic ventilation. Whereas, in pneumonia and atelectasis, HPV is a focal response limited to the diseased lung segment, with global hypoxia, as occurs at high altitude or with sleep apnea, HPV constricts PAs throughout the pulmonary circulation, increasing the PVR (Moudgi et al., 2005).

Vasoconstriction in response to hypoxia can occur in isolated pulmonary arteries, which leads to the conclusion that the oxygen sensor and subsequent constrictor mechanism(s) must be located in either the vascular smooth muscle or the endothelium. The discovery of K^+ channels that are depressed by hypoxia in pulmonary, but not systemic vascular smooth muscle cells, has provided a potential signal mechanism of transduction, which permits to propose a link between reduction in alveolar PO_2, depolarization of the cell membrane, and contraction via voltage-gated Ca^{2+} entry (Post et al., 1992). Several reports have also shown that hypoxia can cause shortening in isolated pulmonary arterial smooth muscle cells (Madden et al., 1992) and this suggests that HPV is a function of the smooth muscle rather than the endothelium. However, other studies have shown that the endothelium is definitely required for sustained vasoconstriction (Demiryurek et al., 1993; Leach et al., 1994; Zhang and Morice, 1994). Although some differences in response might be ascribed to variations among species and variations in artery size (Leach et al.1994), a possibly more important aspect is the time course over which the experiment is conducted.

Most reports, in particular those on isolated cells, describe processes that occur during the first 10-15 min. However, isolated pulmonary arteries show a biphasic response to hypoxia when observed over longer periods (Bennie et al., 1991; Leach et al. 1994; Zhang and Morice, 1994; Robertson et al., 1995). This biphasic response consists of a rapid, transient increase in vascular tone over about 5-10 min (phase 1), which then falls towards the baseline. This is followed by a more slowly developing but sustained increase in tone (phase 2), which reaches a plateau about 40 min later on. The phase 1 of constriction is relatively unaffected by removal of the endothelium, while in most reports phase 2 is abolished (Hoshino et al., 1994; Leach et al. 1994; Zhang and Morice, 1994).

The relative physiological significance of the abovementioned phases is opened to question. Although HPV *in vivo* or in blood-perfused lungs is generally characterized by a rapid rise in pulmonary vascular resistance, this increase in resistance is sustained for long periods. It would seem most likely, therefore, that the second sustained phase of constriction in isolated arteries is more relevant to physiological HPV than the transient first phase. In the whole lung the effects may result in a rapid but sustained increase in resistance. The biphasic response to hypoxia suggests that HPV involves multifactorial mechanisms, which may or may not be interdependent.

HPV is intrinsic to the lung and, although modulated upstream by the endothelium and downstream by calcium sensitization of the contractile apparatus (rho kinase), the core mechanism involves a redox-based O_2 sensor (likely the mitochondria) that generates a diffusible redox mediator (likely H_2O_2) that is withdrawn during hypoxia, leading to hypoxic inhibition of certain voltage-gated K^+ channels (K_v) in pulmonary artery smooth muscle cells (PASMCs). Specific O_2-sensitive K_v channels, including $K_v1.5$ and $K_v2.1$, set membrane potential (E_M) and thus control Ca^{2+} influx, via voltage-gated Ca^{2+} channels, and therefore vascular tone (Moudgi et al., 2005).

Substantial work defining the properties of HPV has been performed by integrative physiologists studying normal and diseased humans. Ignorance of this integrative physiology and overreliance on reductionist models, using vascular cells and rings have created confusion in the quest for the molecular mechanism of HPV. In addition, because HPV is elicited by moderate airway hypoxia, rather than anoxia or low mixed- venous pO_2, it is worthwhile to define "hypoxia" as it pertains to HPV. Ascent to the summit of Mount Everest defines the limit of hypoxia tolerated by humans and thus serves as a practical guide to what constitutes "physiologically relevant" hypoxia. At the summit of Mount Everest, the inspired and arterial PO_2 values are approximately 43 Torr, whereas the arterial pCO_2 is 11 ± 2 Torr and arterial pH is 7.53 (Malconian et al., 1993).

HPV increases PVR by 50-300%. The response to hypoxia onsets in minutes, reaching a maximum within 15 min (Bindslev et al., 1985). In normal volunteers, inhalation of 12.5% O_2

decreases systemic pO_2 to below 50 Torr and increases PVR by 100–150% (Moore et al., 1998). HPV is not potentiated by repeated hypoxic challenges, nor does it decrease when sustained for hours (Dorrington et al., 1997). An interesting case report attests to the potential of segmental HPV to persist chronically. A patient with bronchial obstruction due to an adenoma had persistent, HPV-induced lung hypoperfusion that was normalized by resection of the tumor and restoration of distal airflow (Grant et al., 1980).

In an excellent demonstration that HPV depends on airway and not mixed-venous PO_2, unilateral graded hypoxia (12–5% inspired O_2) was delivered while the contralateral lung received 100% O_2. This reduced the perfusion of the hypoxic lung from a normoxic value of 52 ± 2 to 30 ± 8% of total lung flow, without a significant fall in mixed-venous PO_2 (Hambraeus-Jonzon et al., 1997). In healthy volunteers, 8 h of hypoxia increased PVR from 1.2 ± 0.3 to 2.9 ± 0.3 Wood Units at 2 h and thereafter PVR remained constant, reversing on return to normoxia (Dorrington et al., 1997). Systemic vascular resistance (SVR) decreased in parallel. The intrinsic nature of these opposing responses to hypoxia is demonstrated by the ability to demonstrate simultaneous HPV and renal vasodilatation in the isolated, serially perfused lung-kidney model and even in isolated arterial rings (Michelakis et al., 2002). HPV also occurs in children. In a study of children with congenital heart disease, mild hypoxic ventilation (15% inspired O_2) increased the PVR/SVR ratio from 0.33 to 0.40 (Waldman et al., 1983).

If alveolar pO_2 is maintained above 60 Torr, there is a little pulmonary vasoconstriction to hypoxemia, even when mixed- venous pO_2 is reduced to 10 Torr (Marshall and Marshall, 1983), confirming that alveolar O_2 tension, not blood PO_2, is the major determinant of HPV. Micropuncture studies confirm that the small resistance PAs (<200 μm) are directly exposed to the alveolar PO_2 and are the major site of HPV (Kato and Staub,1966). HPV can be demonstrated in salt-perfused isolated lungs (McMurtry et al., 1976) and resistance PA rings denuded of endothelium (Archer et al., 2004). Indeed, isolated pulmonary artery smooth muscle cell (PASMC) from resistance pulmonary arteries (PAs) constrict to hypoxia. In contrast, smooth muscle cells (SMCs) from carotid arteries or even conduit PAs do not constrict to hypoxia (Madden et al., 1992). This demonstrates that HPV is unique to the PA, particularly the resistance segment of the pulmonary circulation. As in humans, hypoxia dilates most systemic arteries in animals (Hampl et al., 1994).

The persistence of global hypoxia ultimately results in a selective downregulation of acute HPV, despite the occurrence of PH and the finding that constrictor responses to other stimuli are preserved or enhanced (Durmowicz et al., 1993; Reeve et al., 2001). Exposure to hypoxia for only 3 h can elicit this selective suppression of HPV (Greenlees and Tucker,1984). Animals and humans genetically adapted to life at high altitude, such as the yak (Durmowicz et al., 1993) or the native Tibetan (Moore et al., 1998) have weak or absent HPV.

The vascular endothelium is known to produce a wide range of active compounds, including various vasodilators and vasoconstrictors. Vasoconstriction could result from either a reduction in vasodilator activity or an increase in vasoconstrictor activity; several possible mediators have been examined, including nitric oxide (NO), cyclooxygenase and lipoxygenase products, endothelin-1 (ET-1) and serotonin. There is disagreement about the nature of HPV in isolated PA rings. In animals, HPV causes a rapid increase in PVR that gradually reaches a plateau and is sustained, much as occurs in humans. However, in isolated PA rings, some research groups find that HPV is biphasic, consisting of an immediate, endothelium-independent constriction, which peaks in ~10 min (phase I) and a second, slowly developing endothelium-dependent sustained contraction that peaks at ~40 min (phase II) (Ward and Robertson, 1995). On the other hand, Archer et al., 2001 consistently found a monophasic PA constriction in resistance PA rings, even if they are denuded of endothelium. They believe that the role of the endothelium is to modulate HPV. Nitric oxide (NO), produced in response to pulmonary vasoconstriction, suppresses HPV. Endothelin-1 (ET-1), produced in response to hypoxia, enhances HPV (Platoshyn et al., 2000).

One of the problems associated with such examinations is that the release of many of these vasoactive agents is affected by the vascular tone, so that it may be difficult to determine whether changes in a particular agent are due to the enhanced vasoconstriction during hypoxia, or to hypoxia *per se* (Ignarro, 1990; Inagami et al, 1995).

4.1 Molecular mechanisms of pulmonary hypertension

It is now well known that, under physiological conditions, the vascular endothelium produces factors that maintain normal vascular tone and homeostasis. Two of the most important factors produced by the vascular endothelium are the endothelium-derived relaxing and antiproliferative factor NO, and the endothelium-derived vasoconstrictor and mitogenic factor endothelin-1 (ET-1) (Moncada et al., 1991; Yanagisawa, 1994). The interactions between NO and ET-1 in the control of vascular tone have been extensively studied (Lavallee et al., 2001).

Pulmonary vasoconstriction is believed to be an early component of the pulmonary hypertensive process. Excessive vasoconstriction has been related to abnormal function of expression of potassium channels, as well as to endothelial dysfunction. Endothelial dysfunction seems to play an integral role in alveolar hypoxic vasoconstriction. The endothelium mediates the structural changes in the pulmonary vasculature, which includes an altered production of various endothelial vasoactive mediators, such as NO, prostacyclin, endothelin-1 (ET-1), serotonin, and thromboxane. Endothelial dysfunction leads to chronically impaired production of vasodilators such as NO and prostacyclin along with prolonged over expression of vasoconstrictors such as ET-1. These changes affect vascular tone and promote vascular remodeling. Given that most of these mediators affect the growth of smooth muscle cells, an alteration in their production may facilitate the development of pulmonary vascular hypertrophy and the structural remodeling characteristic of pulmonary hypertension (Budhiraja et al., 2004; Humbert et al., 2004).

4.1.1 Nitric oxide

Originally identified as the reactive intermediate by which nitroprusside caused smooth muscle cell relaxation, it was not until nitric oxide (NO) was identified as the endothelium-derived relaxing factor that its role was explored in PH (Gruetter et al., 1979; Ignarro, 1989). NO was found to be a critical vasodilator that could also inhibit platelet aggregation and proliferation of vascular smooth muscle cells. Human studies reported variable production of NO in patients with idiopathic pulmonary arterial hypertension (IPAH). However, important mechanistic insights into the role of NO in the control of pulmonary vascular tone and remodeling originated from animal models, which showed NO-mediated protection against HPV in lungs, inhibition of smooth muscle proliferation and platelet aggregation, and downregulation of ET-1 production (Perrella et al., 1992). NO has broader effects in that it contributes to angiogenesis, endothelial cell survival, and mobilization of bone marrow progenitor cells.

The hypothesized role of endothelial NO deficiency in contributing to PH was further strengthened by the modest but healthy effects of inhaled NO and NO donors such as L-arginine in patients with PH. NO stimulates the production of cGMP starting a regulatory cascade resulting in pulmonary vasodilatation. While inhaled NO is used as a clinical therapy only in patients with primary pulmonary hypertension of the newborn, sildenafil, an oral inhibitor of phosphodiestarase-5, has beneficial effects in both adult and childhood PAH, probably by means of increasing cyclic GMP through decreased breakdown (Sastry et al., 2004).

Synthesis of NO involves incorporation of molecular oxygen, and hypoxia might therefore be expected to reduce NO release. A reduction in NO-mediated relaxation has been proposed as the underlying mechanism for HPV (Rodman et al., 1990), and hypoxia has been shown to inhibit agonist-stimulated release of NO in pulmonary arteries (Demiryurek et al. 1993). Inhibitors of NO synthesis potentiate HPV both *in vivo* and in perfused lungs (Sprague et al., 1992). It has been suggested that endogenous NO opposes HPV and thus limits the reduction in blood flow to the hypoxic alveoli (Sprague et al. 1992). Thus, the NO is clearly a major regulator of pulmonary vascular tone and may be important modulator during hypoxia.

NO is synthesized endogenously by nitric oxide synthase (NOS) enzymes, which convert L-arginine to L-citrulline and NO in the presence of oxygen, NADPH, flavin adenine dinucleotide, flavin adenine mononucleotide, tetrahydrobiopterin, and calmodulin (Knowles and Moncada, 1994). Three NOS enzymes have been so far identified in the lung. Neuronal NOS or NOS1 and endothelial NOS (eNOS) or NOS3 are primarily expressed in neuronal and vascular endothelial cells, respectively, of the normal lung, whereas the inducible NOS (iNOS) or NOS2 is expressed in the airway epithelium (Barnes and Belvisi, 1993; Kobzik et al., 1993; Guo et al., 1995). Basal release of NO by isoform eNOS produces a consistent vasodilator and antimitogenic effect. Although eNOS is constitutively expressed, its expression can be modulated by a variety of chemical, physical, and developmental stimuli (Forstermann et al., 1998).

The effects of eNOS-derived NO are mediated directly and via secondary messengers. In the presence of NO, guanylate cyclase becomes activated and produces cyclic guanosine monophosphate (cGMP) from guanosine triphosphate in the vascular smooth muscle. These two NO dependent routes resulting in calcium sequestration and smooth muscle relaxation (Jia et al., 1996; Moncada, 1993; McDonald and Murad, 1995; Rafikova et al., 2002; Stamler et al., 2001). Endothelial NO-induced vascular smooth muscle relaxation has been termed endothelium dependent. Exogenous NO donors, such as nitroglycerin, can cause endothelium-independent vascular smooth muscle relaxation. In particular, NO seems to be important for maintaining normal blood pressure and matching ventilation-perfusion within the lung in broiler chickens. This concept is supported by the finding of Wang et al. (2002), who found that intravenous infusion of Nv-L-arginine-methyl-ester (L-NAME), which inhibits NO synthesis by both the eNOS and iNOS forms, caused an immediately reduced plasma concentration of NO and continuously increased pulmonary arterial pressure in healthy broilers. However, the L-NAME-induced increase in pulmonary pressure can be reversed by sodium nitroprusside, a nitric oxide donor (Weidong et al., 2002).

Wideman et al (2006) suggested that pulmonary vasodilatation might be affected by the NO produced by iNOS in lungs exposed to an inflammatory stimulus. The endothelium dependent vasodilatation in chickens is partly mediated by NO, as reflected by the finding that L-NAME attenuates the concentration-dependent relaxation response of artery rings to acetylcholine (Martinez-Lemus et al., 1999). It has been considered that the endothelium-dependent relaxation in the pulmonary artery of broilers is impaired, which contributes to the susceptibility of broilers to PH (Martinez-Lemus et al., 1999).

In experimental studies the alteration of eNOS availability in PH was examined by exposing chickens to hypobaric hypoxia (Moreno de Sandino and Hernandez, 2003, 2006) and cold stress (Tan et al., 2007) to induce PH, right ventricular hypertrophy and pulmonary vascular remodeling, similar to that in natural PH cases. Those studies demonstrated that hypoxia-induced as well as cold-induced PH was associated with reduced eNOS expression in the pulmonary arterioles, and that eNOS expression was inversely related to pulmonary vascular remodeling, strengthening the hypothesis of Martinez-Lemus et al. (1999) that impaired NO synthesis contributes to the susceptibility of chickens to PH. Giaid and Saleh (1995) reported decreased eNOS expression in human pulmonary vascular preparations and concluded that the reduction of this vasodilator enzyme contributed to the development of PH. Using eNOS-deficient rats, Steudel et al. (1998) confirmed that impaired eNOS-derived NO enhanced hypoxia-induced PH. NO levels in exhaled breath are reduced in the humans with IPAH, and there is an inverse relationship between NO in exhaled breath and the degree of PH (Kaneko et al., 1998; Machado et al., 2004; Girgis et al., 2005).

The study by Richard et al. (1995) provided evidence that part of the hypertensive response in rats induced by inhibition of NO synthesis, which is generally considered to reflect removal of the tonic vasodilator influence of NO, is in fact due to the unmasking of an endothelin-induced vasoconstrictor response. With the progression of vascular disease and the gradual loss of the ability of vessels to dilate, vasoconstrictor processes can assume a greater importance, thereby causing further vascular dysfunction (Lavallee et al., 2001). In broilers, increased pulmonary pressure accompanied by elevated ET-1 concentration was observed following inhibition of NO synthesis by supplemental L-NAME to the diet (Wang et al., 2002). In this context, it is also probable that reduced production of the NO in hypertensive broilers may be only one manifestation of endothelial dysfunction, and that the vasoconstrictor role of the endothelium-derived vasoconstrictor ET-1 may become progressively important in the development of PH. Indeed, ETA receptor antagonist BQ123 has been shown to effectively prevent cold-induced PH in broilers (Yang et al., 2005).

Supplemental dietary L-arginine has been shown to reduce pulmonary arterial pressure as well as the incidence of PH in chickens exposed to cool environmental temperature without alteration of body weight (Wideman et al., 1995), and further studies revealed that dietary L-arginine supplementation permitted broilers to exhibit flow-dependent pulmonary vasodilatation when a pulmonary artery snare was tightened to force the entire cardiac output through one lung. Those findings were supportive of a NO vasodilator effect. Tan et al (2005a) showed that supplemental L-arginine markedly increased NO production in cold-exposed broilers, coincident with reduced pulmonary blood pressure. This indicates that an increase in endogenous NO synthesis may relax the tone of the resistance vessels in the lung of broilers, thereby permitting the increased blood flow to pass through the lung at a lower pressure. Similarly, intravenous L-arginine was shown to reduce pulmonary arterial pressure in human patients with PH by increasing the endogenous production of NO (Mehta et al., 1995). In an *in vitro* study Eddahibi et al., (1992) provided evidence that L-arginine restores endothelium-dependent relaxation of pulmonary vessels from hypertensive rats.

Although the mechanisms for reduced expression of eNOS in hypertensive broilers remain to be identified, it has been considered reasonable to postulate that endothelium dysfunction significantly contributes to PH development through several mechanisms, including an imbalance between the release of vasoconstrictor agents like ET-1 and vasodilator substances such as prostacycline and NO (Adnot et al., 1991; Inagami et al., 1995: Stewart, 1994; Tozzi and Riley, 1990; Voelkel and Tuder, 1995). A decrease in the amount of endothelium-dependent relaxation has been observed in pulmonary vessels from hypertensive animals, although its precise mechanism in the development of PH has not been established (Dhin-Xuan, et al., 1989, 1992; Martinez-Lemus et al., 1999). Some forms of hypertension might be due to changes in NO synthesis or action in the vasculature (Rees et al., 1989). Differences in endothelial NO synthesis are likely to be the result of various levels of genetically determined susceptibility to chronic hypoxia. Understanding the pathogenesis of PH and its key cellular and molecular mechanisms may allow manipulations to diminish the incidence of PH.

Impairment of NO production in chronic hypoxia occurs in pulmonary hypertensive animals (Maruyama and Maruyama, 1994; Reddy et al., 1996;Tozzi and Riley, 1990) and humans (Cooper et al., 1996; Dinh-Xuan et al., 1992; Dinh- Xuan et al., 1989). However, the cause of this impairment remains unknown. A defect in NOS enzyme could cause reduction of NO production (Cooke et al., 1997; Huang et al., 1995). This hypothesis is supported by previous immunohistochemical analysis showing decreased expression of endothelial NOS (Giaid and Saleh, 1995). Alternatively, there may be inhibition of the enzymatic reaction of NO synthesis, due to deficiency of necessary cofactors or the L-arginine substrate (Ignarro, 1990; Mitzutani and Layon, 1996; Shaul and Wells, 1994). NOS blockade has been shown to worsen hypoxia-induced PH, and administration of NO (in the inhaled air) ameliorates hypoxia-induced PH (Kouyoumdjian et al., 1994). In addition, L-arginine supplementation reduced right ventricular hypertrophy and mortality due to PH in male broilers exposed to low environmental temperatures (Wideman et al., 1995) and intravenous injections of L-arginine reduced pulmonary arterial pressure in pulmonary hypertensive individuals by increasing endogenous production of NO (Mehta et al., 1995). L-arginine ameliorated changes associated with PH in rats, probably by enhancing endogenous NO production (Mitzutani and Layon, 1996).

To determine whether or not exposure to chronic hypoxia and subsequent development of PH induce alterations in endothelial NO production in broiler's pulmonary vascular bed, in our laboratory, we studied the expression of NOS in pulmonary endothelial cells in healthy and hypertensive broilers raised at an altitude of 2638 m above sea level, using a nicotinamide adenine dinucleotide phosphate (NADPH)-diaphorase histochemical staining reaction. In this study, we demonstrated that NOS is present in pulmonary arterial endothelial cells of healthy and pulmonary hypertensive broilers. NOS activity is reduced in pulmonary arterial endothelial cells of pulmonary hypertensive broilers. Pulmonary hypertensive animals had lower numbers of pulmonary arterioles with NADPH-diaphorase-positive-staining endothelial cells than non-hypertensive chickens (healthy chickens) (Figures 4 and 5). Furthermore, the number of arterioles expressing NOS in the endothelial cells was inversely correlated with the degree of PH. The degree of PH was also significantly and inversely associated with NADPH-diaphorase positive staining. In fact, all hypertensive broilers had fewer arterioles expressing NOS in endothelial cells compared with the non-hypertensive broilers. This finding implies that hypertensive chickens show lower NO production than the non-hypertensive ones. Therefore, it is possible that NO participates in the pathogenesis of PH in broilers (Moreno de Sandino and Hernandez, 2003). Low L-arginine in the diet could provoke PH on its own or concomitantly with decreased NOS expression in hypertensive broilers. Although L-arginine content in feed in our study was not quantified, the diet used was presumed to be adequate in this context.

The results of this work are in harmony with previous observations that the degree of PH was significantly and inversely associated with NOS inmunoreactivity (Giaid and Saleh, 1995). Others demonstrated that hypoxia-induced PH is associated with a loss of NO activity in pulmonary vessels (Adnot and Raffestin, 1991). Other mediators, such ET-1, are also likely to be involved in the regulation of pulmonary vascular resistance (Giaid, 1998; Giaid et al., 1993; Stewart, 1994; Stewart et al., 1991). Interactions among mediators and NO may be important.

Endothelial-derived NO production or activity or both are reduced in certain forms of chronic PH in several experimental animal models and in humans. Whether this impairment causes the disease, or merely reflects its severity remains to be elucidated. Hence, NO formation by pulmonary endothelial cells may represent a primary event in the pathogenesis of PH (Moreno de Sandino and Hernández, 2003).

Recent research (Tan et al., 2007) demonstrated that loss of eNOS expression could be prevented by supplemental L-arginine. This finding probably reflects the ability of L-arginine to ameliorate haemodynamic damage to the pulmonary endothelium in hypertensive broilers, and provides a proof that supplemental L-arginine increasing NO production is associated with elevated eNOS expression. Supplemental L-arginine reduced but did not eliminate mortality due to PH (Wideman et al., 1995; Tan et al., 2007), indicating that treatment with L-arginine reduced pulmonary pressure only to a certain extent. In one case, however, supplemental L-arginine did not affect PH mortality (Ruiz-Feria et al., 2001). It is well known that PH in fast-growing broilers is a complex, multi-factorial process. In addition to vascular dysfunction (e.g. remodeling and impaired endothelium-dependent relaxation), causes that may affect pulmonary pressure include an inherently low pulmonary vascular capacity, inadequate gas exchange area for blood cells, and a cardiac output that chronically increases in support of metabolic requirements (Wideman and Tackett, 2000; Wideman, 2001; Hassanzadeh et al., 2005). Therefore, it is difficult to eliminate PH in broilers solely by supplemental L-arginine.

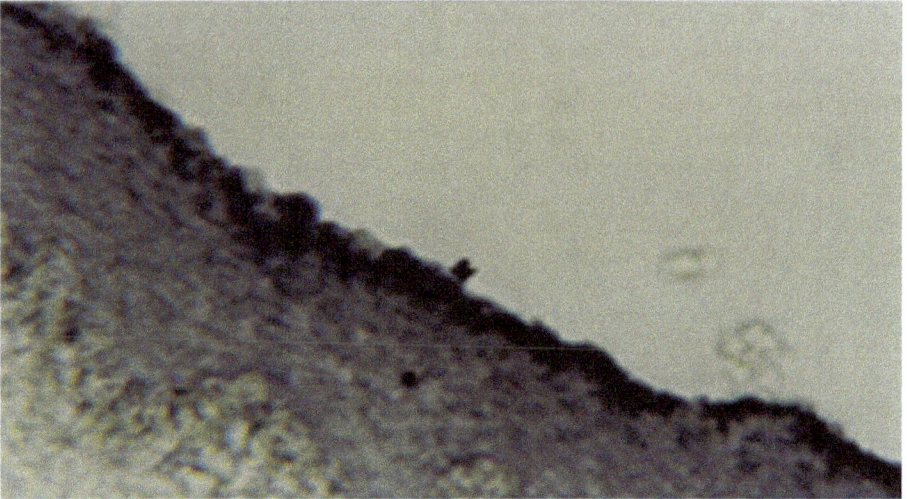

Fig. 4. Endothelium NADPH-diaphorase positive reaction of pulmonary arteriole (Moreno de Sandino and Hernández, 2003).

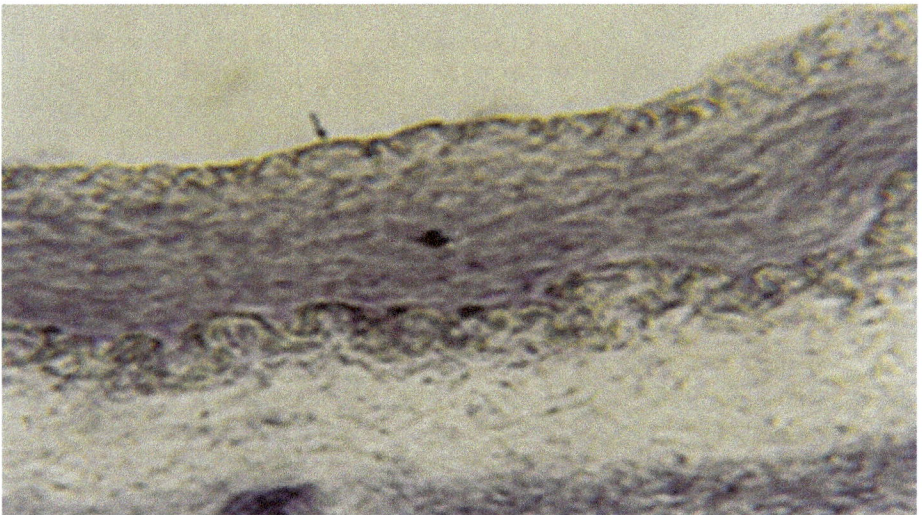

Fig. 5. Endothelium NADPH-diaphorase negative reaction of pulmonary arteriole (Moreno de Sandino and Hernández, 2003).

Several lines of evidence support a major role for NO and in particular for eNOS in the pulmonary circulation:

1. eNOS-deficient mice had mild PH (pulmonary artery pressure 19.0 ± 0.8 compared with 16.4 ± 0.6 mmHg in wild-type mice). In the same study, isolated pulmonary arteries of NOS3-deficient mice failed to show the normal vasodilator response to acetylcholine but were morphologically unaltered (Steudel et al., 1997).

2. In a complementary study by the same group of investigators, mice with congenital deficiency of eNOS (which exhibit major systemic and mild PH under normoxic conditions) developed more severe degrees of PH after a 3- to 6-wk period of hypoxia (11% oxygen). The NOS-deficient mice also showed greater increases in vascular remodeling and right ventricular hypertrophy than wild-type mice, and right ventricular hypertrophy was prevented by breathing at 20 parts per million NO (Steudel et al., 1997).

3. Deletion of the eNOS gene was associated with histological evidence of PH in both male and female mice during fetal life and at birth, but PH and right ventricular hypertrophy persisted only in the adult males. In neither sex did inducible or neuronal NOS compensate for the deletion of eNOS (Miller et al., 2005).

4. Lung tissue from patients with chronic PH showed decreased eNOS expression in vascular endothelium, especially in patients with severe histological abnormalities (i.e., with plexiform lesions); the intensity of the enzyme immunoreactivity correlated inversely with the severity of histological changes. The findings support the conclusion that the reduction of this vasodilator enzyme may contribute to the development of PH (Giaid A and Saleh, 1995).

5. Consistent with the above conclusion, mice deficient in the *de novo* production of tetrahydrobiopterin (BH4), a cofactor for NOS, selectively express a pulmonary hypertensive, but not systemic hypertensive phenotype (Nandi et al., 2005).

6. Inhaled NO attenuated PH and improved lung growth in infant rats after neonatal treatment with a VEGF receptor inhibitor (Tang et al., 2004).

7. In chickens reared at high altitude, NOS expression is lower in the endothelial cells of pulmonary arteries of hypertensive chickens compared with nonhypertensive chickens (healthy subjects) and lower NOS expression was associated with medial smooth muscle thickening (Moreno de Sandino and Hernández, 2003, 2006. See figures 4 and 5)

8. In chickens reared at high altitude, NOS mRNA expression is lower in the lungs of hypertensive chickens compared with nonhypertensive chickens (healthy subjects), and lower NOS mRNA expression was associated with medial smooth muscle thickening (non-published data).

4.1.2 Endothelin- 1

Endothelin (ET-1) is a family of four 21-amino-acid peptides (ET-1, ET-2, ET-3, ET-4). Of the four active endothelins, ET-1 is the predominant isoform in the cardiovascular system, which is generated through the cleavage of prepro-ET-1 to big ET-1 and then to ET-1 by the action of endothelin-converting enzymes (ECE). ET-1 is abundantly expressed in human lung´s vasculature and plays an important role in pulmonary vascular tone regulation (Giaid et al., 1993; Kourembanas et al., 1993). In mammals, both pulmonary vascular endothelial cells and vascular smooth muscle cells synthesize and release ET-1 (Wort et al., 2001). The vascular effects of ET-1 are mediated by two receptor types: ET receptor subtype A (ETA) and ET receptor subtype B (ETB) (Luscher and Barton, 2000). The ETA receptors are expressed on pulmonary vascular smooth muscle cells, while ETB receptors are located on both pulmonary vascular endothelial cells and smooth muscle cells. Stimulation of ETA receptors results in vasoconstriction and cell proliferation, whereas ETB receptors on the endothelial cells mediate clearance of ET-1, inhibition of endothelial cell apoptosis, release of NO and prostacyclin, and inhibit the expression of ECE-1. However, there is evidence that the ETB receptors on smooth muscle cells may also play a major role in mediating ET-1-induced constriction of intrapulmonary conduit and resistance arteries in humans and rats (Wang et al., 2006; Sakurai et al., 1990).

Through its action on the endothelin receptor A (ET_A) on pulmonary artery smooth muscle cells, ET-1 leads to a rapid increase in intracellular calcium and sustained activation of protein kinase C. Early activation of the p42/p44 isoforms of mitogen-activated protein kinase and induction of the early growth response genes c-*fos* and c-*jun* are also observed (Jeffery and Morrell 2002). The mitogenic action of ET-1 on pulmonary artery smooth muscle cells occurs through the ET_A or endothelin receptor B (ET_B) subtype, depending on the anatomic location of cells. For instance, ET_A mediates mitogenesis in cells derived from the main pulmonary artery, whereas in cells from resistance arteries both receptor subtypes may contribute. There is strong evidence that endothelium-derived ET-1 is a major player in the vasodilator/vasoconstrictor imbalance characteristic of PH. Levels of lung and circulating ET-1 are increased in animals and patients with PH of various etiologies (Giaid et al., 1993). These observations indicate that ET-1 is likely to contribute to the vasoactive component of PH, as well as to the abnormal pulmonary vascular remodeling characteristic of the condition. Results of chronic ET receptor antagonist therapy support the relevance of this pathway in PH.

ET-1 is a potent vasoconstrictor peptide, and hypoxia has been demonstrated to increase ET-1 gene expression and secretion in cultured endothelial cells (Kourembanas et al., 1991). A study by Wang et al., (1995) has shown that the ET-1 antagonist BQ-123 can inhibit HPV in fetal lambs, but it is worth noting that the decline to baseline tension on return to normoxia was slow in this preparation. Although a role for ET-1 in HPV cannot be ruled out, it is more likely to be of importance in chronic hypoxia and it may well be involved in mediating some aspects of the pulmonary vascular remodelling seen under these conditions.

Gómez et al (2007, 2008), Davie et al (2002), Giaid et al (1993), Motte et al (2006) and Stewart et al (1991) showed convincing evidence which suggests that local ET-1 synthesis in vascular endothelial cells probably plays an important role in the pathophysiology of PH:

1. ET-1-like immunoreactivity and messenger RNA, rarely present in vascular endothelial cells from control subjects, were abundant in IPAH patients and were associated with medial thickening and intimal fibrosis.
2. There was a strong correlation between the intensity of ET-1-like immunoreactivity and pulmonary vascular resistance in patients with plexogenic pulmonary arteriopathy, but not in those with secondary PH.
3. ET-1 receptor density was considerably greater in smaller pulmonary arteries and lung parenchyma from pulmonary hypertensive patients than in control subjects.
4. ET-1 stimulated DNA synthesis in human PA smooth muscle cells.
5. Inhibition of endogenous ET-1 release or its action attenuated serum-stimulated proliferation of pulmonary vascular smooth muscle cells.
6. ET-1 mRNA expression is higher in the lung of pulmonary hypertensive chickens at high altitude compared with nonhypertensive chickens (healthy subjects), and high ET-1 mRNA expression was associated with medial smooth muscle thickness (Gómez et al., 2007, 2008).

7. In addition, studies have shown enhanced ET-1 and ECE-1 synthesis in humans and experimental animals with primary IPAH (Giaid et al., 1993; Giaid, 1998).

Similarly, increased ET-1 mRNA level in the lung of broilers with PH induced by chronic hypobaric hypoxia was observed in our laboratory; comprehensive gene expression analysis was performed in the lung of broilers under chronic hypobaric hypoxic conditions by using real-time PCR analysis. In this study, it was shown for the first time that ET-1 mRNA expression is higher in the lung of pulmonary hypertensive broilers (PHB) than nonhypertensive broilers (NPHB) (Figures 6,7 and 8; Gómez et al., 2007). This result is in agreement with previous observations made in humans and in induced PH in various animal models (Mortensen and Fink, 1992; Rabelink et al., 1994; Potter et al., 1997; Cardillo et al., 1999), in which it has been shown that ET-1 could be involved in the pathogenesis of PH. ET-1 induces vasoconstriction, promotes fibrosis, has mitogenic potential, and is important in the regulation of vascular tone, arterial remodeling, and vascular injury. However, its role in normal cardiovascular homeostasis and PH is unclear (Touyz and Schiffrin, 2003).

Contrary to previous reports in the lungs of hypoxic rats (Li et al., 1994) and in cells from the pulmonary artery of PH sheep (Balyakina et al., 2002), our work showed a decrease in ETA mRNA levels in the lungs of PHB (Figure 5). Thus, HPB showed high values of mRNA ET-1 and lowest values of mRNA of eNOS, and NHPB had opposite results (data non published). In studies with ET-1 receptors antagonists, differences were found in expression levels, according to the experimental models used (McCulloch and MacLean, 1995; Maxwell et al., 1998; Luscher and Barton, 2000). The distribution and density of ET-1 receptors on vascular SMC varies among species and their location in the corresponding blood vessel (Nishimura et al., 1995; Chen and Oparil, 2000; Balyakina et al., 2002). Nevertheless, the role of ET-1 receptors that mediate the vasoconstrictor response in this animal model requires further study.

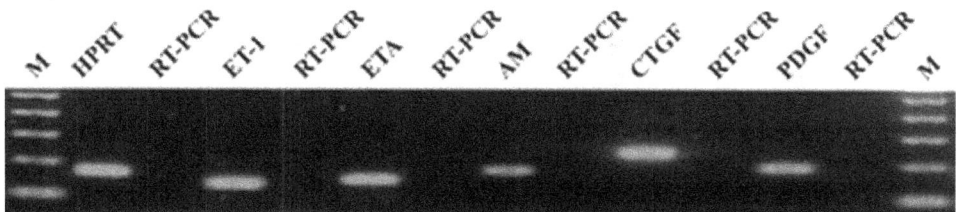

Fig. 6. Representative reverse-transcription PCR (RT-PCR) for hypoxanthine phosphoribosyltransferase (HPRT; 179 bp), endothelin 1 (ET-1; 141 bp), ET receptor type A (ETA; 160 bp), adrenomedullin (AM; 190 bp), connective tissue growth factor (CTGF; 252 bp), and platelet-derived growth factor (PDGF; 200 bp) mRNA in lung samples from nonhypertensive broilers at 24 d old. A 100-bp molecular weight marker (M) was used. The PCR products were separated on 1.5% agarose gel, stained with ethidium bromide and examined with ultraviolet light and visualized with a Gel Doc system (Bio-Rad, Hercules, CA). In addition, negative controls are shown and resulted in no bands after amplification (Gómez et al., 2007).

Several studies have demonstrated the interaction between NO and ET-1 in the vascular endothelium in mammals. NO mitigates the vasopressor activity of ET-1 (Filep et al., 1993), inhibits translation of prepro-ET-1 mRNA (Bodi et al., 1995), augments the degradation of ET-1 protein, and reduces ET-1 formation (Kourembanas et al., 1993). A number of vasculopathies associated with impaired bioavailability of NO are linked to increased ET-1 synthesis (Alonso and Radomski, 2003).

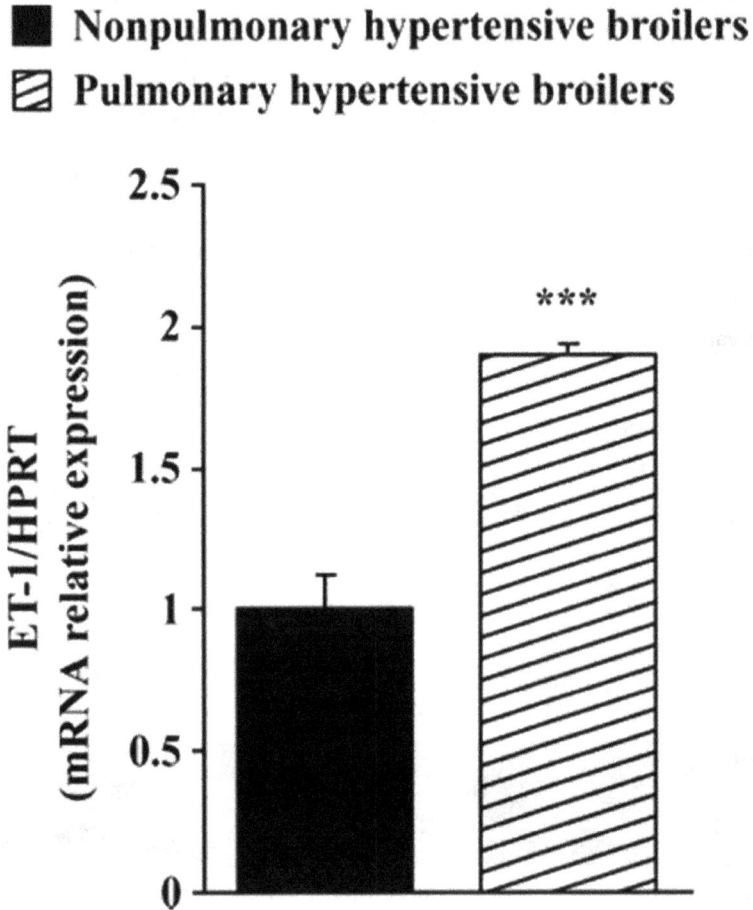

Fig. 7. Comparison by using real-time reverse-transcription PCR analysis of lung endothelin 1 (ET-1) mRNA levels in non-pulmonary hypertensive and pulmonary hypertensive chickens subjected to chronic hypobaric hypoxia. Semiquantitative data of ET-1 mRNA expression levels were normalized to those of the internal control hypoxanthine phosphoribosyltransferase (HPRT). Data are represented as mean ± SEM (n = 15/group). ***$P < 0.001$ (Gómez et al., 2007).

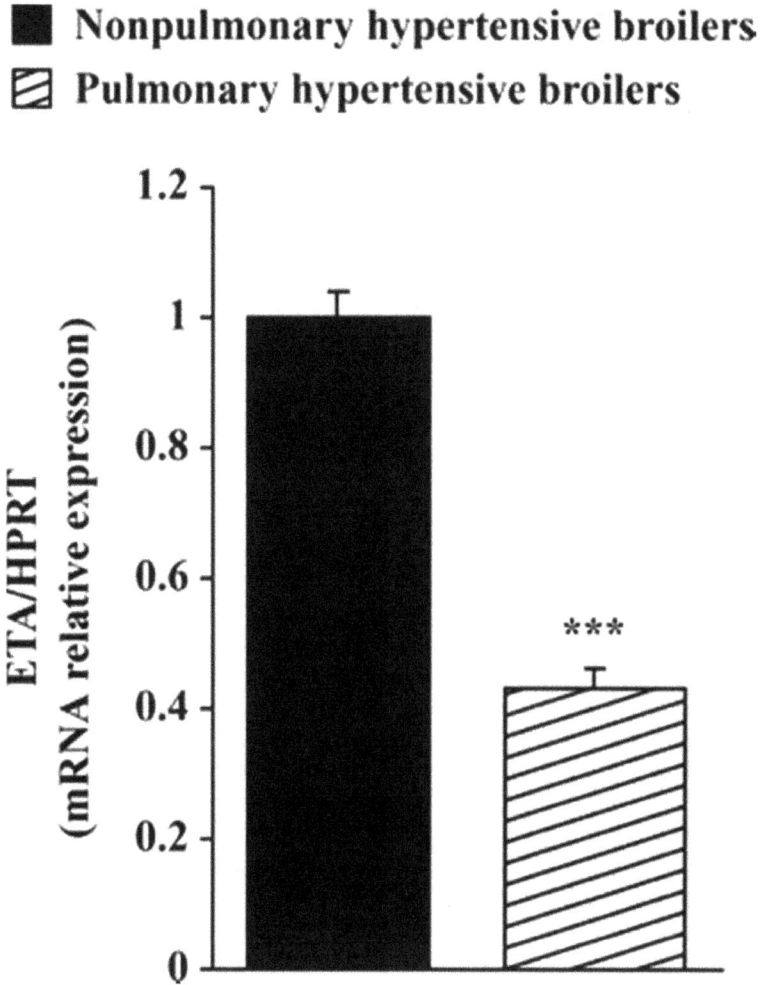

Fig. 8. Relative quantification of the regulation of lung endothelin type A (ETA) mRNA expression in pulmonary hypertensive and non-pulmonary hypertensive chickens subjected to chronic hypobaric hypoxia by using real-time reverse-transcription PCR analysis. Data of ETA mRNA expression levels were normalized to those of the internal control hypoxanthine phosphoribosyltransferase (HPRT). Data are represented as mean ± SEM (n = 15/group). ***P <0.001 (Gómez et al., 2007).

4.1.3 Potassium channels

Lessons relevant to PH can be learned from understanding the mechanism of HPV, although PH also involves cell proliferation and abnormalities of apoptosis (Archer and Rich, 2000). HPV is elicited when hypoxia inhibits one or more voltage-gated potassium channels (Kv) in the pulmonary artery smooth muscle cells of resistance pulmonary arteries. The resulting membrane depolarization increases the opening of voltage-gated calcium channels, raising cytosolic calcium and initiating constriction. The Kv1.5 is downregulated in pulmonary artery smooth muscle cells in humans with PH (Yuan et al., 1998), and both Kv1.5 and Kv2.1 are downregulated in rats with chronic hypoxia-induced pulmonary hypertension (Michelakis et al., 2002).

Furthermore, deoxyribonucleic acid microarray studies have shown downregulation of Kv channel genes in PH lungs (Geraci et al., 2001; Weir and Olschewiski, 2006). The selective loss of these Kv channels leads to pulmonary artery smooth muscle cell depolarization, an increase in the intracellular calcium, and both vasoconstriction and cell proliferation. It is not clear whether these Kv channel abnormalities are genetically determined or acquired. However, it is clear that the appetite suppressants dexfenfluramine and aminorex directly inhibit Kv1.5 and Kv2.1 (Weir et al., 1996). Augmenting Kv pathways should cause pulmonary vasodilation and promote regression of pulmonary remodeling. Drugs including dichloroacetate and sildenafil may enhance the expression and function of these potassium channels.

4-Aminopyridine (4-AP), an inhibitor of K_v channels, but not ATP-sensitive K^+ channels, causes pulmonary vasoconstriction (Hasunuma et al., 1991). Post et al. (1992) showed that hypoxia inhibited K^+ current (I_K) and depolarized membrane (E_M) in canine PASMCs. This initiated extensive research to quantify the contribution of K^+ channels to HPV and determine the molecular identity of the O_2-sensitive K^+ channels. K^+ channels are proteins consisting of four transmembrane-bound α-subunits and four regulatory β-subunits. The ionic pore which determines the channel's intrinsic conductance and ionic specificity is created by the formation of tetramers of α-subunits. The K_v channels also have a voltage sensor in their S4 region. β-Subunits associate with many K^+ channels and alter their expression and kinetics. There are several types of K^+ channel α-subunits, including K_v, inward rectifier, and twin pore channels. The K_v channels have emerged as a possible effector in HPV (Reeve et al., 2001).

K_v channels are important determinants of equilibrium potential of vascular SMCs. Closure of K_v channels decreases the tonic efflux of K^+ that otherwise occurs because of the intra-/extracellular concentration gradient (145/5 mM). Channel closure renders the cell interior relatively more positive (depolarized). At these more positive potentials (positive to –30 mV), the probability of L-type voltage-gated Ca^{2+} channels to open increases. This augments intracellular Ca^{2+} influx (down a 20,000/1 concentration gradient). Although less important than in cardiomyocytes, Ca^{2+} influx also cause release of intracellular stores, so-called calcium-induced calcium release, effectively increasing total calcium levels inside the cell. Increased cytosolic Ca^{2+} activates contraction via the actin-myosin apparatus and also increases the activation of immediate early genes, inducing a proliferative response (Platoshyn et al., 2000). Thus, regulation of K^+ channel activity and the subsequent regulation of Ca^{2+} may be important to maintain the pulmonary circulation's low PVR and the thin-walled morphology of small pulmonary arteries.

Although all K^+ channels are somewhat sensitive to prolonged or severe O_2 deprivation (because most require some basal phosphorylation and thus ATP), certain K^+ channels are specially suited to O_2 sensing, by virtue of their content of key cysteine and methionine groups. Reduction or oxidation of these residues by a redox mediator such as ROS can cause conformational changes in the channel, thereby altering pore function (Archer et al.,1998). In this regard, some K_v channels, including $K_v1.5$, respond to reduction and oxidation by changing their gating and open-state probability (Archer et al., 1998).

Hypoxia and redox agents may alter the function of K^+ channels, directly (Jiang and Haddad, 1994) or by modulating the levels of ROS, a diffusible redox mediator. It is unknown whether the electrophysiological effects of O_2 act directly or through a redox mediator. However, for a channel to respond to a diffusible redox mediator, it probably must be intrinsically redox sensitive.

Nine families of K_v channel have been identified, each with multiple isoforms. These channels activate in a nonlinear fashion with depolarization and many are inhibited by the pore-blocking drug 4-AP. A variety of putative O_2-sensitive channels exist in the PASMCs ($K_v1.2$, $K_v1.5$, $K_v2.1$, $K_v3.1b$, and $K_v9.3$) (Coppock et al., 2001). The importance of $K_v1.5$ and $K_v2.1$, 4-AP-, and redox-sensitive channels is emphasized by two models that manifest selective suppression of HPV: the chronic hypoxic hypertension model and the $K_v1.5$ knockout mouse.

In chronic hypoxia, impairment of HPV results from loss of $K_v1.5$, and to a lesser extent $K_v2.1$, expression with concordant suppression of O_2-sensitive I_K (Reeve et al., 2001). In chronic hypoxia, enhancing expression of $K_v1.5$ via $K_v1.5$ adenoviral gene transfer (Pozeg et al., 2003) restores K_v expression, O_2-sensitive I_K, and HPV. Mice with targeted $K_v1.5$ deletions also have impaired HPV and reduced PASMC O_2-sensitive I_K (Archer et al., 2001).

Archer et al. (2004) showed that preconstriction with the K_v blocker 4-AP eliminates subsequent HPV, although the pulmonary artery constricts vigorously to phenylephrine under the same conditions. The strong parallel between constriction to the selective $K_v1.x$ channel inhibitor correolide and hypoxia suggests that a $K_v1.x$ channel is central to the mechanism of HPV (Archer et al. 2004). Theoretically, correolide can inhibit $K_v1.2$; however, tityustoxin, an inhibitor of $K_v1.2/K_v1.3$, inhibits only a small portion of the hypoxia-sensitive I_K (Archer et al. 2004). Moreover, intracellular dialysis of PASMCs with antibodies against intracellular domains of $K_v1.5$ causes membrane depolarization and the combination of anti-$K_v1.5$ and anti-$K_v2.1$ blunts responsiveness to hypoxia (Archer et al., 1998, Archer et al. 2004). Finally, although mRNA of many K_v channels is more abundant in resistance vs. conduit pulmonary arteries, only $K_v1.5$ protein is expressed more abundantly in resistance pulmonary arteries, which are the main locus for HPV (Archer et al., 2004).

Human $K_v1.5$, cloned from normal pulmonary artery, generates an outward K_v current at -65 mV, which is inhibited by hypoxia (Archer et al., 2004). Thus the consequence of enriched $K_v1.5$ expression in resistance pulmonary arteries is a relative hyperpolarization of resistance vs. conduit pulmonary artery smooth muscle cells (~-60 vs. ~-35 mV) (Archer et al., 2004).

Intracellular Ca^{2+} plays an obligatory role in pulmonary vasoconstriction (Gelband and Gelband, 1997, Salvaterra and Goldman, 1993); the question is the extent to which influx of extracellular Ca^{2+} vs. release of intracellular Ca^{2+} initiates HPV. There is no doubt that, as in all types of smooth muscle cells, release of Ca^{2+} from intracellular pools, particularly the SR, is important to vasoconstriction. As with the differential function of O_2-sensitive K_v channels in pulmonary artery vs. renal arteries, there are differences in handling of intracellular Ca^{2+} between SMCs in these circulations. In PASMCs, inositol triphosphate (IP$_3$) and ryanodine-sensitive Ca^{2+} stores are organized into spatially distinct compartments.

Hypoxia causes intracellular Ca^{2+} increase, reaching maximum level in 1–2 min, and this is sustained during hypoxia, reversing on return to normoxia (Robertson et al., 2000). Urena et al. (1996) found that in conduit pulmonary artery smooth muscle cell, hypoxia reduced basal intracellular Ca^{2+} and decreased Ca^{2+} spikes (Urena et al., 1996), consistent with the lack of significant HPV in conduit pulmonary arteries (Archer et al., 1996). In resistance pulmonary arteries, two subsets of PASMCs were identified, one in which hypoxia increased cytosolic Ca^{2+}, a response mimicked by KCl and inhibited by nifedipine, or the removal of extracellular Ca^{2+}, and another in which hypoxia decreased Ca^{2+} (Urena et al., 1996). These findings of longitudinal heterogeneity in Ca^{2+} homeostasis are in keeping with the previously identified K^+ channel diversity in the pulmonary circulation (Albarwani et al., 1995; Archer et al., 1996). Nonetheless, the predominant source of Ca^{2+} for HPV appears to be extracellular and it enters the PASMCs via the L-type Ca^{2+} channels. For example, in 300-µm pulmonary arteries, hypoxia (PO_2 30–50 Torr) causes vasoconstriction and increases intracellular Ca^{2+} (Harder et al., 1985), both of which were blocked by verapamil, as occurs in humans (Burghuber, 1987) and rodents (McMurtry et al., 1976).

In conclusion, ionic channels play an important role in response to hypoxia in the pulmonary arteries. In addition to responding to membrane depolarization by hypoxia, there is an increase of calcium influx in the pulmonary artery via the L-type Ca channel which signal further release of calcium from the sarcoplasmic reticulum. Clearly, hypoxia increases calcium entry through stored-operated channels (SOCs), enhances calcium sensitivity, and increases vascular smooth muscle contraction and proliferation (Weir et al., 2005; Weir et al., 2006)

5. Pulmonary vascular remodeling

The pulmonary circulation is a low-pressure, high-flow system with a great capacity for recruitment of normally unperfused vessels. As a consequence, the walls of pulmonary arteries are thin, in keeping with their low transmural pressure. PH is a disease of the small pulmonary arteries, characterized by vascular narrowing and thickening, leading to a progressive increase in pulmonary vascular resistance. The consequence of this increased right ventricle afterload is the failure of the after load-intolerant right ventricle. The vascular remodeling is characterized by hypertrophy of the vascular media and the extension of smooth muscle to previously unmuscularized pulmonary arterioles (Hislop and Reid, 1976; Reid, 1979; Stenmark and Mecham, 1997). The process of pulmonary vascular remodeling involves all layers of the vessel wall and is complicated by the cellular heterogeneity which exists within the compartment of the pulmonary arterial wall (Jeffery et al., 2002). Indeed, each cell type (endothelial, smooth muscle, and fibroblast), as well as inflammatory cells and platelets, may play a significant role in PH. There is endothelial cell injury, migration of smooth muscle cells into the subintima, thickening of the medial layer, and increased production of collagen and elastin within the vessel wall (Gibbons and Dzau, 1994). Similar pathological changes are shown in most, if not all, broilers with chronic PH (Enkvetchakul et al., 1995; Xiang et al., 2002). Many factors are involved in the remodeling response in PH in humans and experimental animals (Jeffery and Wanstall, 2001).

In order to determine whether pulmonary arteriolar remodeling is related to eNOS expression in the vascular pulmonary bed of hypoxia-induced PH in broiler chickens, we investigated NOS expression and remodeling in lung vessels of hypertensive and nonhypertensive broilers reared at high altitude (2638 masl). In this study, we demonstrated that normal broilers expressed greater amounts of NOS than PH broilers, and that NOS expression was inversely associated with vascular remodeling. PH broilers had thicker muscular and adventitial layers in pulmonary arterioles when compared with normotensive ones (Figures 9 and 10). We concluded that hypoxia-induced remodeling of pulmonary arterioles in broiler chickens appears to be associated with decreased endothelial NO production (Moreno de Sandino and Hernandez, 2006); the inhibition effect might be associated with decreased NO-induced apoptosis in PASMCs (Tan et al., 2005a). We concluded that the vascular remodeling could be mediated, at least in part, by decreased NO release by endothelial cells (Moreno de Sandino and Hernandez, 2006; Stenmark and Mecham, 1997).

Recent studies demonstrated that supplemental L-arginine inhibited remodeling in hypertensive broilers, an effect associated with NO-induced apoptosis of smooth muscle cells (Tan et al., 2005a) and NO-induced loss of expression of protein kinase C (Tan et al., 2006) in pulmonary arterioles. Other mechanisms involved in this process might include the direct anti-mitogenic effect of NO on smooth muscle cells (Thomae et al., 1995), NO-induced loss of production or expression in vasoconstrictors and mitogens such as ET-1 and platelet-derived growth factor (Kourembanas et al., 1993), and NO-induced loss of MMP activity in the lung (Souza-Costa et al., 2005). However, these mechanisms remain to be studied in broilers.

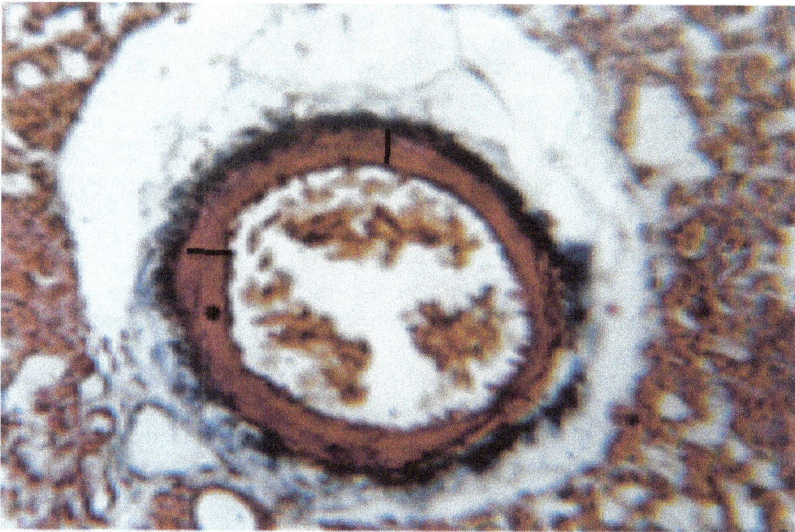

Fig. 9. Non-hypertensive chicken's arteriole. Thin smooth muscular (stained in red and indicated by black lines) and adventitial (dark blue) layers. Masson trichromic-stained.

Hypoxic arterial remodeling includes proliferation and migration of PASMCs. Platelet derived growth factor (PDGF) has also been implicated in these processes. Schermuly et al. (2005) found that administration of STI571, a PDGF receptor inhibitor, reversed pulmonary vascular changes in hypoxia-induced PH. Conversely, we did not find differences in PDGF mRNA expression levels between PH broilers and their controls (Gómez et al., 2007).

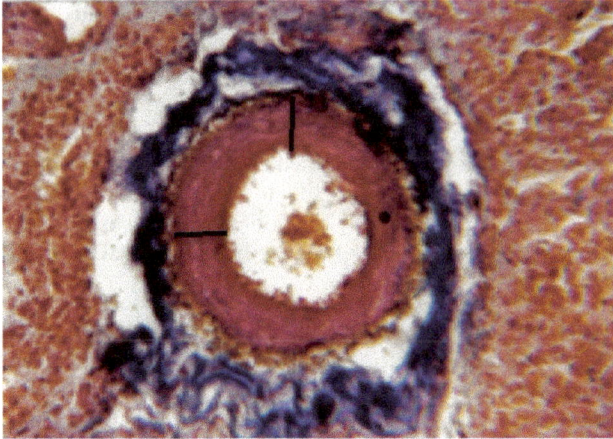

Fig. 10. Hypertensive chicken´s arteriole. Thick smooth muscular (stained in red and indicated by black lines) and surrounding adventitial (stained in dark blue) layers. Masson trichromic stain.

ET-1 participates in remodeling by increasing the connective tissue growth factor (CTGF) mRNA expression, promoter activity, and protein production (Rodriguez-Vita et al., 2005). CTGF regulates cell proliferation and apoptosis, angiogenesis, migration, adhesion, and fibrosis (Brigstock, 1999; Perbal, 2004). In order to determine if CTGF is involved in the PH in chickens, we investigated the CTGFmRNA in hypoxic hypertensive chickens and non hypertensive broilers reared in altitude (2638 masl). We demonstrated an increase in the CTGF mRNA expression levels in hypertensive chickens, which suggests that CTGF could be a mediator of fibrotic effects of ET-1 in hypoxic PH (Gómez et al., 2007). Some investigators suggest that the CTGF might be considered as a new target for therapeutic interventions in PH (Rodriguez-Vita et al., 2005). This is supported by the results of our work (Gómez et al., 2007).

Adrenomedullin (AM) is a potent vasodilator peptide that was originally isolated from human pheochromocytoma (Kitamura et al., 1993). Immunoreactive AM has subsequently been detected in plasma and in a variety of tissues, including blood vessels and lungs (Ichiki et al., 1994; Sakata et al., 1994). It has been reported that there are abundant binding sites for AM in the lungs. Owji et al., 1995; Kakishita et al.,1999; Yoshibayashi et al., 1997 have shown that the plasma AM level increases in proportion to the severity of PH and that circulating AM is partially metabolized in the lungs. Interestingly, AM has been shown to inhibit the migration and proliferation of vascular smooth muscle cells (Horio et al., 1995; Kano et al., 1996). These findings suggest that AM plays an important role in the regulation of pulmonary vascular tone and vascular remodeling. In fact, experimental studies (Heaton et al., 1995; Nossaman et al., 1996) have demonstrated that intralobar arterial infusion of AM induces pulmonary vasodilation in rats and cats. In humans, short-term intravenous infusion of AM significantly decreases pulmonary vascular resistance in patients with congestive heart failure (Nagaya et al., 2000a) or IPAH (Nagaya et al., 2000). Intravenously administered AM also decreases systemic arterial pressure in such patients, as well as in experimental models of PH (Nagaya et al., 1999, 2000, 2005; Nishikimi et al., 2003; Okumura et al., 2004), via a nonselective vasodilation of pulmonary and systemic vascular beds.

Nagaya et al (2003) showed that repeated inhalation of AM inhibited monocrotaline-induced pulmonary hypertension without systemic hypotension and improved survival in rats. Thus, they suggest that the long-term treatment with aerosolized AM may be a new therapeutic strategy for the treatment of PH.

We and others also showed that AM mRNA expression is decreased in pulmonary hypertensive broilers compared with non-hypertensive chickens (Gómez et al., 2007; Nakayama et al., 1998; Wang et al., 2001; Xu et al., 2002).

Adrenomedullin actives the PI3K/Akt-dependent pathway in vascular endothelial cells (Nishimatsu et al., 2001), which is considered to regulate angiogenesis (Jiang et al., 2000). In an *in vitro* study, AM was upregulated by the hypoxia inducible factor-1 under hypoxic conditions (Garayoa et al., 2000). These results suggest that hypoxia simulates AM synthesis, which plays an important regulatory role in pulmonary circulation and vascular remodeling (Wang et al., 2001) and represents a compensatory mechanism as an angiogenic factor promoting neovascularization under hypoxic conditions (Nagaya et al., 2005).

It should be noted that several other molecules appear to participate in the vascular response to hypoxia, such as serotonin (Chapman and Wideman, 2002) and thromboxane (Wideman et al., 1999), nuclear factor, interleukin-6, and early growth response-1 (Semenza, 2000).

Although little is known about the pathogenesis of remodeling in hypertensive broilers, evidence is emerging that there is reduced apoptosis in vascular smooth muscle cells (Tan et al., 2005a) and increased expression of protein kinase C (Tan et al., 2005b), a key enzyme in promoting the proliferation and differentiation of vascular smooth muscle cells and non-muscle cells (Assender et al., 1994; Haller et al., 1995; Wang et al., 1997; Fleming et al., 1998). Additionally, using an immunohistochemical technique, Ozyigit et al. (2005) found that the expression of matrix metalloproteinase (MMP)-2, MMP-9 and tissue inhibitors of metalloproteinase (TIMP)-1 were increased in the lung of broilers with salt-induced PHS, and that MMP-2 was localized mainly in pulmonary vascular endothelium whereas TIMP-1 was localized in the adventitia. MMPs are matrix-degrading enzymes involved in extracellular matrix turnover, smooth muscle cell and endothelial cell migration and proliferation. Increased MMP-2 activity in the pulmonary vessels of hypoxic rats was shown to be associated with the severity of PH (Frisdal et al., 2001). In addition, Herget et al. (2003) reported that inhibition of MMP activity attenuated pulmonary vascular remodeling as well as hypertension in chronically hypoxic rats, and suggested that the increased MMP activity might represent a substantial factor mediating the effect of hypoxia on the development of PH. Another study by Lepetit et al. (2005) demonstrated an imbalance between MMP-3 and TIMP-1 expression and an increase in MMP-2 expression in pulmonary arterial smooth muscle cells from patients with IPAH. These authors speculated that the imbalance between MMP-3 and TIMP-1 might lead to extracellular matrix accumulation and that the increased MMP-2 expression contributes to smooth muscle cell migration and proliferation (Lepetit et al., 2005). In this context, the results from mammals are indicative that the development of pulmonary vascular remodeling in hypertensive broilers may be related to alterations in the expression of MMPs and their TIMPs (e.g., MMP-2 and TIMP-1). However, definitive studies need to be designed to test this hypothesis.

Vascular remodeling will contribute to a sustained elevation in pulmonary arterial pressure and become progressively important as the disease advances because of an increased pulmonary vascular resistance to blood flow and a decreased vascular compliance response. Therefore, inhibiting remodeling may be an important approach for prevention in PH (Jeffery et al., 2001). The development of a resistant genetic strain of commercial chickens to hypobaric hypoxia as a long-term goal should be a coherent strategy to diminish PH in chickens, with a concomitant economic impact. Furthermore, the avian model has been accepted as a model to study PH in mammals. Hence, future research is expected to support pharmacological approaches to be applied in another animal species, including man.

6. References

Adnot S., Raffestin B., Eddhahibi S., Braquet P., Chabrier P. Loss of endothelium-dependent relaxant activity in the pulmonary circulation of rats exposed to chronic hypoxia.J.Clin.Invest. 87: 155-162, 1991.

Albarwani S., Heinert G., Turner J, and Kozlowski RZ. Differential K^+ channel distribution in smooth muscle cells isolated from the pulmonary arterial tree of the rat. Biochem Biophys Res Commun 208: 183–189, 1995.

Alexander AF., Jensen, R. Gross cardiac changes in cattle with high mountain disease and in experimental cattle maintained at high altitudes. Am J Vet Res 20: 680 – 689, 1959.

Alonso, D. and Radomski, MW. The nitric oxide–endothelin-1 connection. Heart Failure Rev, 8: 107–115. 2003.

Archer SL, Huang JMC, Reeve HL., Hampl V., Tolarova S., Michelakis ED., and Weir EK. Differenti.al distribution.n of electrophysiologically distinct myocytes in conduit and resistance arteries determines their response to nitric oxide and hypoxia. Circ Res 78: 431–442, 1996.

Archer SL., Souil E., Dinh-Xuan AT., Schremmer B., Mercier JC., El Yaagoubi A., Nguyen-Huu L., Reeve HL, and Hampl V. Molecular identification of the role of voltage-gated K+ channels, Kv1.5 .and Kv21, in hypoxic pulmonary vasoconstriction and control of resting membrane potential in rat pulmonary artery myocytes. J Clin Invest 101: 2319-2330, 1998.

Archer S., Rich S. Primary pulmonary hypertension: A vascular biology and translational research "work in progress." Circulation 102:2781-2791, 2000.

Archer SL., London B., Hampl V., Wu X., Nsair A, Puttagunta L., Hashimoto K., Waite RE., and Michelakis ED. Impairment of hypoxic .pulmonary vasoconstriction in mice lacking the voltage-gated potassium channel Kv1.5. FASEB J 15: 1801–1803, 2001.

Archer SL., Wu XC., Thebaud B., Nsair A., Bonnet S., Tyrrell B., McMurtry MS., Hashimoto K., Harry G., and Michelakis ED. Preferential expression and function of voltage-gated, O_2-sensitive K+ channels in resistance pulmonary arteries explains regional heterogeneity in hypoxic pulmonary vasoconstriction. Ionic diversity in smooth muscle cells. Circ Res 95: 308–318, 2004.

Areiza, R. Posible papel de la vascularización pulmonar en la resistencia/susceptibilidad a la hipertensión arterial pulmonar en una estirpe comercial de pollos de engorde. Tesis de Doctorado. Universidad Nacional de Colombia, Bogotá. 2010.

Assender JW., Kontny E., and Fredholm BB. Expression of protein kinase C isoforms in smooth muscle cells in various states of differentiation. FEBS Letters, 342, 76_80, 1994.

Balyakina, EV., Chen, D., Lawrence, ML., Manning, S., Parker, RE., Shappell., SB., and Meyrick, B. ET-1 receptor expression and distribution in L1 and L2 cells from hypertensive sheep pulmonary atery. Am J Physiol Cell Mol Physiol 283: L42-51, 2002.

Bartsch, P., H. Mairbaurl, M. Maggiorini, and E. R. Swenson. 2005. Physiological aspects of high-altitude pulmonary edema. J. Appl. Physiol. 98:1101–1110, 2005.

Barnes, P.J. and Belvisi, M.G. Nitric oxide and lung disease. Thorax 48:1034-1043, 1993.

Bennie RE., Packer CS., Powell DR., Jin N., and Rhoades RA. Biphasic contractile response of pulmonary artery to hypoxia. American J of Physiol 261:L156-163, 1991.

Bernal, L., Noguera, I., Hernández, A.. Comparación morfométrica e histológica del corazón, hígado, tiroides y adrenales en pollos ascíticos y sanos. Rev. Med. Vet. Zoot. 37:5-19, 1984.

Bindslev L., Jolin A., Hedenstierna G., Baehrendtz S., and Santesson J. Hypoxic pulmonary vasoconstriction in the human lung: effect of repeated hypoxic challenges during anesthesia. Anesthesiology 62: 621–625, 1985.

Bodi, I., Bisphoric, NH., Discher, DJ., Wu, X., and Webster, KA. Cell specificity and signaling pathway of endothelin-1 gene regulation by hypoxia. Cardivascular Res 30: 975-984. 1995.

Bradford J., and Dean H. The pulmonary circulation. J Physiol 16: 34–96, 1894.

Brigstock D.R. The connective tissue growth factor/cysteine-rich 61/nephroblastoma overexpressed (CCN) family. Endocr. Rev. 20:189–206, 1999.

Brimioulle S., LeJeune P., and Naeije R. Effects of hypoxic pulmonary vasoconstriction on pulmonary gas exchange. J Appl Physiol 81: 1535–1543, 1996.

Budhiraja R., Tuder RM., Hassoun PM. Endotelial dysfunction in pulmonary hypertension. Circulation, 109: 159-165, 2004.

Burghuber OC. Nifedipine attenuates acute hypoxic pulmonary vasoconstriction in patients with chronic obstructive pulmonary disease. Respiration 52: 86–93, 1987.

Burton RR., Smith AH. Effect of policytemia and chronic hypoxia on heart mass in the chicken. J. Appl. Physiol. 22 (15): 782-785, 1967.

Burton RR., Besch EL, Smith AH.. Effect of chronic hypoxia on the pulmonary arterial blood pressure of the chicken. Am. J. Physiol. 214 (6): 1438-1444, 1967.

Camacho-Fernández, D. López, C., Ávila, E., J. Arce, J. Evaluation of Different Dietary Treatments to Reduce Ascites Syndrome and Their Effects on Corporal Characteristics in Broiler Chickens. J Appl Poult Res 11: 164-174, 2002.

Cárdenas, D., Hernández, A. , Osuna, O. Algunos valores hematimétricos y de proteínas totales en pollos Arbor Acres sanos y ascíticos en la Sabana de Bogotá. Rev. ACOVEZ. 9:42-46, 1985

Cardillo C., Kilcoyne CM., Waclawiw M., Cannon RO III, and Panza JA. Role of endothelin in the increased vascular tone of patients with essential hypertension. Hypertension 33:753–758, 1999.

Chen YF. and Oparil S. Endothelin and pulmonary hypertension. J. Cardiovasc. Pharmacol. 35:S49–S53, 2000.

Chapman ME., and Wideman RF Jr. Hemodynamic responses of broiler pulmonary vasculature to intravenously infused serotonin. Poult. Sci. 81:231–238, 2002.

Cogo, A., R. Fischer, and R. Schoene. Respiratory diseaes and high altitude. High Alt. Med. Biol. 5:435–444, 2004.

Colmenares, H., Hernández, A., Sandino, M., Useche, J. Diferentes grados de reacción eritropoyética a la hipoxia en pollos de engorde. En: Resúmenes. XVII Congreso

Nacional de Medicina Veterinaria y Zootecnia. Popayán- Cauca, Colombia. p. 21, 1990.

Coppock EA., Martens JR., and Tamkun MM. Molecular basis of hypoxia-induced pulmonary vasoconstriction: role of voltage-gated K+ channels. Am J Physiol Lung Cell Mol Physiol 281: L1–L12, 2001.

Cooke J., and Dzau J. Nitric oxide synthase: role in the genesis of vascular disease. Annu Rev Med 48:489-509, 1997.

Cooper CJ., Landzberg MJ., Anderson TJ., Charbonneau MA., Creager P., and Selwyn AP. Role of nitric oxide in the local regulation of pulmonary vascular resistance in humans. Circulation 93:266-271, 1996.

Cueva S., Sillau H., Valenzuela A., Ploog HP. High altitude induced pulmonary hypertension and right heart failure in broiler chickens. Res. Vet. Sci. 16 (6): 370-374, 1974.

Currie, R. J. Ascites in poultry: Recent investigations. Avian Pathol. 28:313–326, 1999.

Dalmau, E.A. Estudio morfológico y morfométrico en el pulmón y posibles correlaciones con parámetros hematimétricos, volumen pulmonar e índice cardíaco en pollos de engorde sanos y con ascitis de origen hipóxico. Tesis de M.Sc. Universidad Nacional. Bogotá, 1997.

Davie N., Haleen SJ., Upton PD., Polak JM., Yacoub MH., Morrell NW., and Wharton J. ET$_A$ and ET$_B$ receptors modulate the proliferation of human pulmonary artery smooth muscle cells. *Am J Respir Crit Care Med* 165: 398–405, 2002.

Demiryurek, A. T., Wadsworth, R. M., Kane, K. A. and Peacock, A. J. The role of endothelium in hypoxic constriction of human pulmonary artery rings. American Review of Respiratory Disease 147, 283-290, 1993.

Dinh-Xuan AT., Higenbottam TW., Pepke-Zaba J., Clelland CA., and Wallwork J. Reduced endothelium dependent relaxation of cystic fibrosis pulmonary arteries. Eur J Pharmacol 163:401-403, 1989.

Dinh-Xuan AT., Higenbottam TW., Wallwork J. Relationship between chronic hypoxia and in vitro pulmonary relaxation mediated by endfothelium derived relaxing factors in human chronic obstructive lung disease. Angiology. 43:350-356, 1992.

Dorrington KL., Clar C., Young JD., Jonas M, Tansley JG., and Robbins PA. Time course of the human pulmonary vascular respon.se to 8 hours of isocapnic hypoxia. Am J Physiol Heart Circ Physiol 273: H1126–H1134, 1997.

Durmowicz AG., Hofmeister S., Kadyraliev TK.; Aldashev,A.A.; Stenmark,K.R. Functional and structural adaptation of the yak pulmonary circulation to residence at high altitude. J Appl Physiol 74(5): 2276-2285, 1993.

Eddahibi, S., Adnot S., Carville C., Blouquit Y., and Raffestin B. L-arginine restores endothelium-dependent relaxation in pulmonary circulation of chronically hypoxic rats. Am J Physiol 26: L194-L200, 1992.

Enkvetchakul B., Beasley J., and Bottje W. Pulmonary arteriole hypertrophy in broilers with pulmonary hypertension syndrome (ascites). Poul. Sci. 74:1676-1682, 1995.

Filep, JG., Foldes-Flip, E., Rousseau, A., Sirois, P., and Fournier, A. Vacular response of enfothelin-1 following inhibition of nitric oxide synthesis in the conscious rat. Br J Pharmacol 110: 1213-1221. 1993.

Fleming I., MacKenzie SJ., Vernon RG., Anderson NG., Houslay MD., and Kilgour E. Protein kinase C isoforms play differential roles in the regulation of adipocyte differentiation. The Biochemical Journal 333:719-727, 1998.

Forstermann U., Boissel JP., and Kleinert H. Expressional control of the "constitutive" isoforms of nitric oxide synthase (NOS I and NOS III). The FASEB Journal 2:773-790, 1998.

Frisdal E., Gest V., Vieillard-Baron A., Levame M., Lepetit H., Eddahibi S., Lafuma C., Harf A., Adnot S. , and Dortho MP. Gelatinase expression in pulmonary arteries during experimental pulmonary hypertension. The European Respiratory Journal 18:838-845, 2001.

Garayoa M., Martinez A., Lee S., Pio R., An WG., Neckers L., Trepel J., Montuenga LM., Ryan H., Johnson R., Gassmann M. and Cuttitta F. Hypoxia-inducible factor-1 (HIF-1) up-regulates adrenomedullin expression in human tumor cell lines during oxygen deprivation: A possible promotion mechanism of carcinogenesis. Mol. Endocrinol. 14:848-862, 2000.

Gelband CH and Gelband H. Ca^{2+} release from intracellular stores is an initial step in hypoxic pulmonary vasoconstriction of rat pulmonary artery resistance vessels. Circulation 96: 3647-3654, 1997.

Geraci MW., Moore M., Gesell T., et al. Gene expression patterns in the lungs of patients with primary pulmonary hypertension: A gene microarray analysis. Circ Res 88:555-562, 2001.

Giaid A and Saleh D. Reduced expression of endothelial nitric oxide synthase in the lungs of patients with pulmonary hypertension. N Engl J Med 333: 214-221, 1995.

Giaid A., Yanagisawa M., Langleben D., Michel RP., Levy R., Shennib H., Kimura S., Masaki T., Duguid WP. and Stewart DJ. Expression of endothelin-1 in the lungs of patients with pulmonary hypertension. The New England Journal of Medicine, 328:1732-1739, 1993.

Giaid A. Nitric oxide and endothelin-1 in pulmonary hypertension. Chest 114:208-212, 1998.

Gibbons GH. and Dzau VJ. The emerging concept of vascular remodelling. T,he New England J Med 330, 1431_1438, 1994.

Girgis RE., Champion HC., Diette GB., Johns RA., Permutt S. and Sylvester JT. Decreased exhaled nitric oxide in pulmonary arterial hypertension: response to bosentan therapy. Am J Resp Crit Care 172: 352-357, 2005.

Glogowska, M, P.S. Richardson, P.S J.G. Widdicombe, J.G., Winning, A.J. The role of the vagus nerves, peripheral chemoreceptors and other afferent pathways in the genesis of augmented breaths in cats and rabbits. Respir Physiol 16(2): 179-196, 1972.

Gómez AP., Moreno MJ., Iglesias A., Coral PX. and Hernandez A. Endothelin 1, its endothelin type a receptor, connective tissue growth factor, platelet-derived growth factor, and adrenomedullin expression in lungs of pulmonary hypertensive and nonhypertensive chickens. Poultry Science 86:909-916, 2007.

Gómez, AP., Moreno MJ., Baldrich RM., AND Hernández A. " Endothelin-1 Molecular Ribonucleic Acid Expression in Pulmonary Hypertensive and nonhypertensive Chickens. Poultry Science 87: 1395-1401, 2008.

Graham, R.S., and Milsom, K.M. Control of breathing and adaptation to high altitude in the bar-headed goose Am J Physiol Regul Integr Comp Physiol 293: R379–R391, 2007.

Grant JL., Naylor RW., and Crandell WB. Bronchial adenoma resection with relief of hypoxic pulmonary vasoconstriction. Chest 77: 446–449, 1980.

Greenlees KJ., and Tucker A. Hypoxic pressor responses in lungs from rats acutely exposed to simulated high altitude. Respiration 45: 169–174, 1984.

Grover FR., Wagner WW., McMurtry IV., Reeves JT. Pulmonary circulation; the cardiovascular system. In: Handbook of physiology, Vol III, part 1. American Physiological Soc, sec 2, vol 3 part 1:103-106, 1983.

Gruetter CA., Barry BK., McNamara DB., Gruetter DY., Kadowitz PJ., Ignarro L. Relaxation of bovine coronary artery and activation of coronary arterial guanylate cyclase by nitric oxide, nitroprusside and a carcinogenic nitrosoamine. J Cyclic Nucl Prot 5:211–224, 1979.

Guo FH., De Raeve HR., Rice TW., Stuehr DJ., Thunnissen FB., and Erzurum, S.C. Continuous nitric oxide synthesis by inducible nitric oxide synthase in normal human airway epithelium in vivo. P Natl Acad Sci-Biol 92:7809-7813, 1995.

Guzmán, L, Sandino de M, Hernández, A. Hipertensión arterial pulmonar en pollos de engorde inoculados experimentalmente con mycoplasma gallisepticum. Rev Col Cienc Pec 14 (supl):55, 2001.

Haller H., Lindschau C., Quass P., Distler A., and Luft FC. Differentiation of vascular smooth muscle cells and the regulation of protein kinase C. Circ Res, 76:22-29, 1995.

Hambraeus-Jonzon K., Bindslev L., Mellgard AJ., and Hedenstierna G. Hypoxic pulmonary vasoconstriction in human lungs. A stimulus-response study. Anesthesiology 86: 308–315, 1997.

Hampl V., Weir EK., and Archer SL. Endothelium-derived nitric oxide is less important for basal tone regulation in the pulmonary than the renal vessels of adult rat. J Vasc Med Biol 5: 22–30, 1994.

Harder DR., Madden JA., and Dawson C. Hypoxic induction of Ca^{2+}-dependent action potentials in small pulmonary arteries of the cat. J Appl Physiol 59: 1389–1393, 1985.

Hassanzadeh, M., Gilanpour, H., Charkhkar, S., Buyise, J., Decuypere, E. Anatomical parameters of cardiopulmonary system in three different lines of chickens: further evidence for involvement in ascites syndrome. Avian Pathol 34(3): 188-193, 2005.

Hasunuma K, Rodman D., and McMurtry I. Effects of K^+ channel blockers on vascular tone in the p.erfused rat lung. Am Rev Respir Dis 144: 884–887, 1991.

Heaton J, Lin B, Chang JK, Steinberg S, Hyman A, and Lippton H. Pulmonary vasodilation to adrenomedullin: a novel peptide in humans. Am J Physiol Heart Circ Physiol 268: H2211–H2215, 1995.

Herget J., Novotna J., Bibova J., Povysilova V., Vankova M., and Hampl V. Metalloproteinase inhibition by Batimastat attenuates pulmonary hypertension in chronically hypoxic rats. Am J of Physiol Lung Cellular and Molecular Physiol 285:L199-208, 2003.

Hernández, A. 1982. Influencia de la altitud, el sexo, la raza y el nivel energético de la ración en la incidencia de la ascitis de origen hipóxico en pollos de engorde. Rev. Fac. Med. Vet. Zoot. Universidad Nacional de Colombia, Bogotá, 35:1.

Hernández, A. 1984. Disminución de la incidencia de la ascitis aviar de origen hipóxico en el incremento de la temperatura en los galpones. XIV Cong. Nal. de Med. Vet. y Zoot. Cartagena. Memorias p. 6

Hernández, A. Hypoxic ascites in broilers: A review of several studies done in Colombia. Avian Dis. 31:658- 663, 1987.

Hislop, A, and Reid L. New findings in pulmonary arteries of rats with hypoxia-induced pulmonary hypertension. Br J Exp Pathol 57: 542-554, 1976.

Horio T, Kohno M, Kano H, Ikeda M, Yasunari K, Yokokawa K, Minami M, and Takeda T. Adrenomedullin as a novel antimigration factor of vascular smooth muscle cells. *Circ Res* 77: 660–664, 1995.

Hoshino Y., Morison K.J., and Vanhoutte PM. Mechanisms of hypoxic vasoconstriction in the canine isolated pulmonary artery: role of endothelium and sodium pump. Am J of Physiol 267:L120-127, 1994.

Huang PL., Hyang LZ., and Mashimo H. Hypertension in mice lacking the gene for endothelial nitric oxide synthase. Natue 377:239-242, 1995.

Huchzermeyer, F.W, Cilliers, J., Diasla-Vigne, A., Celestina, D. Broiler pulmonary hypertension syndrome. I. Increased right ventricular mass in broilers experimentally infected with Aegyptanella pullorum, Ondestepoort J. Vet Res. 54: 113, 1987.

Huchzermeyer FM., De Ruyck A.N, Vanark H. Broiler pulmonary hypertension syndrome. III. Comercial broiler strains differ in their susceptibility. Onderstepoort J. Vet. Res. 55: 5-9, 1988.

Humbert M., Silbon O., Simonneau G. Treatment of pulmonary arterial hypertension. N Engl J Med 351:1425-1436, 2004.

Ichiki Y., Kitamura K., Kangawa K., Kawamoto M., Matsuo H., and Eto T. Distribution and characterization of immunoreactive adrenomedullin in human tissue and plasma. FEBS Lett 338: 6–10, 1994.

Ignarro LJ. Endothelium-derived nitric oxide: actions and properties. Faseb J. 3: 31-36, 1989.

Ignarro LJ. Biosyntesis and metabolism of endothelium - derived nitric oxide. Ann. Rev. Pharmacol.Toxicol.30: 535-560, 1990.

Inagami T., Mitsuhide N., Hoover R. Endothelium as an endocrine organ. Annu Rev. Physiol 57: 171-189, 1995.

Jeffery TK., and Wanstall JC. Pulmonary vascular remodeling: a target for therapeutic intervention in pulmonary hypertension. Pharmacology and Therapeutics, 92, 1_20, 2001.

Jeffery TK., Morrell NW. Molecular and cellular basis of pulmonary vascular remodeling in pulmonary hypertension. Prog Cardiovasc Dis. 45:173–202, 2002.

Jia L., Bonaventura C., Bonaventura J., and Stamler JS. S-Nitrosohaemoglobin: a dynamic activity of blood involved in vascular control. Nature 380:221-226, 1996.

Jiang C and Haddad GG. A direct mechanism for sensing low oxygen levels by central neurons. Proc Natl Acad Sci USA 91: 7198–7201, 1994

Jiang BH., Zheng JZ., Aoki M., and Vogt PK. Phosphatidylinositol 3-kinase signaling mediates angiogenesis and expression of vascular endothelial growth factor in endothelial cells. Proc. Natl. Acad. Sci. USA 97:1749–1753, 2000.

Kakishita M., Nishikimi T., Okano Y., Satoh T., Kyotani S., Nagaya N., Fukushima K., Nakanishi N., Takishita S., Miyata A., Kangawa K., Matsuo H., and Kunieda T. Increased plasma levels of adrenomedullin in patients with pulmonary hypertension. *Clin Sci (Lond)* 96: 33–39, 1999.

Kanazawa F., Nakanishi K., Osada Y., Kanamaru N., Ohrui M., Uenoyama Y., Masaki Y., Kanatani S., Hiroi S., Tominaga A., Yakata-Suzuki S., Matsuyama S., and Kawai T. Expression of endothelin-1 in the brain and lung of rats exposed to permanent hypobaric hypoxia. Brain Res. 1036:145–154, 2005.

Kaneko FT., Arroliga AC., Dweik RA., Comhair SA., Laskowski D., Oppedisano R., Thomassen MJ. and Erzurum SC. Biochemical reaction products of nitric oxide as quantitative markers of primary pulmonary hypertension. Am J of Resp and Critical Care Medicine, 158 , 917 _923, 1998.

Kano H., Kohno M., Yasunari K., Yokokawa K., Horio T., Ikeda M., Minami M., Hanehira T., Takeda T., and Yoshikawa J. Adrenomedullin as a novel antiproliferative factor of vascular smooth muscle cells. J Hypertens 14: 209–213, 1996.

Kato M and Staub N. Response of small pulmonary arteries to unilobar alveolar hypoxia and hypercapnia. Circ Res 19: 426–440, 1966.

Kitamura K., Kangawa K., Kawamoto M., Ichiki Y., NakamuraS., Matsuo H., and Eto T. Adrenomedullin: a novel hypotensive peptide isolated from human pheochromocytoma. Biochem Biophys Res Commun 192: 553–560, 1993.

Knowles RG., and Moncada S. Nitric oxide synthases in mammals. The Biochemical Journal 298: 249 -258, 1994.

Kobzik L., Bredt DS., Lowenstein C.J., Drazen J., Gaston B., Sugarbaker D., and Stamler JS. Nitric oxide synthase in human and rat lung: immunocytochemical and histochemical localization. Am J of Resp Cell and Molecular Biology 9:371-377, 1993.

Kourembanas, S., Marsden, P.A., Mcquillan, L.P., Faller, D.V. Hypoxia induces endothelin gene expression and secretion in cultured human endothelium. J. Clin. Invest. 88:1054–1057, 1991.

Kourembanas S., McQuillan LP., Leung GK. and Faller DV. Nitric oxide regulates the expression of vasoconstrictors and growth factors by vascular endothelium under both normoxia and hypoxia. The Journal of Clinical Investigation 92: 99-104, 1993.

Kouyoumdjian C., Adnot S., Levame M., Eddahibi S., Bousbaa H., Raffestin B. Continuous inhalation of nitric oxide protects against development of pulmonary hypertension in chronically hypoxic rats. J Clin Invest 94:578-584, 1994.

Lavallee, M., Takamura, M., Parent, R. and Thorin, E. Crosstalk between endothelin and nitric oxide in the control of vascular tone. Heart Failure Reviews, 6 , 265 _276, 2001.

Lahiri, S., Roy, A., Baby, S.M., Hoshi, T., Semenza, G.L., Prabhakar, N.R. Oxygen sensing in the body. Prog Biophys Mol Biol 91(3):249-86, 2006.

Leach RM., Robertson TP., Twort CH. and Ward JP. Hypoxic vasoconstriction in rat pulmonary and mesenteric arteries. American J of Physiol 266:L223-231, 1994.

Lepetit H., Eddahibi S., Fadel E., Frisdal E., Munaut C., Noel A., Humbert M., Adnot S., D'Ortho MP., and Lafuma C. Smooth muscle cell matrix metalloproteinases in idiopathic pulmonary arterial hypertension. Europ Respir J 25:834-842, 2005.

Li H., Chen SJ., Chen YF., Meng QC., Durand J., Oparil S., and Elton TS. Enhanced endothelin-1 and endothelin receptor gene expression in chronic hypoxia. J. Appl. Physiol. 77:1451-1459, 1994.

Luscher TF. and Barton M. Endothelins and endothelin receptor antagonists: therapeutic considerations for a novel class of cardiovascular drugs. Circulation 102 :2434-2440, 2000.

Machado RF., Londhe Nerkar MV., Dweik RA., Hammel J., Janocha A., Pyle J., Laskowski D., Jennings C., Arroliga AC.and Erzurum SC. Nitric oxide and pulmonary arterial pressures in pulmonary hypertension. Free Radical Biology and Medicine 37:1010-1017, 2004.

Madden JA., Vadula MS., and Kurup VP. Effects of hypoxia and other vasoactive agents on pulmonary and cerebral artery smooth muscle cells. Amer J Physiol 263:L384-393,1992.

Malconian MK., Rock PB., Reeves JT., Cymerman A., and Houston CS. Operation Everest II: gas tensions in expired air and arterial blood at extreme altitude. Aviat Space Environ Med 64: 37–42, 1993.

Marshall C and Marshall B. Site and sensitivity for stimulation of hypoxic pulmonary vasoconstriction. J Appl Physiol 55: 711–716, 1983.

Martinez-Lemus LA., Hester RK., Becker EJ., Jeffrey JS, an Odom TW. Pulmonary artery endothelium-dependent vasodilation is impaired in a chicken model of pulmonary hypertension. The Am J of Physiol 277:R190 -R197, 1999.

Maruyama J., Maruyama K. Impaired nitric oxide dependent responses and their recovery in hypertensive pulmonary arteries of rats. Am. J. Physiol. 266(Heart Cir. Physiol. 35): H2476-H2488, 1994.

Maxwell, M. H., Robertson, G. W. World Broiler Acites Survey. Poultry International. 36, 16-30, 1997.

Maxwell, M. J., R. G. Goldie, and P. J. Henry. Altered ETB–but not ETA–receptor density and function in sheep airway smooth muscle cells in culture. Am J Physiol 274:L951–L957, 1998.

McCulloch KM., and MacLean MR. Endothelin B receptor-mediated contraction of human and rat pulmonary resistance arteries and the effect of pulmonary hypertension on endothelin responses in the rat. J. Cardiovasc. Pharmacol. 26(Suppl 3):S169-S176, 1995.

McDonald LJ., and Murad F. Nitric oxide and cGMP signalling. Advances in Pharmacology 34:263-275, 1995.

McMurtry I., Davidson B., Reeves J, and Grover R. Inhibition of hypoxic pulmonary vasoconstriction by calcium antagon.ists in isolated rat lungs. Circ Res 38: 99–104, 1976.

Mehta S., Stewart DJ., Langleben D., Levy RD. Short-term pulmonary vasodilation with L-arginine in pulmonary hypertension. Circ. 92: 1539-1545, 1995.

Mejía, G. Influencia del frío en la incidencia de la ascitis de orígen hoipóxico en pollos de engorde. Medicina Veterinaria. Universidad Nacional. Bogotá, 1982.

Meyrick, B., and L. Reid. The effect of continued hypoxia on rat pulmonary arterial circulation. An ultrastructural study. Lab. Invest. 38:188–200, 1978.

Michelakis E., Hampl V., Nsair A, Wu X., Harry G., Haromy A., Gurtu R., and Archer S. Diversity in mitochondrial function. explains differences in vascular oxygen sensing. Circ Res 90: 1307–1315, 2002.

Miller AA, Hislop AA, Vallance PJ, and Haworth SG. Deletion of the eNOS gene has a greater impact on the pulmonary circulation of male than female mice. Am J Physiol Lung Cell Mol Physiol 289: L299–L366, 2005.

Mitani Y., Maruyama K., Sakurai M. Prolonged administration of L-arginine ameliorates chronic pulmonary hypertension and pulmonary vascular remodeling in rats. Circulation. 96: 689-697, 1997.

Mizutani T., Layon J. Clinical applications of nitric oxide. Chest. 110: 506-524, 1996.

Moncada S., Palmer RM., and Higgs EA. Nitric oxide: physiology, pathophysiology, and pharmacology. Pharmacol Reviews 43:09-142, 1991.

Moncada S. The L-arginine nitric oxide pathway. The New England Journal of Medicine 329:2002-2012, 1993.

Monge C., Leon-Velarde F. Physiological adaptation to high altitude: oxygen transport in mammals and birds. Physiol. Rev. 71(4): 1135-1171, 1991.

Moore LG., Niermeyer S., and Zamudio S. Human adaptation to high altitude: regional and life-cycle perspectives. Am J Phys Anthropol Suppl 27: 25–64, 1998.

Moreno de Sandino M., and Hernandez A. Nitric oxide synthase expression in the endothelium of pulmonary arterioles in normal and pulmonary hypertensive chickens subjected to chronic hypobaric hypoxia. Avian Dis, 47:1291-1297, 2003.

Moreno de Sandino M., and Hernandez A. Pulmonary arteriole remodeling in hypoxic broilers expressing different amounts of endothelial nitric oxide synthase. Poultry Science 85:899-901, 2006.

Mortensen LH., and Fink GD. Salt-dependency of endothelin-induced, chronic hypertension in conscious rats. Hypertension 19:549–554, 1992.

Motte S., McEntee K., and Naeije R. Endothelin receptor antagonists. Pharmacol Ther 110: 386–414, 2006.

Moudgil R., Michelakis ED., and Archer S. Hypoxic pulmonary vasoconstriction J Appl Physiol 98: 390-403, 2005.

Nakayama, M., K. Takahashi, O. Murakami, K. Shirato, and S. Shibahara. Induction of adrenomedullin by hypoxia and cobalt chloride in human colorectal carcinoma cells. Biochem. Biophys. Res. Commun. 243:514–517, 1998.

Nagaya N., Mori H., Murakami S.,Kangawa, K. and Kitamura S. Adrenomedullin: Angiogenesis and gene therapy. Am. J. Physiol. Regul. Integr. Comp. Physiol. 288:R1432–R1437, 2005.

Nagaya N., Nishikimi T., Horio T., Yoshihara F., Kanazawa A., Matsuo, H. and Kangawa K. Cardiovascular and renal effects of adrenomedullin in rats with heart failure. Am. J. Physiol. 276:R213–R218, 1999.

Nagaya N., Satoh T., Nishikimi T., Uematsu, M., Furuichi S., Sakamaki F., Oya H., Kyotani S., Nakanishi N., Goto Y., Masuda Y., Miyatake K., and Kangawa. K Hemodynamic, renal, and hormonal effects of adrenomedullin infusion in patients with congestive heart failure. Circulation 101:498–503, 2000.

Nagaya N, Nishikimi T., Uematsu M., Satoh T., Oya H., Kyotani S., Sakamaki F., Ueno K., Nakanishi N., Miyatake K., and Kangawa K. Hemodynamic and hormonal effects of adrenomedullin in patients with pulmonary hypertension. Heart 84:653–658, 2000a.

Nagaya N., Okumura H., Uematsu M., Shimizu W., Ono F., Shirai M., Mori H., Miyatake K., and Kangawa K. Repeated inhalation of adrenomedullin ameliorates pulmonary hypertension and survival in monocrotaline rats. Am J Physiol Heart Circ Physiol 285: H2125–H2131, 2003.

Nandi M., Miller A., Stidwill R., Jacques TS., Lam AAJ., Haworth S., Heales S., and Vallance P. Pulmonary hypertension in GTP-cyclohydrolase 1-deficient mouse. Circulation 111: 2086–2090, 2005.

Nishikimi T., Yoshihara F., Mori Y., Kangawa K., and Matsuoka H. 2003. Cardioprotective effect of adrenomedullin in heart failure. Hypertens. Res. 26(Suppl.):S121–S127, 2003.

Nishimatsu H., Suzuki E., Nagata D., Moriyama N., Satonaka H., Walsh K., M. Sata M., Kangawa K., Matsuo H., Goto A., Kitamura T., and Hirata Y. Adrenomedullin induces endothelium-dependent vasorelaxation via the phosphatidylinositol 3-kinase/Akt-dependent pathway in rat aorta. Circ. Res. 89:63–70, 2001.

Nishimura, J., H. Aoki, X. Chen, T. Shikasho, S. Kobayashi, and H. Kanaide. Evidence for the presence of endothelin ETA receptors in endothelial cells in situ on the aortic side of porcine aortic valve. Br. J. Pharmacol. 115:1369–1376, 1995.

Nossaman BD., Feng CJ., Kaye AD., DeWitt B., Coy DH., Murphy WA., and Kadowitz PJ. Pulmonary vasodilator responses to adrenomedullin are reduced by NOS inhibitors in rats but not in cats. Am J Physiol Lung Cell Mol Physiol 270: L782–L789, 1996.

Okumura H., Nagaya N., Itoh T., Okano I., Hino J., Mori K., Tsukamoto Y., Ishibashi-Ueda H., Miw S., Tambara K., Toyokuni S., Yutani C., and Kangawa K. Adrenomedullin infusion attenuates myocardial ischemia/reperfusion injury through the phosphatidylinositol 3-kinase/Akt-dependent pathway. Circulation 109:242–248, 2004.

Owji AA, Smith DM, Coppock HA, Morgan DG, Bhogal R, Ghatei MA, and Bloom SR. An abundant and specific binding site for the novel vasodilator adrenomedullin in the rat. *Endocrinology* 136: 2127–2134, 1995.

Ozyigit MO., Kahraman MM. and Sonmez G. The identification of matrix metalloproteinases and their tissue inhibitors in broiler chickens by immunohistochemistry. Avian Pathology 34:509-516., 2005.

Paliege, A., Rosenberger, C., Bondke, A., Sciesielski, L., Shina, A., Heyman, S.N., Flippin, L.A., Arend, M., Klaus, S.J., Bachmann, S. Hypoxia-inducible factor-2alpha-expressing interstitial fibroblasts are the only renal cells that express erythropoietin under hypoxia-inducible factor stabilization. Kidney Int 77(4):312-318, 2010.

Pakdel A, Van Arendonk JA, Vereijken AL, Bovenhuis H. Genetic parameters of ascites-related traits in broilers: effect of cold and normal temperature conditions. Br Poult Sci 46(1): 35 – 42, 2005.

Pan JQ, Tan X, Li JC, Sun WD, Wang, XL. Effects of early feed restriction and cold temperature on lipid peroxidation, pulmonary vascular remodelling and ascites morbidity in broilers under normal and cold temperature. Br Poult Sci 46(3): 374–381, 2005.

Pavlidis, H. O., Balog, J. M., Stamps, L. K., Hughes, J. D., Huff, W. E., Anthony, N. B. Divergent Selection for Ascites Incidence in Chickens. Poultry Science. 86: 2517 – 2529, 2007.

Perbal B. CCN proteins: Multifunctional signalling regulators. Lancet 363:62–64, 2004.

Perrella MA, Edell ES, Krowka MJ, Cortese DA, Burnett JC Jr. Endothelium-derived relaxing factor in pulmonary and renal circulations during hypoxia. Am J Physiol 263:R45–R50, 1992.

Platoshyn O., Golovina VA, Bailey CL., Limsuwan A., Krick S., Juhaszova M., Seiden JE., Rubin LJ., and Yuan JX. .Sustained membrane depolarization and pulmonary artery smooth muscle cell proliferation. Am J Physiol Cell Physiol 279: C1540–C1549, 2000.

Post JM., Hume JR., Archer SL and Weir EK. Direct role for potassium channel inhibition in hypoxic pulmonary vasoconstriction. Ame J Physiol 262, C882-890,1992.

Potter CF., Dreshaj IA., Haxhiu MA., Stork EK., Chatburn RL., and Martin RJ. Effect of exogenous and endogenous nitric oxide on the airway and tissue components of lung resistance in the newborn piglet. Pediatr. Res. 41:886–891, 1997.

Pozeg, Z.I., Michelakis, E.D., McMurtry, M.S., Thebaud, B., Wu, X., Dyck, J.R.B. Hashimoto, K., Wang, S., Moudgil, R., Harry, G., Sultanian, R., Koshal, A., and Archer, S.L. Circulation 107: 2037-2044. 2003.

Pulido, M. Ascitis aviar de orígen hipóxico: evaluación del daño cardíaco mediante la técnica electrocardiográfica y las posibles relaciones con los valores del índice cardíaco, hematocrito y hemoglobina. Tesis de M.Sc. Universidad Nacional. Bogotá, 1996.

Rabelink TJ., Kaasjager KA, Boer P., Stroes EG, Braam B., and Koomans HA. Effects of endothelin-1 on renal function in humans: Implications for physiology and pathophysiology. Kidney Int. 46:376–381, 1994, 1994.

Rafikova O., Rafikov R., and Nudler E. (2002). Catalysis of S-nitrosothiols formation by serum albumin: the mechanism and implication in vascular control. Proceedings of the National Academy of Sciences of the United States of America 99:5913-5918, 2002.

Reddy VM., Wong J., Liddicoat JR., Johengen M., Chang R., Fineman JR. Altered endothelium-dependent responses in lambs with pulmonary hypertension and increased pulmonary blood flow. Am.J.Physiol. 271(40): H562-H570, 1996.

Reeve HL., Michelakis E., Nelson DP., Weir EK., and Archer SL. Alterations in a redox oxygen sensing mechanism in chronic hypoxia. J Appl Physiol 90: 2249–2256, 2001.

Rees DD., Palmer RM., Moncada S. Rle of endothelium-derived nitic oxide in the regulation of blood pressure. Proc Natl Acad Sci 86:3375-3378, 1989.

Reeves, JT., and R.F. Grover. Insights by Peruvian scientists into the pathogenesis of human chronic hypoxic pulmonary hypertension. J. Appl. Physiol. 98:384–389, 2005.

Reid LM. The pulmonary circulation: Remodeling in growth and disease. The 1978 J. Burns Amberson lecture. Am. Rev. Respir. Dis. 119:531–546, 1979.

Reid, L. M. The pulmonary circulation: Remodeling in growth and disease. The 1978 J. Burns Amberson lecture. Am. Rev. Respir. Dis. 119:531–546, 1979

Remillard CV., and Yuan JX. High altitude pulmonary hypertension: Role of K+ and Ca2+ channels. High Alt. Med. Biol. 6:133–146, 2005.

Rhodes J. Comparative physiology of hypoxic pulmonary hypertension: Historical clues from brisket disease. J. Appl. Physiol. 98:1092–1100, 2005.

Richard V., Hogie M., Clozel M., Loffler B., and Thuillez C. In vivo evidence of an endothelin-induced vasopressor tone after inhibition of nitric oxide synthesis in rats. Circulation 91 , pp. 771-775, 1995.

Robertson TP., Aaronson PI. and Ward JPT. Hypoxic intracellular Ca^{2+} in pulmonary arteries: evidence for PKC-independent Ca^{2+} sensitization. American J of Physiol 268:H301-307, 1995.

Robertson TP., Hague D, Aaronson PI., and Ward JP. Voltage-independent calcium entry in hypoxic pulmona.ry vasoconstriction of intrapulmonary arteries of the rat. J Physiol 525: 669-680, 2000

Rodman DM., Yamaguchi T., Hasunuma K., O'Brien RF. And McMurtry I. F. Effects of hypoxia on endothelium-dependent relaxation of rat pulmonary artery. Am J Physiol 258:L207-214, 1990.

Rodriguez-Vita, J., M. Ruiz-Ortega, M. Ruperez, V. Esteban, E. Sanchez-Lopez, J. J. Plaza, and J. Egido. Endothelin-1, via ETA receptor and independently of transforming growth factor-ß, increases the connective tissue growth factor in vascular smooth muscle cells. Circ. Res. 97:125-134, 2005.

Ruiz-Feria CA., Kidd MT. and Wideman RF. Plasma level of L-arginine, ornithine, and urea and growth performance of broilers fed supplemental L-arginine during cool temperature exposure. Poult Sci 80:358-369, 2001.

Sakata J., Shimokubo T., Kitamura K., Nishizono M., Iehiki Y., Kangawa K., Matsuo H., and Eto T. Distribution and characterization of immunoreactive rat adrenomedullin in tissue an plasma. FEBS Lett 352: 105-108, 1994.

Sakurai T., Yanagisawa M., Takuwa Y., Miyazaki H., Kimura S., Goto K., and Masaki T. Cloning of a cDNA encoding a nonisopeptide-selective subtype of the endothelin receptor. Nature 348:732-735, 1990.

Salvaterra CG., and Goldman WF. Acute hypoxia increases cytosolic calcium in cultured pulmonary arterial myocytes. Am J Physiol 264, L323-328, 1993.

Sastry BK, Narasimhan C, Reddy NK, Raju BS. Clinical efficacy of sildenafil in primary pulmonary hypertension: a randomized, placebo-controlled, double-blind, crossover study. J Am Coll Cardiol 43:1149-1153, 2004.

Shaul PW., and Wells. Oxigen modulates nitric oxide production selectively in fetal pulmonary endothelial cells. Am J Respir Cell Mol Biol 11:432-438, 1994.

Schermuly RT., Dony E., Ghofrani HG., Pullamsetti S., Savai R., Roth M., Sydykov A., Lai YJ., Weissman N., Seeger W., and Grimminger F. Reversal of experimental pulmonary hypertension by PDGF inhibition. J. Clin. Invest. 115:2811-2821, 2005.

Semenza GL. Oxygen-regulated transcription factors and their role in pulmonary disease. Respir. Res. 1:159-162, 2000.

Sillau, A.H., Montalvo, C. Pulmonary hypertension and the smooth muscle of the pulmonary arterioles in chickens at high altitudeComp Biochem Physiol 71:125-13, 1982.

Souza-Costa DC., Zerbini T., Palei AC., Gerlach RF., and Tanus- Santos JE. L-arginine attenuates acute pulmonary embolism- induced increases in lung matrix metalloproteinase-2 and matrix metalloproteinase-9. Chest 128:3705-3710, 2005.

Sprague RS., Thiemermann C. and Vane JR. Endogenous endothelium-derived relaxing factor opposes hypoxic pulmonary vasoconstriction and supports blood flow to hypoxic alveoli in anesthetized rabbits. Proceedings of the National Academy of Sciences of the USA 89, 8711-8715, 1992.

Stamler JS., Lamas S., and Fang FC. Nitrosylation: the prototypic redox-based signaling mechanism. Cell 106:675-683, 2001.

Stenmark KR., and Mecham RP. Cellular and molecular mechanisms of pulmonary vascular remodeling. Annu. Rev. Physiol. 59:89–144, 1997.

Steudel W., Ichinose F., Huang PL., Hurford WE., Jones RC., Bevan JA., Fishman MC., and Zapol WM. Pulmonary vasoconstriction and hypertension in mice with targeted disruption of the endothelial nitric oxide synthase (NOS 3) gene. Circ Res 81: 34–41, 1997.

Steudel W., Scherrer-Crosbie M., Bloch KD., Weimann J., Huang PL., Jones RC., Picard MH. and Zapol WM. Sustained pulmonary hypertension and right ventricular hypertrophy after chronic hypoxia in mice with congenital deficiency of nitric oxide synthase 3. The Journal of Clinical Investigation 101:2468-2477, 1998.

Stewart DJ. Endothelial disfunction in pulmonary vascular disorders. Arzneim-Forsch. Drug Res 44:451-454, 1994.

Stewart DJ., Levy RD., Nacek P., and Gleben D. Increase plasma endothelin-1 in pulmonary hypertension: marker or mediator of disease? Ann Inter Med 114:464-469, 1991.

Tan X., Pan JQ., Li JC., Liu YJ., Sun WD., and Wang XL. L-arginine inhibiting pulmonary vascular remodelling is associated with promotion of apoptosis in pulmonary arterioles smooth muscle cells in broilers. Res Vet Sci, 79:203-209, 2005a.

Tan X., Liu YJ., Li JC., Pan JQ., Sun WD., and Wang XL. Activation of PKCa and pulmonary vascular remodelling in broilers. Res Vet Sci 79:131-137, 2005b.

Tan X., Sun WD., Li JC., Pan JQ., and Wang XL. Changes in pulmonary arterioles protein kinase Ca expression associated with supplemental L-arginine in broilers during cool temperature exposure. Br Poult Sci 47:230-236, 2006.

Tan X., Sun WD., Li JC., Pan JQ., Liu YJ., Wang JY. and Wang, XL. L-arginine prevents reduced expression of endothelial nitric oxide synthase (NOS) in pulmonary arterioles of broilers exposed to cool temperatures. Vet J 173:151-157, 2007.

Tang JR., Markham NE., Lin YJ., McMurtry IF., Maxey A., Kinsella JP., and Abman SH. Inhaled nitric oxide attenuates pulmonary hypertension and improves lung growth in infant rats after neonatal treatment with a VEGF receptor inhibitor. Am J Physiol Lung Cell Mol Physiol 287: L344–L351, 2004.

Tarquino, C., Hernández, A., Moreno, J.C. y Useche, J. Influencia de la ascitis en pollo de engorde alimentados con dietas de bajo y alto contenido energético. En: Trabajos científicos. Resúmenes. XVII Congreso Nacional de Medicina Veterinaria y Zootecnia. Popayán- Cauca. Colombia. p. 24, 1990.

Thomae KR., Nakayama DK., Billiar TR., Simmons RL., Pitt BR., and Davies,P. The effect of nitric oxide on fetal pulmonary artery smooth muscle growth. The Journal of Surgical Research 59:337-343, 1995.

Thompson, BT., Hassoun, PM., Kradin, RL., and Hales, CA. Acute and chronic hypoxic pulmonary hypertension in guinea pigs. J Appl Physiol 66:920-928, 1989.

Touyz RM., and Schiffrin EL. Role of endothelin in human hypertension. Can. J. Physiol. Pharmacol. 81:533–541, 2003.

Tozzi C., and Riley DJ. Impaired endothelium-dependent relaxation of pulmonary artery rings is restored after recovery from hypoxic pulmonary hypertension. Abstract Am J Rev Respir Dis 141:A350- A360, 1990.

Urena J, Franco-Obregon A., and Lopez-Barneo J. Contrasting effects of hypoxia on cytosoli.c Ca^{2+} spikes in conduit and resistance myocytes of the rabbit pulmonary artery. J Physiol 496: 103–109, 1996.

Useche, J., Hernández, A., Herrán, W. Morfometría cardiopulmonar en pollos de engorde ascíticos. Rev. Col. Cien. Pec. 3:213-223, 1981.

Vásquez, I.C., Efecto de la edad, tiempo de permanencia y desarrollo pulmonar en la incidencia de hipertensión arterial pulmonar en pollos de engorde. Tesis de Maestría.Universidad Nacional. Bogotá. 2010.

VoelkeL NF., Tuder RM. Cellular and molecular mechanisms in the pathogenesis of severe pulmonary hypertension. Eur. Resp. J. 8: 2129-2138, 1995.

Voelkel NF, Tuder RM, Weir EK. Pathophysiology of primary pulmonary hypertension. Rubin L, Rich S. Primary Pulmonary Hypertension. New York, NY: Marcel Dekker. 83-129, 1997.

Von Euler U and Liljestrand G. Observations on the pulmonary arterial blood pressure in the cat. Acta Physiol Scand 12: 301-320, 1946.

Waldman JD., Lamberti JJ., Mathewson JW., Kirkpatrick SE., Turner SW., George L., and Pappelbaum SJ. Congenital heart disease and pulmonary artery hypertension. I. Pulmonary vasoreactivity to 15% oxygen before and after surgery. J Am Coll Cardiol 2: 1158-1164, 1983.

Wang Y., Coe Y., Toyoda 0. and Coceani, F. Involvement of endothelin-1 in hypoxic pulmonary vasoconstriction in the lamb. J of Physiol 482:421-434, 1995.

Wang S., Desai D., Wright G., Niles RM., and Wright GL. Effects of protein kinase C alpha over-expression on A7r5 smooth muscle cell proliferation and differentiation. Exper Cell Res 236:117-126, 1997.

Wang S., Yu Z., and Liu K. Synthesis and release of pulmonary tissue adrenomedullin on hypoxic pulmonary hypertension in rats and its significance. Zhonghua Jie He He Hu Xi Za Zhi 24:725-727, 2001.

Wang J., Wang X., Xiang R. , and Sun W. Effect of L-NAME on pulmonary arterial pressure, plasma nitric oxide and pulmonary hypertension syndrome morbidity in broilers. Br Poult Sci 43:615-620, 2002.

Wang X., Tong M., Chinta S., Raj JU., and Gao Y. Hypoxia induced reactive oxygen species downregulate ETB receptor-mediated contraction of rat pulmonary arteries. Am J Physiol Lung Cellular and Molecular Physiology 290:L570-L578, 2006.

Ward JP., and Robertson TP. The role of the endothelium in hypoxic pulmonary vasoconstriction. Exp Physiol 80: 793-801, 1995.

Weber, R.E., Jessen, T.H., Malte, H., Tame, J. Mutant hemoglobins (alpha 119-Ala and beta 55-Ser): functions related to high-altitude respiration in geese. J Appl Physiol 75: 2646-2655, 1993.

Weidong S., Xiaolong W., Jinyong W., and Ruiping X. Pulmonary arterial pressure and electrocardiogram in broiler chickens infused intravenously with L-NAME, an inhibitor of nitric oxide synthase, or sodium nitroprusside (SNP), a nitric oxide donor. British Poult Sci 43:306-312, 2002.

Weir EK, Reeve HL, Huang JMC, et al. Anorexic agents aminorex, fenfluramine, and dexfenfluramine inhibit potassium current in rat pulmonary vascular smooth muscle and cause pulmonary vasoconstriction. Circulation 94:2216–2220, 1996.

Weir EK., Lopez-Barneo J., Buckler KJ., Archer SL. Acute oxygen sensing mechanisms. N Engl J Med 353: 2942-2955, 2005.

Weir EK., Archer SL. Hypoxic pulmonary vasoconstriction is not mediated by increased production of reactive oxygen species. J Appl Physiol 101:995-998, 2006.

Weir E., Olschewski A. Role of ion channels in acute and chronic responses of the pulmonary vasculature to hypoxia. Cardiovascular Res 71(4):630-641, 2006

Wideman RF., Kirby YK., Ismail M., Bottje WG., Moore R., and Vardeman RC. Supplemental L-arginine attenuates pulmonary hypertension syndrome (ascites) in broilers. Poult Sci 74:323-330, 1995.

Wideman RFJr., Maynard P., and Bottje W. Thromboxane mimics the pulmonary but not systemic vascular responses to bolus HCl injections in broiler chickens. Poult. Sci. 78:714-721, 1999.

Wideman RF. And Tackett CD. Cardio-pulmonary function inbroilers reared at warm or cool temperatures: effect on acute inhalation of 100% oxygen. Poult Sci 79:257-264, 2000.

Wideman RF. Pathophysiology of heart/lung disorders: pulmonary hypertension syndrome in broiler chickens. World Poultry Sci J 57:289-307, 2001.

Wideman RF., Bowen OT., Erf GF., and Chapman ME. Influence of aminoguanidine, an inhibitor of inducible nitric oxide synthase, on the pulmonary hypertensive response to microparticle injections in broilers. Poult Sci 85:511-527, 2006.

Wort SJ., Woods M., Warner TD., Evans TW. and Mitchell JA. Endogenously released endothelin-1 from human pulmonary artery smooth muscle promotes cellular proliferation. Am J Respir Cell and Mol Biol 25:104-110, 2001.

Xiang RP., Sun WD., Wang JY. and Wang XL. Effect of vitamin C on pulmonary hypertension and muscularisation of pulmonary arterioles in broilers. Br Poult Sci, 43:705 -712, 2002.

Xu P., Dai A., and Zhou H. Expression of adrenomedullin and its receptor in lungs of rats with hypoxia-induced pulmonary hypertension. Zhonghua Jie He He Hu Xi Za Zhi 25:465-469, 2002.

Yang Y., Qiao J., Wu Z., Chen Y., Gao M., Ou D., and Wang H. Endothelin-1 receptor antagonist BQ123 prevents pulmonary artery hypertension induced by low ambient temperature in broilers. Biological and Pharmaceutical Bulletin 28:2201-2205, 2005.

Yanagisawa, M. The endothelin system: a new target for therapeutic intervention. Circulation 89:1320-1322, 1994.

Yoshibayashi M, Kamiya T, Kitamura K, Saito Y, Kangawa K, Nishikimi T, Matsuoka H, Eto T, and Matsuo H. Plasma levels of adrenomedullin in primary and secondary pulmonary hypertension in patients 20 years of age. Am J Cardiol 79: 1556–1558, 1997.

Yuan JX, Wang J, Juhaszova M, Gaine SP, Rubin LJ. Attenuated K+ channel gene transcription in primary pulmonary hypertension. Lancet 351:726–727, 1998.

Zhang F., and Morice AH. Effect of levcromakalim on hypoxia-, KCl- and prostaglandin F2ainduced contractions in isolated rat pulmonary artery. J Pharmacol Exper Therap 271, 326-333, 1994.

Zhang, H., Wu, C.X., Chamba, Y., Ling, Y. Blood Characteristics for High Altitude Adaptation in Tibetan Chickens. Poult Sci 86(7): 1384 - 1389. 2007.

7

Inadequate Myocardial Oxygen Supply/Demand in Experimental Pulmonary Hypertension

B. J. van Beek-Harmsen, H. M. Feenstra and W. J. van der Laarse
Department of Physiology, Institute for Cardiovascular Research,
VU University Medical Center Amsterdam
The Netherlands

1. Introduction

Right ventricular (RV) hypertrophy is an adaptive response to chronic pulmonary hypertension, but can progress to chronic or advanced RV heart failure. The treatment of pulmonary hypertension is improving but remains unsatisfactory (Humbert et al., 2010). A better understanding of the transition from hypertrophy to RV failure may lead to new insights in the treatment of pulmonary hypertension.

The increased workload of the right heart due to pulmonary hypertension increases oxygen consumption of right ventricular cardiomyocytes because the mitochondria have to operate at a higher rate. Hypertrophy can normalize right ventricular wall stress, thereby also normalizing the rate of oxygen consumption by mitochondria. However, hypertrophy may cause hypoxia in cardiomyocytes because intracellular diffusion distances for oxygen increase and capillary density decreases when the myocytes enlarge. Increased diffusion distances imply that the interstitial oxygen tension preventing core hypoxia in cardiomyocytes (PO_{2crit}) increases, whereas reduced capillary density likely reduces interstitial PO_2. In addition to the increased power output of the right ventricular myocytes, the rate of oxygen consumption of the cells also increases because their mechanical efficiency decreases (Wong et al., 2010). These changes can lead to oxidative stress (Redout et al., 2007) and may lead to apoptosis of RV cardiomyocytes (Ecarnot-Laubriet et al., 2002).

Whether or not hypoxia occurs in hypertrophied cardiomyocytes is a matter of debate because measurement of core PO_2 in cardiomyocytes in vivo is technically impossible. Previous reports, in which myoglobin saturation was measured to estimate mean intracellular PO_2 in the left heart, suggest that hypoxic cores in cardiomyocytes are absent (Bache et al., 1999; Kreuzer et al., 2001). However, Hill et al. (1989) demonstrated that supplemental oxygen reduces hypertrophy in experimental pulmonary hypertension.

We use calibrated histochemistry to obtain the physiological parameters required to evaluate oxygen demand and supply at the cellular level in hypertrophied right ventricular myocardium of pulmonary hypertensive rats (des Tombe et al., 2002). To investigate whether the cardiomyocytes adapt to hypoxia, we determined the expression of the hypoxia inducible transcription factor HIF 1α (Wang & Semenza, 1995) by quantitative immunohistochemistry in cardiomyocyte nuclei.

2. Calculation of PO$_2$'s

The mean extracellular oxygen tension required to drive oxygen from the interstitial space into cardiomyocytes preventing hypoxic cores (PO$_{2crit}$) is calculated from a Hill-type diffusion model including myoglobin-facilitated diffusion (Murray, 1974):

$$PO_{2crit} = (VO_{2max} CSA - 4\pi D_{Mb}[MbO_2]_R)/4\pi K_{O2} \tag{1}$$

where VO$_{2max}$ is the maximum rate of oxygen consumption of the cardiomyocyte, CSA is the cross-sectional area of the cardiomyocyte, D$_{Mb}$ is the radial diffusion coefficient of myoglobin in the cardiomyocyte, [MbO$_2$]$_R$ is the concentration of oxygenated myoglobin at the sarcolemma of the cardiomyocyte and K$_{O2}$ is Krogh's diffusion coefficient for oxygen in heart muscle. [MbO$_2$]$_R$ can be calculated from:

$$[MbO_2]_R = PO_{2crit} Mb_{tot}/(PO_{2crit} + P_{50}) \tag{2}$$

where Mb$_{tot}$ is the total myoglobin concentration in the cardiomyocyte and P$_{50}$ is the oxygen tension at which 50% of myoglobin is oxygenated. Substitution of equation 2 into equation 1 allows the calculation of PO$_{2crit}$. CSA, VO$_{2max}$ and myoglobin concentration were determined as described below. The values for the other parameters were taken from the literature: D$_{Mb}$ = 2.0 10^{-5} mm^2 s^{-1} (Papadopoulos et al., 2001), K$_{O2}$ = 1.5 nM mm^2 s^{-1} hPa^{-1} (van der Laarse et al., 2005), and P$_{50}$ = 8.7 hPa. The latter value was calculated from P$_{50}$ of rat myoglobin and the temperature dependency of P$_{50}$ (Gayeski & Honig, 1991; Enoki et al., 1995; Schenkman et al., 1997).

Assuming that oxygen supply is limiting VO$_{2max}$ by a negligible percentage in normal muscle (Spriet et al., 1986; Mootha et al., 1997), it is possible to calculate the permeability of the capillary endothelium and the interstitial space for oxygen using Fick's law, because in the steady state the flux of oxygen entering the cardiomyocytes equals the flux of oxygen crossing the capillary endothelium. This flux per unit myocyte length is:

$$CSA\ VO_{2max} = D_{cap} (PO_{2cap}-PO_{2crit}) \tag{3}$$

where D$_{cap}$ is the permeability of capillary endothelium and interstitial space (in nmol mm^{-1}$_{myocyte}$ s^{-1} hPa^{-1}), and PO$_{2cap}$ is the average capillary oxygen tension. PO$_{2cap}$-PO$_{2crit}$ is the minimum driving force required to prevent hypoxia in the cardiomyocytes. The average capillary PO$_2$ used in the calculation in normal myocardium is 66 hPa, which equals P$_{50}$ of rat blood (Schmidt-Nielsen & Larimar, 1958; Gray & Steadman, 1964) and approximates the mean of capillary arterial and venous PO$_2$. We assume that D$_{cap}$ is proportional to the number of capillaries per cardiomyocyte (for discussion, see Bekedam, 2010). The permeability in normal myocardium was used to calculate PO$_{2cap}$ in hypertrophied myocardium, taking changes in CSA VO$_{2max}$, capillaries per cell and PO$_{2crit}$ into account.

3. Animals and histochemical methods

3.1 Preparations

All experiments were approved by the local Animal Ethics Committee. Male Wistar rats (n = 33) were used for this study. At 180 g body mass, 18 rats were injected s.c. with 40 mg monocrotaline (MCT) per kg body mass, to induce pulmonary hypertension (Okumura et al., 1992). Body mass was determined daily. The body mass change (in %/day) was calculated as the mean of the last three days. Untreated, age-matched rats served as controls. Right ventricular systolic pressure of monocrotaline-injected rats in our laboratory increases after the injection from 25 (SEM 0.9) mmHg in control (CNTR) to 45 (SEM 4.6) mmHg after two weeks (MCT2) and to 64 (SEM 2.8) mmHg after 4 weeks (MCT4, Henkes et al., 2007). We did not measure pulmonary arterial pressure in the rats used in the present experiments because the measurement and the anaesthesia may interfere with HIF 1α expression (YY Wong and WJ van der Laarse, unpublished results). After 2 or 4 weeks, 6 or 12 MCT rats and 6 or 9 control rats, respectively, were anaesthetized with halothane and the lungs and heart were excised. The heart was perfused with Tyrode solution (120 mM NaCl, 5 mM KCl, 1.2 mM $MgSO_4$, 2.0 mM Na_2HPO_4, 27 mM $NaHCO_3$, 1 mM $CaCl_2$, 10 mM glucose and 20 mM 2,3-butanedione monoxime, equilibrated with 95% O_2 and 5% CO_2; pH 7.3-7.4 at 10°C) to slow down metabolism and remove the blood and a biopsy was taken from the right ventricular wall within 10 min after excision. The biopsy was frozen in liquid nitrogen (van der Laarse & Diegenbach, 1988). Sections, 5 μm thick, were cut in a cryostat, air-dried for 30 min and incubated for succinate dehydrogenase (SDH) activity or stored at -80°C until use. The wet mass of the lungs and the dry mass after freeze-drying were determined.

3.2 Calibrated enzymehistochemistry

SDH activity was demonstrated as described (des Tombe et al., 2002). The incubation medium consisted of 37.5 mM sodium phosphate buffer, pH 7.6, 75 mM sodium succinate, 5 mM sodium azide, and 0.4 mM tetranitro blue tetrazolium. Sections were incubated at 37°C in the dark for 7 min. To calculate the extracellular oxygen tension required to prevent a hypoxic core in the cardiomyocyte (PO_{2crit}), an estimate of VO_{2max} (in nmol mm^{-3} s^{-1} = mM s^{-1}) was calculated from the absorbance of the formazan precipitate measured in the section, based on the proportional relationship between VO_{2max} and SDH activity under hyperoxic conditions *in vitro*: VO_{2max} = 2.9 mM s^{-1} per unit of absorbance at 660 nm (des Tombe et al., 2002; van der Laarse et al., 2005).

The sections for the determination of the myoglobin concentration and cytosolic cytochrome c were vapour-fixed with formaldehyde as described (van Beek-Harmsen et al., 2004, van Beek-Harmsen & van der Laarse, 2005). Myoglobin peroxidase activity was determined as described (Lee-de Groot et al., 1998), in a medium consisting of 59 ml 50 mM Tris(hydroxymethyl)aminomethane and 80 mM KCl, pH 8.0, 25 mg ortho-tolidine (Sigma T8533, St Louis, MI) dissolved in 2 ml 96% ethanol (at 50°C) and 1.43 ml 70% tertiary-butyl-hydroperoxide (Fluka Chemie 19995, Buchs, Switzerland). The myoglobin concentration was determined using gelatine sections with known concentrations of myoglobin. The concentration was calculated from the absorbance using an extinction coefficient of 363 mM^{-1} cm^{-1} (van Beek-Harmsen et al., 2004).

3.3 Immunohistochemistry of HIF 1α, cytochrome c, and collagen type IV

Incubations were carried out at room temperature (22-25°C). Sections for HIF 1α and collagen type IV were fixed in 4% formaldehyde in 150 mM NaCl, 10 mM Na_2HPO_4, 1.5 mM KH_2PO_4 (PBS), pH 7.4, for 10 min. sections for cytochrome c were fixed as indicated above. Sections were incubated with 1:100 dilution of anti-HIF 1α (H-206, Santa Cruz Biotechnology, Santa Cruz, CA), anti-collagen type IV (Rockland, Gilbertsville PA), or anti-cytochrome c (Santa Cruz) for 1h, followed by incubation with a secondary biotin-labelled anti-rabbit antibody in a 1:100 dilution (Vector Laboratories, Burlingame, CA) for 30 min. Endogenous peroxidase activity was quenched using 0.3% hydrogen peroxide in methanol for 30 min. Subsequently, following the manufacturers guidelines, the sections were incubated with Vectastain ABC reagent (Vector Laboratories). Each step was followed by rinsing in PBS containing 0.05% (v/v) Tween 20. Peroxidase activity was demonstrated in a solution containing 3 mg 3,3'-diaminobenzidine in 30 µl dimethyl sulphoxide, 10 ml 0.05 M Tris(hydroxymethyl)aminomethane, 10 mM imidazole and 10 mM sodium azide, pH 7.6. Hydrogen peroxide was added before use (final concentration 0.003%).

3.4 Microdensitometry and morphometry

Staining intensities and morphometry were quantified using a DMRB microscope (Leica, Wetzlar, Germany) fitted interference filters at 660 nm for SDH activity (Pool et al., 1979) and 436 nm for myoglobin (Lee-de Groot et al., 1998), cytochrome c (van Beek-Harmsen et al., 2005), and HIF 1α. Images were obtained using a 40x objective, and a monochrome Charge-Coupled Device camera (Sony XC 77CE, Towada, Japan), connected to a LG-3 frame grabber (Scion, Frederick, MD) in an Apple Macintosh computer. Images were analysed using NIH Image 1.61 (http://rsb.info.nih.gov/nih-image/). Grey values were transformed to absorbance values using calibrated grey filters. Morphometry was calibrated using a slide micrometer taking the pixel to aspect ratio into account.

Cytochrome c release in cardiomyocytes or in the interstitial space was categorized as 0: no release, 1: some release in one or two areas of the section, 2: maximum release in more than two areas of the section, 3: maximum release detectable in the entire section.

HIF 1α was measured by using the threshold option in NIH Image to measure the absorbance and size of the stained nuclei. The total staining of a nucleus was calculated as the product of absorbance and size. The mean absorbance of positive nuclei was multiplied by the fraction of positive nuclei to obtain the mean HIF 1α expression in the heart.

The number of capillaries per cardiomyocyte was determined after incubation with anti-collagen type IV (Madsen & Holmskov, 1995) in two areas of a section where cardiomyocytes were cut perpendicularly to their longitudinal axis.

The sarcomere length was determined using a 100x phase contrast objective in areas of the section where the cardiomyocytes were cut along their longitudinal axis. This value was used to normalise the cross-sectional area to a sarcomere length of 2 µm, assuming that the volume of cardiomyocytes does not change when the cells contract. The volume of cytoplasm per nucleus was determined in sections fixed for 10 min in 4% formaldehyde in 0.1 M sodium phosphate buffer, pH 7.4, and stained with hematoxylin and eosin (Loud & Anversa, 1984; des Tombe et al., 2002). The number of cardiomyocyte nuclei in the right ventricular free wall was determined from the volume of the wall (calculated as wet mass/1.04). The volume of interstitial space was subtracted, and the volume occupied by cardiomyocytes was divided by the volume of cytoplasm per nucleus to obtain the number of cardiomyocyte nuclei.

3.5 Statistics

Values are given as mean (standard deviation, SD). Students t-test with equal or unequal variances was used to determine differences between groups. $P<0.05$ was considered significant.

4. Results

4.1 Lung and body mass

Fig. 1 shows lung masses and the change in body mass of control and MCT-injected rats. The wet mass of the lung was slightly but significantly increased after two weeks, as was the change in body mass. The wet/dry mass of the lung in MCT2 was higher than control 5.64 (SD 0.42) and 5.22 (SD 0.34), respectively, indicating oedema in MCT2. The wet/dry mass of MCT4 rats was intermediate between control and MCT2 (5.33, S.D. 0.31; not different from control or MCT2). After 4 weeks, both wet and dry lung mass were significantly higher than control and MCT2, and the body mass decreased by 2% per day on average. However, the change in body mass in MCT4 rats was rather variable, as indicated by the large standard deviation (Fig. 1C); the range was +3.0 to –8.5 %per day.

The changes in lung and body mass are indicative of the severity of pulmonary hypertension (Mouchaers et al., 2007; Handoko et al, 2009).

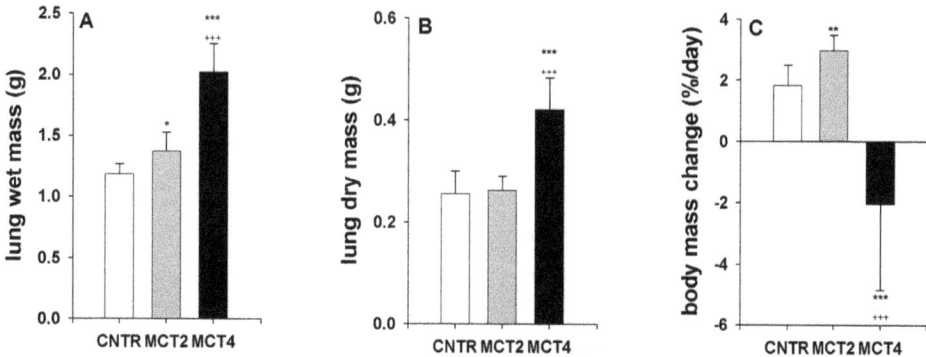

Fig. 1. A: Lung wet mass, B: lung dry mass and C: body mass change of control and monocrotaline-injected rats after 2 (MCT2) and 4 (MCT4) weeks. The body mass change is the mean value over the last three days. * P<0.05, ** P<0.01, *** P<0.001: difference between MCT and control. +++ P<0.001: difference between MCT2 and MCT4. Controls at 2 and 4 weeks are similar and were pooled.

4.2 Right myocardial histology and histochemistry

The histology is shown in Fig 2. Hematoxylin and eosin staining clearly shows hypertrophy of cardiomyocytes of the MCT4 rat, and also shows considerable heterogeneity of the cross-sectional area of cardiomyocytes in the hypertrophic heart and many interstitial cells, which are leucocytes (Handoko et al. 2009).

SDH activity was distributed fairly evenly in controls whereas it clusters in hypertrophic heart. Myoglobin shows a similar distribution as SDH activity in control and hypertrophic hearts. This staining was lost when sections were preincubated in saline before fixation, indicating that the peroxidase activity is not structurally bound (result not shown).

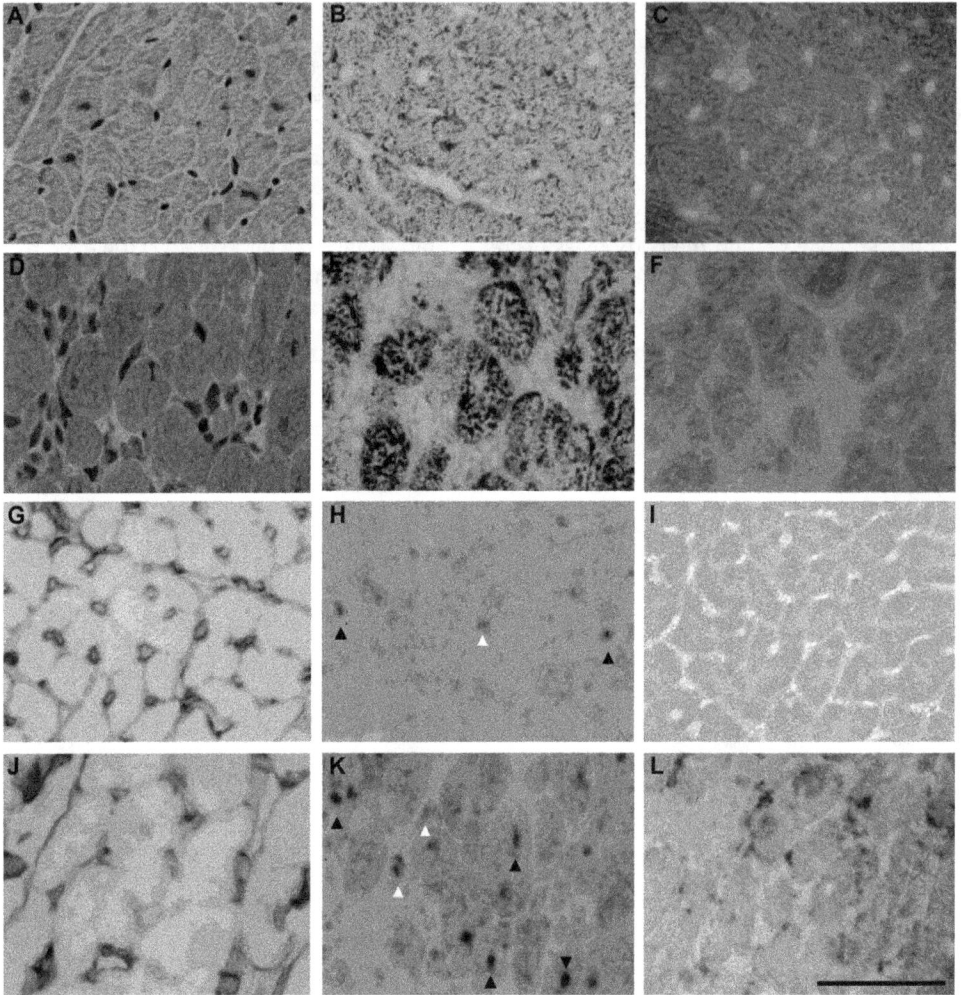

Fig. 2. Sections of a control and of a MCT-injected rat after 4 weeks. A,D: hematoxylin and eosin; B,E: SDH activity; C,F: Myoglobin concentration, G,J: Collagen type IV (capillaries); H,K: HIF 1α expression; black arrow heads point at cardiomyocyte nuclei, white arrow heads point at nuclei in interstitial cells; I,L: cytochrome c. Top and third row: control; second and bottom row: MCT4. Bar 50 μm.

The sections incubated for collagen type IV show a decrease of capillary density expressed per unit of area in the hypertrophic heart, indicating that maximum oxygen supply per unit mass of the hypertrophic myocardium was reduced, and intracellular diffusion distances were increased. HIF 1α staining was very weak in control cardiomyocyte nuclei, whereas intensive nuclear staining as well as expression in interstitial cells was present in MCT4 rats.

Cytochome c release was absent in controls. In MCT rats, cytochrome c was detected in a variable fraction of RV cardiomyocytes and could also be present in the interstitial space.

4.3 Oxygen demand and supply

The oxygen demand of the right heart can increase threefold due to the increase in pulmonary artery pressure (Handoko et al., 2009) and by a similar factor due to a decrease of mechanical efficiency (Wong et al., 2010). Fig. 3 shows the parameters relevant to oxygen demand and supply. Four weeks after monocrotaline the mean cross-sectional area of cardiomyocytes was significantly increased, whereas the mean SDH activity was similar to control. The maximum rate of oxygen uptake per unit of cardiomyocyte length ($VO_{2max}CSA$, in pmol mm^{-1} s^{-1}) was increased, whereas the myoglobin concentration was slightly decreased in MCT4. These changes increased PO_{2crit}. The number of capillaries per cardiomyocyte in MCT4 is slightly higher compared to MCT2, but not different from control.

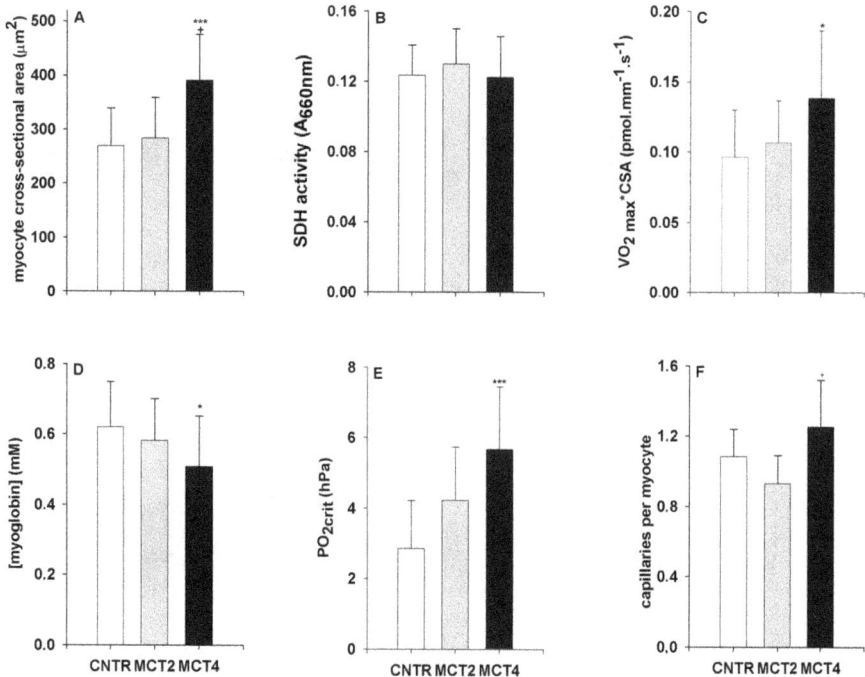

Fig. 3. Right ventricular cardiomyocyte characteristics of control rats (CNTR) and monocrotaline-injected rats after 2 (MCT2) and 4 weeks (MCT4). A: cardiomyocyte cross-sectional area (CSA); B SDH activity given as absorbance value at 660 nm; C: oxygen uptake per mm cardiomyocyte, calculated from data in A and B; D: myoglobin concentration; E: PO_{2crit} (see text); F: the number of capillaries per cardiomyocyte. *P<0.05, *P<0.001: difference between MCT and control; +P<0.05, +++P<0.001: difference between MCT2 and MCT4.

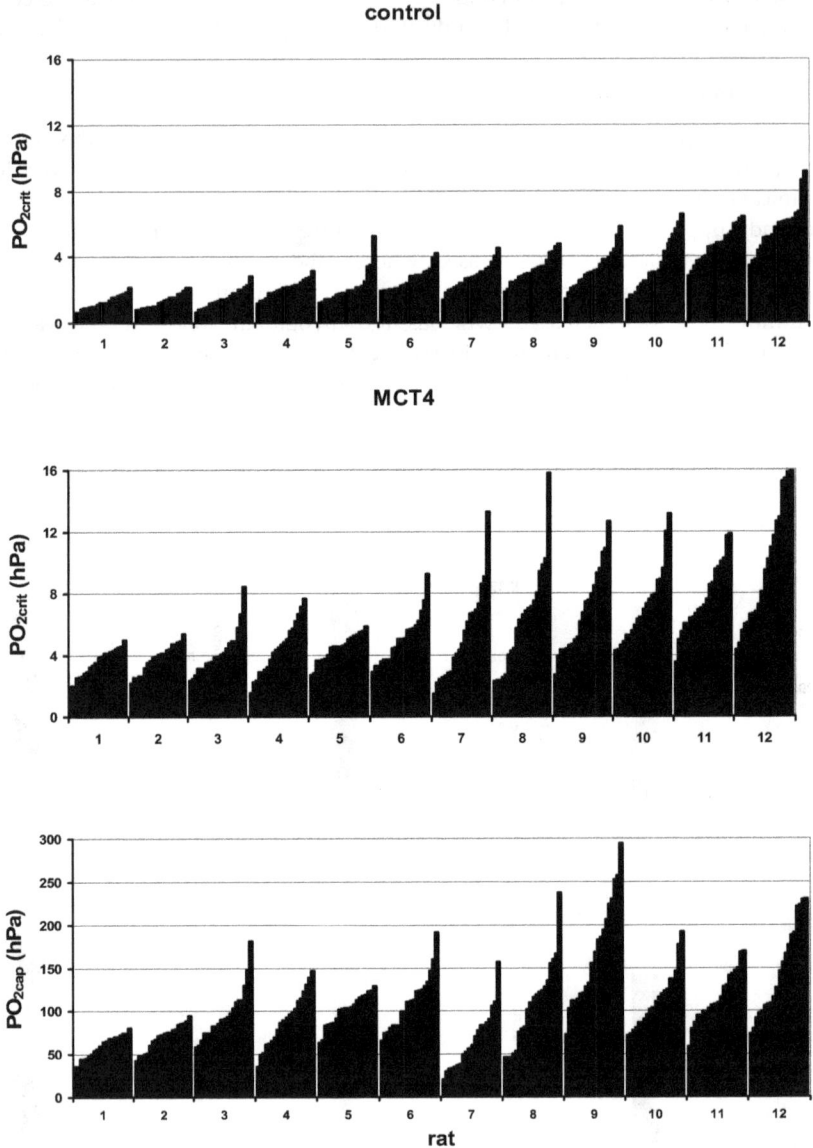

Fig. 4. PO_{2crit} of individual cardiomyocytes of 12 control rats (upper panel), and 12 MCT4 rats (middle panel), and required capillary PO_2 in the MCT 4 rats (lower panel). 12 control rats were randomly selected and sorted by ascending mean PO_{2crit}. PO_{2crit} of 20 cardiomyocytes in each rat are shown, also sorted by ascending PO_{2crit}. PO_{2crit} was calculated using equations 1 and 2. This value was used to calculate the mean capillary PO_2 required to prevent hypoxia in MCT4 cardiomyocytes using CSA VO_{2max}, PO_{2crits} from the middle panel, and the number of capillaries per cardiomyocyte (see text).

Fig. 4 shows the distributions of PO_{2crit} of individual cardiomyocytes. Individual rats differed with respect to PO_{2crit}, with mean PO_{2crit} ranging from 1.2 to 5.7 hPa; the overall mean was 2.8 hPa in control. In MCT4 rats, mean PO_{2crit} increased to 5.7 hPa mainly due to an increase in myocyte cross sectional area and slightly due to a decrease of the myoglobin concentration (Fig 3AD). However, the lowest PO_{2crit} values found in MCT4 rats were within the normal range observed in controls. The hypertrophic process increased the range of PO_{2crit} in MCT4 rats considerably, from 2 to 16 hPa. The control rats were used to calculate capillary permeability using Fick's law (equation 3). The permeability for oxygen normalised by the number of capillaries per myocyte (Fig. 3F) equalled 1.31 (SEM 0.17) fmol mm^{-1}_{cap} s^{-1} hPa^{-1}. This value was used to calculate mean capillary PO_2 in MCT4 rats. It can be inferred from the lower panel of Fig. 4 that a substantial fraction of the cardiomyocytes becomes hypoxic when the mitochondria are maximally activated and mean capillary PO_2 equals 66 hPa. The highest required capillary PO_2's found in MCT4 rats are well above normal arterial PO_2 (about 133 hPa), indicating that the risk of oxygen supply limitation is substantial in MCT4 rats, especially during exercise.

4.4 Cytosolic cytochrome c and the number of cardiomyocyte nuclei

It can be expected that the cardiomyocytes try to adapt to hypoxia. Indeed, Fig. 5 shows that HIF 1α in cardiomyocyte nuclei was significantly increased in MCT4. Cytosolic cytochrome c was detected in cardiomyocytes of one out of six MCT2 rats and in nine out of twelve MCT4 rats. Interstitial cytochrome c was detected in two MCT2 rats and in eight MCT4 rats, indicating that HIF 1α expression cannot prevent mitochondrial dysfunction. Release of cytochrome c can lead to apoptosis of cardiomyocytes, but surprisingly the numbers of cardiomyocyte nuclei in the right ventricular free wall of control and experimental groups were similar.

4.5 Correlation analyses

Correlation analyses were carried out on the mean values of the parameters measured in MCT-injected animals, 2 and 4 weeks pooled (n = 18). As shown in Fig 4B, the correlation of HIF 1α expression and PO_{2crit} is significant (r = 0.64, P=0.004) but the explained variance of HIF 1α expression only 41% (r^2 = 0.41). The change of body mass - a decrease of body mass is indicative of the severity of heart failure in MCT injected rats - correlated with volume of cytoplasm per cardiomyocyte nucleus (r = -0.48, P = 0.046), lung wet mass (r = -0.74, P <0.001) and lung dry mass (r = -0.79, P<0.001).

HIF 1α expression correlated strongly with the coefficient of variation of spatially integrated SDH activity (or $VO_{2max}CSA$, Fig 3C: r = 0.80, P <0.001), indicating an increase of HIF 1α expression with an increase of the variability of the maximum oxygen consumption per myocyte. There were no correlations between cytosolic cytochrome c or the presence of cytochrome c in the interstitial space and PO_{2crit} or HIF 1α expression.

5. Discussion

5.1 Hypoxic cores in hypertrophied cardiomyocytes

The results demonstrate heterogeneous responses of most myocardial parameters to MCT-induced pulmonary hypertension, not only between rats within experimental groups, but also between individual cardiomyocytes in a heart. The heterogeneity indicates that individual cardiomyocytes react differently to MCT-induced increased workload. Furthermore, the heterogeneity is strongly related to HIF 1α expression. PO_{2crit} increases in most MCT rats, and correlates with the expression of HIF 1α in nuclei of cardiomyocytes. The upper value of PO_{2crit} is similar to coronary sinus PO_2 during maximum exercise, 20 hPa (swine: Merkus et al., 2003; dog: Tune et al., 2004). End capillary venous PO_2 in the RV myocardium of MCT rats is not known. It can be lower than 20 hPa, because myocardial blood flow is heterogeneous (Zuurbier et al., 1999), arterial PO_2 in awake, freely moving MCT rats is reduced (to 88 ± 7 hPa (Hill et al., 1989), and because interstitial PO_2 must be lower than capillary PO_2 to extract oxygen. The present results provide an explanation for reduced survival induced by training in progressive pulmonary hypertensive rats (Handoko et al., 2009), because repeated increases of the workload of the right ventricle can lead to hypoxia-reoxygenation injury.

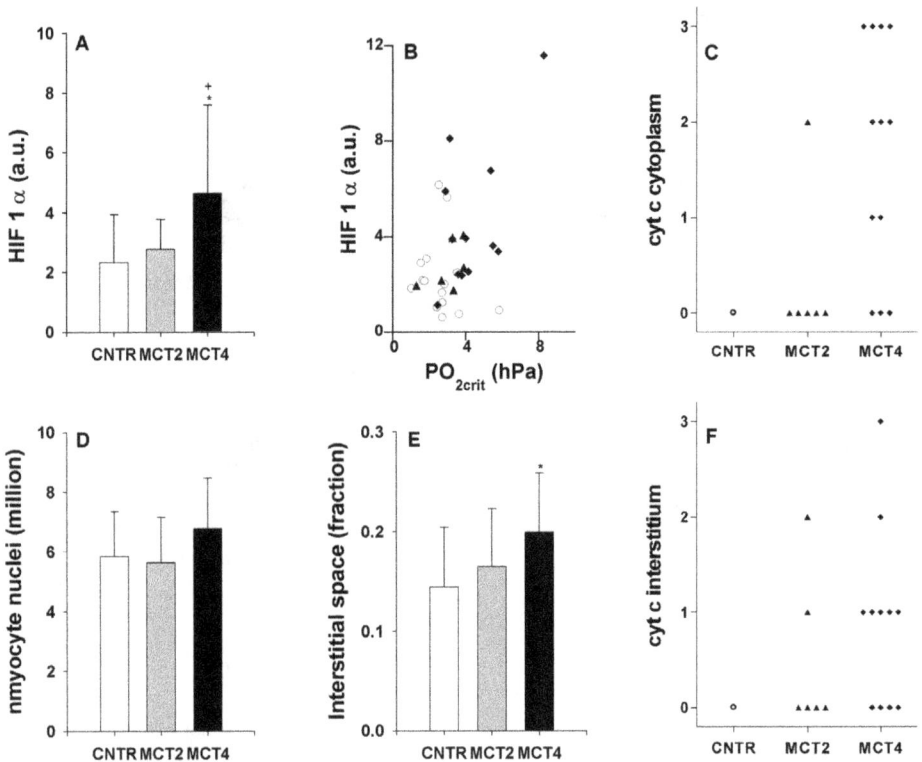

Fig. 5. A: Expression of HIF 1α in arbitrary units (a.u.) in nuclei of right ventricular cardiomyocytes of control (CNTR) and monocrotaline-injected rats after 2 (MCT2) and 4 (MCT4) weeks. B: HIF 1α expression in individual rats related to PO_{2crit}. ○: control, ▲: MCT2; ♦ MCT4, C: cytochrome c detected in cardiomyocyte cytoplasm; all 15 controls are negative; D: the number of cardiomyocyte nuclei in the right ventricular free wall; E: interstitial space; F: presence of cytochrome c in interstitium. * P<0.05: difference from control, + P<0.05: different from MCT2.

5.2 Oxygen consumption and cytochrome c release

The effect of cytochrome c release on the rate of oxygen consumption and PO_{2crit} is not known. We previously found (van der Laarse et al., 2005) that the maximum rate of oxygen consumption of myocardial trabecula dissected from the right ventricular wall of MCT4 rats is not different from control, whereas the rate of oxygen consumption at rest is much higher than control. It is a possibility that the high rate of oxygen consumption of quiescent hypertrophied trabeculae is due to cytochrome c release because cytosolic cytochrome c can oxidize cytosolic NADH (La Piana et al., 2005). This will reduce the efficiency of metabolic recovery, i.e. lower ATP/O_2. It is unlikely therefore, that the release of cytochrome c would cause a decrease of VO_{2max} and PO_{2crit} in failing myocardium. It is a possibility that mitochondrial damage is the reason for the reduced mechanical efficiency in observed in papillary muscles (Wong et al., 2010).

Bache et al. (1999) concluded that changes in energy rich phosphate concentrations that occur during high workload of hypertrophic hearts were not due to limited myocardial oxygenation using ^{1}H nuclear magnetic resonance to monitor myoglobin desaturation *in situ* in the anaesthetised dog. In these studies, however, coronary sinus PO_2 was about 40 hPa. Because this PO_2 is twice the value measured in exercising animals (see above), it is not surprising that myoglobin remained saturated with oxygen in these experiments. This argument may also hold for a similar study in normal rat myocardium by Kreutzer et al. (2001), in which coronary sinus oxygen content was 2.8 mM during dopamine infusion (34% of control, corresponding to PO_2 = 44 hPa; Gray et al., 1964).

The release of cytochrome c from the mitochondria is a first sign of failure of cardiomyocytes to adapt to overload. It could already be observed two weeks after the monocrotaline injection when hypertrophy started to develop. We did not identify a single factor or a combination of factors that could fully explain the release, possibly because relevant factors were excluded in the analyses. For instance, arterial PO_2 was not taken into account and interstitial cytochrome c may have been removed from the heart by lymph or blood (Radhakrishnan et al., 2007).

5.3 Cytochrome c release and the number of cardiomyocyte nuclei

The amount of cytochrome c released in different cardiomyocytes in one heart can vary from no to total release (van Beek-Harmsen & van der Laarse, 2005). Cytochrome c release did not induce apoptosis judging from the number of cardiomyocyte nuclei in the right ventricular free wall. This is surprising because we previously found a 40% decrease of the number of cardiomyocyte nuclei (des Tombe et al., 2002). Ecarnot-Laubriet et al. (2002) found apoptotic nuclei in the right ventricular myocardium of MCT-injected Wistar rats after 3 weeks but used a 1.5 times higher dose, 60 mg MCT/kg body mass. The reason for not finding a reduction of the number of cardiomyocyte nuclei in the present study could be that the occurrence of apoptosis in MCT-injected rats is dose-dependent and critically depends on type of rat strain, and food and housing conditions. This requires further study. We conclude that in the present experiments apoptosis is not the cause of the transition from hypertrophy to heart failure.

5.4 Myoglobin

The myoglobin concentration in hypertrophied cardiomyocytes decreased. It may be that the capacity to synthesize myoglobin (e.g. the increased cytoplasm/nucleus ratio or the availability of iron (Rohbach et al., 2007) is the limiting factor, or that degradation of myoglobin in hypertrophied cardiomyocytes is increased, e.g. due to H_2O_2 production. We previously found higher myoglobin concentrations in hyperthyroid rats compared to MCT-injected rats (Lee-de Groot et al., 1998).

Transcription of the myoglobin gene is thyroid hormone (Gianocco et al., 2004) and vascular endothelial growth factor (VEGF) dependent (van Weel et al., 2004). Myocardial overload can lead to a hypothyroid state due to induction of deiodinase (Simonides et al., 2008), while VEGF expression is regulated by HIF 1α. (Forsythe et al., 1996). It has been shown that HIF 1α in pressure overloaded mouse heart can be inhibited by p53 (Sano et al., 2007). Whether or not p53 plays a role in the monocrotaline-induced pulmonary hypertension model remains to be investigated. Myoglobin mRNA is reduced in dog and bovine dilated myocardium (O'Brien et al., 1995; Weil et al, 1997), but is increased in pressure overloaded mouse heart (Lindsey et al., 2007). These results indicate that myoglobin expression may critically depend on different types of interacting factors. Increasing the myoglobin concentration in hypertrophied cardiomyocytes is an important therapeutic target because it can lower PO_{2crit} and thereby increase oxygen extraction from capillaries.

5.5 Limitations

The values of PO_{2crit} and PO_{2cap} presented above are underestimates because the model calculation of PO_{2crit} assumes zero-order kinetics. Rumsey et al. (1990) showed that the Michaelis constant for oxygen of isolated rat heart mitochondria is 0.45 hPa at rest. However, any deviation from zero-order kinetics increases PO_{2crit}, impairing oxygen extraction from capillaries. The Michaelis constant may also increase due to inhibition of complex IV by nitric oxide (Cooper & Brown, 2008). This could increase intracellular PO_2 at the expense of reduced ADP phosphorylation and cardiac output. The calculation of capillary and interstitial permeability is based on assuming a reasonable mean capillary PO_2 but this permeability has not been verified. The calculation of capillary PO_2 in MCT4 rats is based on the assumption that capillary permeability in control and pulmonary hypertensive rats is the same. This is a simplification because capillary circumference may increase, thereby increasing the endothelial diffusion area, whereas the permeability can decrease because the capillary basement menbrane thickens. These changes require further study and direct measurements of capillary permeability for oxygen are required. The translation of the present results to clinical applications will require the demonstration of similar changes in pulmonary hypertensive patients. Preliminary results indicate that this is the case (van Beek-Harmsen et al., 2007; Ruiter et al., 2011).

5.6 Conclusions

We conclude that hypertrophying cardiomyocytes in MCT-injected pulmonary hypertensive rats adapt to hypoxia. However, the changes observed in the hypertrophied myocardium of MCT rats will lead to hypoxic cores in cardiomyocytes with high $VO_{2max}CSA$ or PO_{2crit} when the mitochondria are maximally activated. The adaptation cannot prevent cytochrome c release from mitochondria. The results indicate that an increase of the number of capillaries per cardiomyocyte is required to normalize the oxygen supply/demand ratio in the hypertrophied RV myocardium and that an increase of the myoglobin concentration is required to normalize PO_{2crit}. When PO_{2crit} cannot be normalized, interstitial PO_2 has to increase to prevent core hypoxia in hypertrophied cardiomyocytes, or intramyocyte capillaries (Kobayashi et al., 1999) have to be induced.

6. References

Bache, R.J., Zhang, J., Murakami, Y., Zhang, Y., Cho, Y.K., Merkle, H., Gong, G., From, H.L. & Ugurbil K. (1999). Myocardial oxygenation at high work states in hearts with left ventricular hypertrophy. *Cardiovascular Research* 42: 616-626.

Bekedam, M.A. (2010). Skeletal muscle in chronic heart failure. Thesis VU University Amsterdam, The Netherlands.

des Tombe, A.L., van Beek-Harmsen, B.J., Lee-de Groot, M.B.E. & van der Laarse, W.J. (2002). Calibrated histochemistry applied to oxygen supply and demand in hypertrophic myocardium. *Microscopy Research and Technique* 58: 412-420.

Cooper, C.E. & Brown G.C. (2008). The inhibition of mitochondrial cytochrome oxidase by the gasses carbon monoxide, nitric oxide, hydrogen cyanide and hydrogen sulfide: chemical mechanism and functional significance. *Journal of Bioenergetics and Biomembranes* 40: 533-539.

Ecarnot-Laubriet, A., Assem, M., Poirson-Bichat, F., Moisant M, Bernard ,C., Lecour, S., Solary, E., Rochette, L. & Teyssier, J-R. (2002). Stage-dependent activation of cell-cycle and apoptosis mechanisms in the right ventricle by pressure overload. *Biochemica Biophysica Acta* 1586: 233-242.

Enoki, Y., Matsumura, K., Ogha, Y., Kohuki, H. & Hattori, M. Oxygen affinities (P50) of myoglobins from four vertebrate species (*Canis familiaris, Rattus norvegius, Mus musculus, and Gallus domesticus*) as determined by a kinetic and an equilibrium method. *Compatarive Biochemistry and Physiology* B110: 193-199.

Forsythe, J.A., Jiang, B-H., Iyer, N.V., Agani, F., Leung, S.W., Koos, R.D. & Semenza, G.L. (1996). Activation of Vascular endothelial growth factor gene transcription by hypoxia-inducible factor 1. *Molecular Cell Biology* 16: 4604-4613.

Gayeski, T.E.J. & Honig, C.R. (1991). Intracellular PO2 in individual cardiomyocytes in dogs, cats, rabbits, ferrets and rats. *American Journal of Physiology Heart and Circulatory Physiology* 260: H522-H531.

Gianocco, G., DosSantos, R.A. & Nunes, M.T. (2004). Thyroid hormone stimulates myoglobin gene expression in rat cardiac muscle. *Molecular and Cellular Endocrinology* 226: 19-26.

Gray, L.H. & Steadman, J.M. (1964). Determination of the oxyhemoglobin dissociation curves for mouse and rat blood. *Journal of Physiology* 175: 161-171.

Handoko, M.L., de Man F.S., Happé, C.M., Schalij, I., Musters, R.J.P., Westerhof, N., Postmus, P.E., Paulus, W.J., van der Laarse W.J. & Vonk-Noordegraaf, A. (2009) Opposite effects of training in rats with stable and progressive hypertension. *Circulation* 120: 42-49.

Hill, N.S., Jederlinic, P.& Gagnon, J. (1989). Supplemental oxygen reduces right ventricular hypertrophy in monocrotaline-injected rats. *Journal of Applied Physiology* 66: 1642-1648.

Humbert, M., Sitbon, O., Chaouat, A., Bertocchi, M., habib, G., Gressin, V., Yaïci, A., Weitzenblum, E., Cordier, J-F., Chabot, F., Dromer, D., Pison, C., Reynaud-Gaubert, M., Haloun, A., Laurent, M., Hachulla, E., Cottin, V., Degano, B., Jaïs, X., Montani, D., Souza, R. & Simmoneau, G. (2010). Survival in patients with idiopathic, familial, and anorexigen-associated pulmonary arterial hypertension in the modern management era. *Circulation* 122: 156-163.

Kobayashi, M., Kawamura, K., Honma, M., Masuda, H., Suzuki, Y. & Hasegawa, H. (1999). Tunnel capillaries of cardiac myocyte in pressure-overload rat heart – an ultrastructural three-dimensional study. *Microvascular Research* 57: 258-272.

Kajihara H (1970). Electron microscopic observations of hypertrophied myocardium of rat produced by injection of monocrotaline. *Acta Pathologica Japonica* 20: 183-206.

Kreutzer, U., Mekhamer, Y., Chung, Y. & Jue, T. (2001). Oxygen supply and oxidative phosphorylation limitation in situ. *American Journal of Physiology Heart and Circulatory Physiology* 280: H2030-H2037.

La Piana, G., Marzulli, D., Gorgoglione. V. & Lofrumento, N.E. (2005). Porin and cytochrome oxidase containing contact sites involved in the oxidation of cytosolic NADH. *Archives of Biochemistry and Biophysics* 436: 91-100.

Lee-de Groot, M.B.E., des Tombe, A.L. & van der Laarse, W.J. (1998). Calibrated histochemistry of myoglobin concentration in cardiomyocytes. *Journal of Histochemistry and Cytochemistry* 46:1077-1084.

Lindsey, M.L., Goshorn, D.K., Comte-Wolters, S., Hendrick, J.W., Hapke, E., Zile, M.R. & Schey, K. (2006). A multidimensional proteomic approach to identify hypertrophy-associated proteins. *Proteomics* 6: 2225-2235.

Loud, A.V.& Anversa, P. (1984). Morphometric analysis of biological processes. *Laboratory Investigation* 50: 250-261.

Madsen, K. & Holmskov, U. (1995). Capillary density measurements in skeletal muscle using immunohistochemical staining with anti-collagen type IV antibodies. *European Journal of Applied Physiology* 71: 472-474.

Merkus, D., Haitsma, D.B., Fung, T., Assen, Y.J., Verdouw, P.D. & Duncker, D.J. (2003). Coronary blood flow regulation in exercising swine involves parallel rather than redundant vasodilator pathways. *American Journal of Physiology Heart and Circulatory Physiology* 285: H424-H433.

Mootha, V.K., Arai, A.E. & Balaban, R.S. (1997) Maximum oxidative phosphorylation capacity of the mammalian heart. *American Journal of Physiology Heart and Circulatory Physiology* 272: H769-H775.

Mouchaers, K.T.B., Henkes, I.R., Vliegen, H.W., van der Laarse, W.J., Swenne, C.A., Maan, A.C., Draisma, H.H.M., Schalij, I., van der Wall, E.E., Schalij, M.J. & Vonk-Noordegraaf, A. (2007) Early changes in rat hearts with developing pulmonary arterial hypertension can be detected with 3-dimensional electrocardiography. *American Journal of Physiology Heart and circulatory Physiology* 293: H1300-H1307.

Murray, J.D. (1974). On the role of myoglobin in tissue respiration. *Journal of Theoretical Biology* 47: 115-127.

O'Brien, P.J., Duke, A.L., Shen, H. & Shohet, R.V. (1995). Myocardial mRNA content and stability, and enzyme activities of Ca-cycling and aerobic metabolism in canine dilated cardiomyopathies. *Molecular and Cellular Biochemistry* 142: 139-150.

Okumura, K., Kondo, J., Shimizu, K., Yoshino, M., Toki, Y., Hashimoto, H. & Ito, T. (1992). Changes in ventricular 1,2-diacylglycerol content in rats following monocotaline treatment. *Cardiovascular Research* 26: 626-630.

Papadopoulos, S., Endeward, V., Revesz-Walker, B., Jürgens, K.D.& Gros, G. (2001). Radial and longitudinal diffusion of myoglobin in single living heart and skeletal muscle cells. *Proceedings of the National Academy of Sciences* 98: 5904-5909.

Pool, C.W., Diegenbach, P.C. & Scholten, G. (1979) Quantitative succinate dehydrogenase histochemistry. I. A methodological study on mammalian and fish muscle. *Histochemistry* 64: 251-262.

Radhakrishnan, J., Wang, S., Ayoub, I.M., Korarova, J.D., Levine, R.F. & Gazmuri, R.J. (2007). Circulating levels of cyochrome c after resuscitation from cardiac arrest: a marker of mitochondrial injury and predictor of survival. *American Journal of Physiology Heart and Circulatory Pysiology* 292: H767-H775.

Redout, E.M., Wagner, M.J., Zuidwijk, M.J., Boer , C., Musters, R.J.P., van Hardeveld,, C., Paulus, W.J. & Simonides, W.S. (2007). Right-ventricular failure is associated with increased mitochondrial complex II activity and production of reactive oxygen species. *Cardiovascular Research* 75: 770-781.

Rohbach, P., Cairo, G., Gelf, C., Bernuzzi, F., Pilegaard, H., Viganò Santambrogio, P., Cerretelli, P., Calbet, J.A.L., Montereau, S. & Lundby, C. (2007). Strong iron demand during hypoxia-induced erythropoiesis is associated with down-regulation of iron-related proteins and myoglobin in human skeletal muscle. *Blood* 109: 4724-4731.

Ruiter G., Wong, Y, de Man, F., Postmus, P., Westerhof, N., Niessen, H., van der Laarse, W. & Vonk-Noordegraaf, A. (2011). Right ventricular myoglobin decrease in human pulmonary hypertension. ATS 2011 Denver: https://cms.psav.com

Rumsey, W.L., Schlosser, C., Nuutinen, E.M., Robiolio, M. & Wilson, D.F. (1990). Cellular energetics and the oxygen dependence of respiration in cardiac myocytes isolated from adult rat. *Journal of Biological Chemistry* 265: 15392-15399.

Sano, M., Minamino, T., Toko, H., Miyauchi, H., Orimo, M., Qin, Y., Akazawa, H., Taneto, K., Kayama, Y., Harada, M., Shimizu, I., Asahara, T., Hamada, H., Tomita, S., Molkentin, J.D., Zou, Y. & Komuro, I. (2007). p53-induced inhibition of Hif-1 causes cardiac dysfunction during pressure overload. *Nature* 446: 444-448

Schenkman, K.A., Marble, D.R., Burns, D.H. & Feigl, E.O. (1997) Myoglobin oxygen dissociation by multiwavelength spectroscopy. *Journal of Applied Phyisology* 82: 86-92.

Schmidt-Nielsen, K. & Larimar J.L. (1958). Oxygen dissociation curves of mammalian blood in relation to body size. *American Journal of Physiology* 195: 424-428.

Simonides, W.S., Mulcahhey, M.A., Redout, E.M., Muller, A., Zuidwijk, M.J., Visser, T.J., Wassen, F.W., Crescenti, A., da Silva, W.S., Harney, J., Engel, F.B., Obregon, M.J., Larsen, P.R., Bianco, A.C. & Huang, S.A. (2008). Hypoxia-inducible factor induces local thyroid hormone inactivation during hypoxic-ischemic disease in rats. *Journal of Clinical Investigation* 118: 975-983.

Spriet, L.L., Gledhill, N., Froese, A.B. & Wilkes DL (1986) Effect of graded erythrocythemia on cardiovascular and metabolic responses to exercise. *Journal of Applied Physiology* 61, 1942-1948.

Tune, J.D., Richmond, K.N.,Gorman, M.W., Olsson, R.A. & Feigl, E.O (2000). Adenosine is not responsible for local metabolic control of coronary blood flow in dogs during exercise. *American Journal of Physiology Heart and Circulatory Physiology* 278: H74-H84.

van Beek-Harmsen, B.J., Bekedam, M.A., Feenstra, H.M., Visser, F.C. & van der Laarse, W.J. (2004). Determination of myoglobin concentration and oxidative capacity in cryostat sections of human and rat skeletal muscle fibres and rat cardiomyocytes. *Histochemistry and Cell Biology* 121: 335-342.

van Beek-Harmsen, B.J. & van der Laarse, W.J. (2005). Immunohistochemical determination of cytosolic cytochrome c concentration in cardiomyocytes. *Journal of Histochemistery and Cytochemistry* 53: 803-807.

van Beek-Harmsen, B.J., de Man, F.S., Vonk-Noordegraaf, A., Boonstra, A., Niessen, J.W.M., & van der Laarse, W.J. (2007). Cytochrome c release from mitochondria in cardiomyocytes of pulmonary hypertensive patients. ERS 2007 Stockholm: www.ers-education.org

van der Laarse, W.J., des Tombe, A.L., van Beek-Harmsen, B.J., Lee-de Groot, M.B.E. & Jaspers, R.T. (2005). Krogh's diffusion coefficient for oxygen in isolated Xenopus skeletal muscle fibres and rat myocardial trabeculae at maximum rates of oxygen consumption. *Journal of Applied Physiology* 99: 2173-2180.

van der Laarse, W.J. & Diegenbach, P.C. (1988). Method of quenching of muscle fibres affects apparent succinate dehydrogenase activity. *Histochemical Journal* 20: 624-644.

van Weel, V., Deckers, M.M.L., Grimbergen, J.M., van Leuven, K.J.M., Lardenoye, J.H.P., Schlingemann, R.O., van Nieuw Amerongen, G.P., van Bockel, J.H., van Hinsbergh, V.W.M. & Quax, P.H.A. (2004). Vascular endothelial growth factor overexpression in ischemic skeletal muscle enhances myoglobin expression in vivo. *Circulation Research* 95: 58-66

Wang, G.L. & Semenza, G.L. (1995). Purification and characterization of hypoxia-inducible factor 1. *Journal of Biological Chemistry* 203: 1253-1263.

Weil, J., Eschenhagen, T., Magnussen, O., Mittmann, C., Orthey, E., Scholtz, H., Schäfer, H. & Scholtysik G. (1997). Reduction of myocardial myoglobin in bovine dilated cardiomyopathy. *Journal of Molecular and Cellular Cardiology* 29: 743-751.

Wong, Y.Y., Handoko, M.L., Mouchaers, K.T.B., de Man, F.S., Vonk-Noordegraaf, A. & van der Laarse, W.J. (2010). Reduced mechanical efficiency of rat papillary muscle related to degree of hypertrophy of cardiomyocytes. *American Journal of Physiology Heart and Circulatory Phyiology* 298: H1190-H1197.

Zuurbier, C.J., van Iterson, M. & Ince, C. (1999). Functional heterogeneity of oxygen supply-consumption ratio in the heart. *Cardiovascular Research* 44: 488-497.

Part 3

Clinical Evaluation and Diagnostic Approaches for Pulmonary Hypertension

8

Dyspnea in Pulmonary Arterial Hypertension

Dimitar Sajkov, Karen Latimer and Nikolai Petrovsky
Australian Respiratory and Sleep Medicine Institute (ARASMI)
Flinders Medical Centre and Flinders University, Flinders Drive, Bedford Park
Australia

1. Introduction

Dyspnea is a complex sensation involving interaction of physiological, psychological, social, and environmental factors. Dyspnea in general is common across cardio-vascular and respiratory conditions and it is often difficult to clinically differentiate the exact cause of dyspnea in patients with heart or lung disease. Pulmonary hypertension in the absence of heart or lung disease, a condition called pulmonary arterial hypertension (PAH), is due to endothelial dysfunction and remodelling of small pulmonary arteries. Progressive dyspnea on exertion is a cardinal sign of PAH, which is often first diagnosed when in advanced stages. Improved understanding of pathogenic mechanisms underlying PAH and the related dyspnea should translate into new treatment options for symptom control and to prevent disease progression. This chapter reviews the current understanding of the etiology and pathogenesis of PAH and recent advances in management of this debilitating condition.

2. Pulmonary hypertension: Definition, classification and assessment of severity

Pulmonary hypertension was first described by Ernst von Romberg (von Romberg, 1891) and manifests as an increase in blood pressure in the pulmonary artery, vein, or capillaries. Elevated pulmonary vascular resistance and pressure lead to dyspnea, dizziness and fainting, all of which are exacerbated by exertion. Pulmonary hypertension leads to a progressive decrease in exercise tolerance, and ultimately to heart failure, with a median life expectancy from diagnosis of only 2.8 years. Pulmonary hypertension was previously defined as a mean pulmonary arterial pressure of 25 mmHg or more at rest, and/or 30 mmHg or more on light to moderate exercise. However, this definition has recently been revised with the exercise criterion in the previous definition being removed due to the difficulty of defining an exact upper limit of normal for pulmonary pressures during exercise. According to the most recent Dana Point revised classification (Simonneau et al., 2009; Galiè et al., 2009b), pulmonary hypertension is classified into five major groups: 1) pulmonary arterial hypertension (PAH), 2) pulmonary hypertension due to left heart disease, 3) pulmonary hypertension due to chronic lung disease and/or hypoxia, 4) pulmonary hypertension due to chronic thromboembolic disease and 5) pulmonary hypertension with unclear or multifactorial etiologies (Table 1).

1. PAH

      1.1 Idiopathic PAH (IPAH)

      1.2 Heritable

            1.2.1 BMPR2

            1.2.2 ALK-1, endoglin (with or without hereditary haemorrhagic telangiectasia)

            1.2.3 Unknown

      1.3 Drugs and toxins induced

      1.4 Associated with (APAH)

            1.4.1 Connective tissue diseases

            1.4.2 HIV infection

            1.4.3 Portal hypertension

            1.4.4 Congenital heart disease

            1.4.5 Schistosomiasis

            1.4.6 Chronic haemolytic anaemia

      1.5 Persistent pulmonary hypertension of the newborn

1' Pulmonary veno-occlusive disease and/or pulmonary capillary haemangiomatosis

2. Pulmonary hypertension due to left heart disease

      2.1 Systolic dysfunction

      2.2 Diastolic dysfunction

      2.3 Valvular disease

3. Pulmonary hypertension due to lung diseases and/or hypoxia

      3.1 Chronic obstructive pulmonary disease

      3.2 Interstitial lung disease

      3.3 Other pulmonary diseases with mixed restrictive and obstructive pattern

      3.4 Sleep-disordered breathing

      3.5 Alveolar hypoventilation disorders

      3.6 Chronic exposure to high altitude

      3.7 Developmental abnormalities

4. Chronic thromboembolic pulmonary hypertension

5. PH with unclear and/or multifactorial mechanisms

      5.1 Haematological disorders: myeloproliferative disorders, splenectomy

      5.2 Systemic disorders: sarcoidosis, pulmonary Langerhans cell histiocytosis, lymphangioleiomyomatosis, neurofibromatosis, vasculitis

      5.3 Metabolic disorders: glycogen storage disease, Gaucher disease, thyroid disorders

      5.4 Others: tumoural obstruction, fibrosing mediastinitis, chronic renal failure on dialysis

BMPR2: bone morphogenetic protein receptor, type 2; ALK-1: activin receptor-like kinase 1 gene; APAH: associated pulmonary arterial hypertension; PAH: pulmonary arterial hypertension. (Simonneau et al., 2009)

Table 1.Classification of Pulmonary Hypertension

PAH is defined by a mean pulmonary arterial pressure at rest equal or greater than 25 mm Hg in the presence of a normal pulmonary capillary wedge pressure ($\leq$ 15 mm Hg) and forms a distinct subgroup of pulmonary hypertension. PAH incorporates a number of different groups including familial/heritable PAH, idiopathic PAH and PAH associated with connective tissue disease, congenital heart disease, portal hypertension, or human immuno-deficiency virus (HIV) infection. Clinical severity of PAH is expressed in World Health Organisation (WHO) functional classes (FC), which mainly describe the severity of dyspnea experienced by patient (Barst et al., 2004) (Table 2). Assessment of severity is important as it guides clinical management and helps to determine prognosis (D'Alonzo et al., 1991). In untreated patients with PAH, historical data showed a median survival of 6 years for WHO-FC I and II, 2.5 years for WHO-FC III, and just 6 months for WHO-FC IV (D'Alonzo et al., 1991). Extremes of age (<14 yrs or >65 yrs), falling exercise capacity, syncope, haemoptysis and signs of RV failure all confer a worse prognosis in PAH. Patients with PAH in WHO-FC III or IV benefit from specific disease-modifying treatments and data to support improved outcomes from treatment of earlier stages of PAH are emerging.

Class	Symptomatic profile
Class I	Patients with pulmonary hypertension but without resulting limitation of physical activity. Ordinary physical activity does not cause dyspnea or fatigue, chest pain or near syncope
Class II	Patients with pulmonary hypertension resulting in slight limitation of physical activity. They are comfortable at rest. Ordinary physical activity causes undue dyspnea or fatigue, chest pain or near syncope
Class III	Patients with pulmonary hypertension resulting in marked limitation of physical activity. They are comfortable at rest. Less than ordinary activity causes undue dyspnea or fatigue, chest pain or near syncope
Class IV	Patients with pulmonary hypertension with inability to carry out any physical activity without symptoms. These patients manifest signs of right heart failure. Dyspnea and/or fatigue may even be present at rest. Discomfort is increased by any physical activity.

Table 2. WHO Classification of functional status of patients with pulmonary hypertension

3. Dyspnea and exercise intolerance in pulmonary arterial hypertension

Dyspnea is a complex sensation comprising at least three distinct sensations including air hunger, work/effort, and chest tightness. Dyspnea on exertion is a hallmark of PAH. The mechanism of dyspnea in pulmonary hypertension is complex and depends on the underlying condition and co-morbidities. It has been hypothesised that in pulmonary hypertension associated with pulmonary thromboembolism pressure, receptors or C fibers in the pulmonary vasculature or right atrium mediate the sensation of dyspnea (Manning & Schwartzstein, 1995). This mechanism may also operate in PAH since the severity of dyspnea in these patients is disproportionate to the impairment of left ventricular function, respiratory mechanics and gas exchange. In PAH dyspnea on exertion is usually associated with little or no abnormalities in lung mechanics measured at rest (e.g., normal spirometry and lung volumes), while lung gas exchange may be abnormal (e.g., reduced diffusing lung capacity for carbon monoxide (DLco) (Chandra et al., 2010). Therefore, it is likely that exertional dyspnea in PAH results from complex interactions of signals from the central nervous system (i.e. autonomic centers in the brain stem and the motor cortex) and receptors in the upper airway, lungs, right atrium, pulmonary vessels and chest wall (Manning et al., 1995; O'Donnell et al, 2009). Cardiopulmonary exercise testing (CPET), which measures pulmonary gas exchange during exercise, demonstrates significant oxygen transport abnormalities, such as a decrease in peak oxygen uptake ($V'O_2$), a decreased slope of the increase in $V'O_2$-work rate relationship and a low lactic threshold (Palange et al, 2007). In addition, patients with PAH often have a low V'_E and a normal breathing reserve at peak exercise. This reflects the fixed high physiological dead space consequent to reduced pulmonary perfusion. The alveolar-arterial O_2 difference is often widened during exercise; a right-to-left shunt may contribute to arterial hypoxemia during exercise in a proportion of patients with co-existent patent foramen ovale. Excessive V'_E at low absolute work rates may also reflect the influence of a premature lactic academia. Finally, the breathing pattern tends to be more rapid and shallow than normal; this pattern is not explained by restrictive mechanics and may result from activation of vagal-innervated mechanoreceptors in the right atrium, pulmonary vasculature and pulmonary interstitium. Importantly, with CPET it is possible to detect an abnormal increase in exercise ventilatory response relative to carbon dioxide output ($V'_E/V'CO_2$) that is associated with a proportional and sustained reduction in end-tidal carbon dioxide partial pressure ($P_{ET}CO_2$) (Riley et al., 2000). The degree of ventilatory and gas exchange inefficiency during exercise (i.e., the increase in $V'_E/V'CO_2$ and the drop in $P_{ET}CO_2$) correlates with the severity of the disease, and the level of $P_{ET}CO_2$ reduction may be a useful non-invasive screening tool for the selection of PAH patients for right heart catheterization (Yasunoby et al., 2005). Interestingly, differences in ventilatory and gas exchange adaptations to cycling and walking exercise have been described in PAH; walking, in particular, is more severely limited by high ventilatory response, arterial O_2 desaturation and dyspnea sensation compared to cycling (Valli et al., 2008).

Right heart catheterization with measurement of pulmonary artery pressure and cardiac output has traditionally been used to assess the severity of PAH and the response to interventions. However, catheterization is invasive and cumbersome, largely restricted to tertiary referral centers and not suitable for regular follow-up. Therefore, exercise testing has been used in its place as a surrogate marker to monitor disease severity and prognosis. Wensel et al. studied the prognostic value of $V'O_2$ peak in patients with PAH and reported that patients with $V'O_2$ peak $\leq$ 10.4 ml/min/kg have a 50% risk of early death at 1 year and 85% at 2 years (Wensel et al., 2002). Since CPET is not always available, field walking tests have been utilized to assess the degree of exercise intolerance in PAH (Steel, 1996). The degree of exercise impairment is judged by the measurement of distance covered during a fixed time period. The six minute walking test (6MWT), in which patients are free to choose the most convenient walking speed, is the most popular walking test (American Thoracic Society [ATS], 2002). The distance achieved in the 6MWT has been used as a primary endpoint in most randomised controlled trials of modern PAH therapies (Galiè et al., 2002). The 6MWT has good reproducibility and some studies have demonstrated a significant correlation between the 6MWT distance and peak oxygen uptake ($V'O_2$ peak) measured during standard incremental protocols (Myamoto et al., 2000). Walk distance and oxygen desaturation during 6MWT in patients with PAH relate well to $V'O_2$ peak and appear to have a prognostic value (Myamoto et al., 2000; Paciocco et al., 2001). Unexplained dyspnea on exertion is the main symptom in the early stages of PAH and causes exercise intolerance. In PAH exercise intolerance correlates with the severity of the disease (Sun et al., 2002). Furthermore, the reduction of pulmonary vascular resistance and/or pulmonary arterial pressure with treatment (see below) is paralleled by changes in WHO FC and improvement in dyspnea on exertion as measured by the 6MWT.

4. Management of dyspnea in pulmonary hypertension

Treatment is determined by whether the pulmonary hypertension is arterial, venous, hypoxic, or thromboembolic and is first directed to the primary cause. Since pulmonary venous hypertension (Group 2) is synonymous with congestive heart failure, therapy of dyspnea aims to optimize left ventricular function through use of diuretics, beta blockers, and ACE inhibitors, and where relevant repair/replace dysfunctional heart valves. Similarly, in patients with lung disease and/or hypoxia (Group 3) therapy of dyspnea is usually directed at the underlying cause and correction of hypoxia.

PAH (Group 1) has no underlying cardiac or respiratory cause and most often is associated with scleroderma or idiopathic. While lifestyle changes, digoxin, diuretics, oral anticoagulants, and oxygen therapy were long considered appropriate treatments for PAH-associated dyspnea, these have never been proven to be beneficial in a randomized, prospective manner. As there is currently no cure, therapy of dyspnea in PAH is targeted at symptom control with the aim being to ease dyspneic symptoms thereby allowing patients to become more active, and to use treatments to reduce pulmonary vascular resistance and pressures and thereby slow disease progression.

As outlined in subsequent sections, four major classes of medications are available for treatment of PAH-associated dyspnea (Fig. 1) (Humbert et al., 2004b). Calcium channel blockers reduce contractility of pulmonary arterial smooth muscle thereby reducing pulmonary vascular resistance. Prostacyclin analogues induce pulmonary vasodilation by supplementing inadequate endothelial prostacyclin caused by under-activity of endothelial prostacyclin synthase. Endothelin receptor antagonists block the vasoconstrictor effects of endothelin on pulmonary smooth muscle. Phosphodiesterase 5 (PDE5) inhibitors promote the vasodilation activity of the nitric oxide pathway by reducing conversion of cyclic guanylate monophosphate (a nitric oxide second messenger) to 5'-guanylate monophosphate (an inactive product). By reducing pulmonary arterial pressures and resistance, these treatments reduce dyspnea and improve exercise tolerance in patients with PAH.

4.1 Calcium channel blockers

High-dose calcium channel blockers only showed benefit for symptom relief in about 10% of patients with idiopathic PAH, who achieved reduction in their mean pulmonary arterial pressure and pulmonary vascular resistance by > 20% as measured by Swan-Ganz catheterization during acute vasodilator challenge. In the absence of measurable improvement in pulmonary arterial pressure, calcium channel blockers are not indicated.

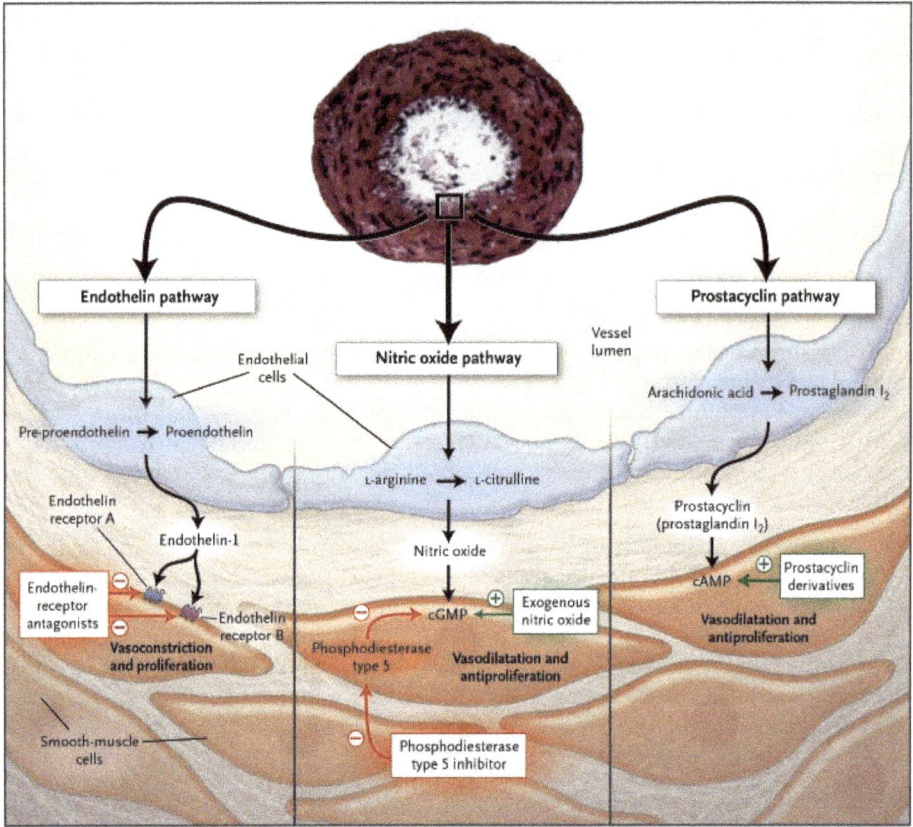

Fig. 1. Therapeutic Targets for Pulmonary Arterial Hypertension
Three major pathways involved in abnormal proliferation and contraction of the smooth-muscle cells of the pulmonary artery in patients with pulmonary arterial hypertension are shown. These pathways correspond to important therapeutic targets in this condition and play a role in determining which of four classes of drugs -- endothelin-receptor antagonists, nitric oxide, PDE5 inhibitors, and prostacyclin derivatives -- will be used. At the top of the figure, a transverse section of a small pulmonary artery (<500 μm in diameter) from a patient with severe pulmonary arterial hypertension shows intimal proliferation and marked medial hypertrophy. Dysfunctional pulmonary-artery endothelial cells (blue) have decreased production of prostacyclin and endogenous nitric oxide, with an increased production of endothelin-1 -- a condition promoting vasoconstriction and proliferation of smooth-muscle cells in the pulmonary arteries (red). Therapies interfere with specific targets in smooth-muscle cells in the pulmonary arteries. In addition to their actions on smooth-muscle cells, prostacyclin derivatives and nitric oxide have several other properties, including antiplatelet effects. Plus signs denote an increase in the intracellular concentration; minus signs blockage of a receptor, inhibition of an enzyme, or a decrease in the intracellular concentration; and cGMP cyclic guanosine monophosphate.

The criteria for vasoreactivity have recently changed. Only patients whose *mean* pulmonary artery pressure falls by > 10 mm Hg to < 40 mm Hg with an unchanged or increased cardiac output when challenged with adenosine, epoprostenol, or nitric oxideare considered "vasoreactive". Of these, only 50% may have sustained response to calcium channel blockers (Rich & Brundage, 1987; Sitbon et al., 2005) and can be treated with dihydropiridine calcium channel blockers (i.e. nifedipine, felodipine or amlodipine) or diltiazem. Verapamil is contraindicated because of its negative inotropic effect.

4.2 Prostacyclin analogues

Prostacyclin is a potent pulmonary vasodilator and inhibits platelet aggregation. It is a metabolite of arachidonic acid produced in the normal vascular endothelium. Reduced expression of prostacyclin synthase in patients with PAH causes prostacyclin deficiency. Epoprostenol is a potent, short-acting prostacyclin analogue that induces pulmonary vasodilation and is approved for treatment of patients with PAH in WHO FC III or IV. Epoprostenol is administered by continuous intravenous infusion through an indwelling central line. Unfortunately, it is expensive, inconvenient (patients need to carry a continuous infusion pump) and has significant dose-dependent adverse effects including flushing, headache, jaw and lower extremity muscular pain, diarrhea, nausea, and rash. Patients with PAH may live at distance from the nearest tertiary care facility and a well-established setting for ensuring continuous supply and supervision is critical, as sudden interruption of the epoprostenol infusion may cause rebound severe PAH and death. Despite the side effects and inconveniences with administration, epoprostenol has solid clinical evidence of efficacy in PAH. It has been shown to reduce dyspnea, improve exercise capacity, quality of life and survival in patients with PAH (Badesch et al., 2000; Barst et al., 1996; McLaughlin et al., 2002; Sitbon et al., 2002). Three-year survival of patients with PAH treated with epoprostenol was 63% (McLaughlin et al., 2002; Sitbon et al., 2002). Most patients experienced optimal benefit from epoprostenol at a stable dose of 25 to 40 ng/kg per minute, after incremental increases over the course of 6 -12 months from an initial dosage of 2 to 6 ng/kg per minute.

Treprostinil is a prostacyclin analogue that is stable at room temperature and has a longer half-life than epoprostenol (3-4 hours). This allows it to be given intravenously or via a small subcutaneous catheter with a continuous pump. Treatment by either route improves the 6MWT distance in patients with PAH in WHO FC III or IV (Simonneau et al., 2002; Tapson et al., 2006). Three-year survival of patients with idiopathic PAH treated with subcutaneous treprostinil monotherapy has been reported as 71% (Barst et al., 2006a). Whilst short-term efficacy of intravenous treprostinil may equal epoprostenol; comparative survival data are lacking. The adverse effect profile of treprostinil is similar to epoprostenol. Frequent, severe pain at the site of infusion may limit the treprostinil dose that can be administered subcutaneously. This limitation may reduce treprostinil's efficacy because the effect on 6MWT distance is dose-dependent, and higher doses may require intravenous administration. Other clinical trials of treprostinil inhaled and oral formulations are ongoing. Some patients treated with epoprostenol may be switched to intravenous treprostinil with maintenance of 6MWT distance; although a larger dose of treprostinil is required (Gomberg-Maitland et al., 2005).

Iloprost is an inhaled prostacyclin analogue that was shown to improve dyspnea, exercise capacity and hemodynamics in patients with PAH. In a randomized, placebo-controlled, 12-week study, iloprost produced a placebo-corrected increase in 6MWT distance of 36 m in 207 patients with symptomatic idiopathic PAH, PAH associated with connective tissue disease or appetite suppressants, or pulmonary hypertension related to inoperable chronic thromboembolic disease (Olschewski et al., 2002). Long-term maintenance of improved exercise capacity and hemodynamics was observed with iloprost use (Hoeper et al., 2000). Adverse effects of iloprost are similar to other prostacyclin analogues and include flushing, headache, and cough. A major downside for patients is that iloprost's short duration of action necessitates frequent 10-minute inhalations, 6 to 9 times per day.

4.3 Endothelin receptor antagonists (ERA)

By binding to endothelin receptors A and B, endothelin-1 triggers pulmonary vasoconstriction and stimulates vascular smooth muscle and fibroblast proliferation. Endothelin-1 levels are increased in PAH, and correlate with disease severity, suggesting that blockade of endothelin-1 should have beneficial effects. Bosentan is an orally-active, dual ERA that improves exercise capacity, quality of life, hemodynamics, and time to clinical worsening in PAH (Channick et al., 2001; Rubin et al., 2002). Two-year survival of patients with idiopathic PAH in whom bosentan was used as first-line therapy was 87% (McLaughlin et al., 2005; Provencher et al., 2006). Bosentan is currently approved for treatment of PAH patients in WHO FC III or IV. Adverse effects of bosentan include flushing, edema, nasal congestion, mild anemia, and teratogenicity. Dose-dependent elevation of liver transaminases occurs in about 10% of patients on bosentan, requiring monthly monitoring of liver function.

Ambrisentan and sitaxentan are ERA with relative selectivity for the endothelin receptor subtype A. Treatment with sitaxentan was efficacious for patients with PAH with low incidence of liver toxicity in initial reports (Barst et al., 2006b; Benza et al., 2008). However, it was recently removed from the market due to case reports of severe hepatitis and liver toxicity. Ambrisentan is another ERA with safer liver toxicity profile. It has been shown to improve symptoms, exercise capacity, and hemodynamics (Galiè et al., 2005a). Adverse effects of ambrisentan include flushing, edema, nasal congestion, and teratogenicity. Although associated with a low incidence of liver enzyme elevations, monthly liver function monitoring is still required (McGoon et al., 2009).

4.4 Phosphodiesterase 5 Inhibitors

Sildenafil, originally commercialized for erectile dysfunction, is a potent, highly specific inhibitor of PDE5 that has been shown to improve symptoms and functional capacity in PAH patients (Galiè et al., 2005b). Adverse effects associated with sildenafil include headache, flushing, dyspepsia, nasal congestion, and epistaxis. Nitrates are contraindicated in patients taking PDE5 inhibitors because the additive effects of the drugs can cause life-threatening hypotension.

Tadalafil, a long-acting PDE5 inhibitor, is the most recent oral agent for treatment of PAH (Rosenzweig, 2010). The Pulmonary Arterial Hypertension and Response to Tadalafil (PHIRST) clinical trial examined the efficacy and tolerability of tadalafil for the treatment of

PAH over a period of 16 weeks (Galiè et al., 2009a). Tadalafil 40 mg showed significant improvement over placebo for six of eight SF-36 domains and EQ-5D index scores. Also, the tadalafil 40-mg group showed significant improvement over placebo on the 6MWT distance (p < 0.001), but no clear relationship was found between 6MWT distance and health-related quality of life (HRQoL). Results suggest that tadalafil may significantly improve HRQoL and exercise capacity in patients with PAH.

4.5 Combination treatments

Combinations of disease-modifying agents of various classes seems a logical next step in PAH management and is becoming standard care in many PAH centres. Clinical trial evidence for combination therapy is encouraging (Humbert et al., 2004a; McLaughlin et al., 2006; O'Callaghan & Gaine, 2007; Simonneau et al., 2008). The relatively small BREATHE-2 study (Humbert et al., 2004a) showed a trend to haemodynamic improvement with combination epoprostenol-bosentan as compared to epoprostenol alone. The STEP-1 study (Simonneau et al., 2008) addressed the safety and efficacy of 12 weeks therapy with inhaled iloprost plus bosentan and reported a non-significant increase of 26 m in the post-inhalation 6MWT distance (p=0.051). There was no improvement in pre-inhalation haemodynamics in the iloprost group after 12 weeks of treatment, but time to clinical worsening was significantly prolonged in the iloprost group (0 events *versus* 5 events in the placebo group; p = 0.02). In contrast, the COMBI trial which also studied the benefits of inhaled iloprost added to bosentan, was stopped prematurely after a planned interim analysis failed to show an effect on 6MWT distance or time to clinical worsening (Hoeper et al., 2006). The TRIUMPH trial studied the effects of inhaled treprostinil in patients already treated with bosentan or sildenafil (McLaughlin et al., 2010). The primary end-point, change in 6MWT distance at peak exposure, improved by 20 m compared with placebo (p<0.0006). At trough exposure, *i.e.* after >4 hours post-inhalation, the difference was 14 m in favour of the treprostinil group (p<0.01). There were no significant differences in Borg dyspnea index, functional class and time to clinical worsening. The PACES trial addressed the effects of adding sildenafil to epoprostenol in 267 patients with PAH (Simonneau et al., 2008) and showed significant improvements after 12 weeks in 6MWT distance and time to clinical worsening.

Additional data are available for the combination of ERA and PDE5 inhibitors. In the subgroup of patients enrolled in the EARLY study (Galiè et al., 2008) (bosentan in WHO FC II PAH patients already on treatment with sildenafil), the haemodynamic effect of the addition of bosentan was comparable with that achieved in patients without background sildenafil treatment. A pharmacokinetic interaction has been described between bosentan and sildenafil, which act as inducers or inhibitors of cytochrome P450 CYP3A4, respectively. The co-administration of both results in a decline of sildenafil and increase in bosentan plasma levels (Paul et al., 2005). So far there is no indication that these interactions are associated with reduced safety (Humbert et al., 2007), but whether the clinical efficacy of sildenafil is significantly reduced is still controversial. No pharmacokinetic interactions have been reported between sildenafil and the two other available ERAs, sitaxentan and ambrisentan. In the PHIRST study (Galiè et al., 2009a) the combination of tadalafil and bosentan resulted in an improvement of exercise capacity of borderline statistical significance.

Avoid pregnancy (I-C)
Influenza and pneumococcal immunisation (I-C)
Supervised rehabilitation (IIa-B)
Psycho-social support (IIa-C)
Avoid excessive physical activity (III-C)

General measures and supportive therapy

Diuretics (I-C)
Oxygen# (I-C)
Oral anticoagulants:
IPAH, heritable PAH and PAH due to anorexigens (IIa-C)
APAH (IIb-C)
Digoxin (IIb-C)

Expert referral (I-C)

Acute vasoreactivity test
(I-C for IPAH)
(IIb-C for APAH)

Vasoreactive   Nonvasoreactive

WHO-FC I-III
CCB (I-C)

Sustained response
(WHO-FC I-II)

YES   NO

Continue CCB

Initial therapy			
Recommendation-evidence	WHO-FC II	WHO-FC III	WHO-FC IV
I-A	Ambrisentan, bosentan, sildenafil	Ambrisentan, bosentan, sitaxentan, sildenafil epoprostenol *i.v.*, iloprost inhaled	Epoprostenol *i.v.*
I-B	Tadalafil¶	Tadalafil¶ Treprostinil s.c., inhaled¶	
IIa-C	Sitaxentan	Iloprost *i.v.*, treprostinil *i.v.*	Ambrisentan, bosentan, sitaxentan, sildenafil, tadalafil¶, iloprost inhaled, and *i.v.* treprostinil s.c., *i.v.*, inhaled¶, initial combination therapy
IIb-B		Beraprost	

Inadequate clinical response

Inadequate clinical response

Sequential combination therapy (IIa-B)+

ERA

+   +

Prostanoids   +   PDE-5 I

BAS (I-C) and/or lung transplantation (I-C)

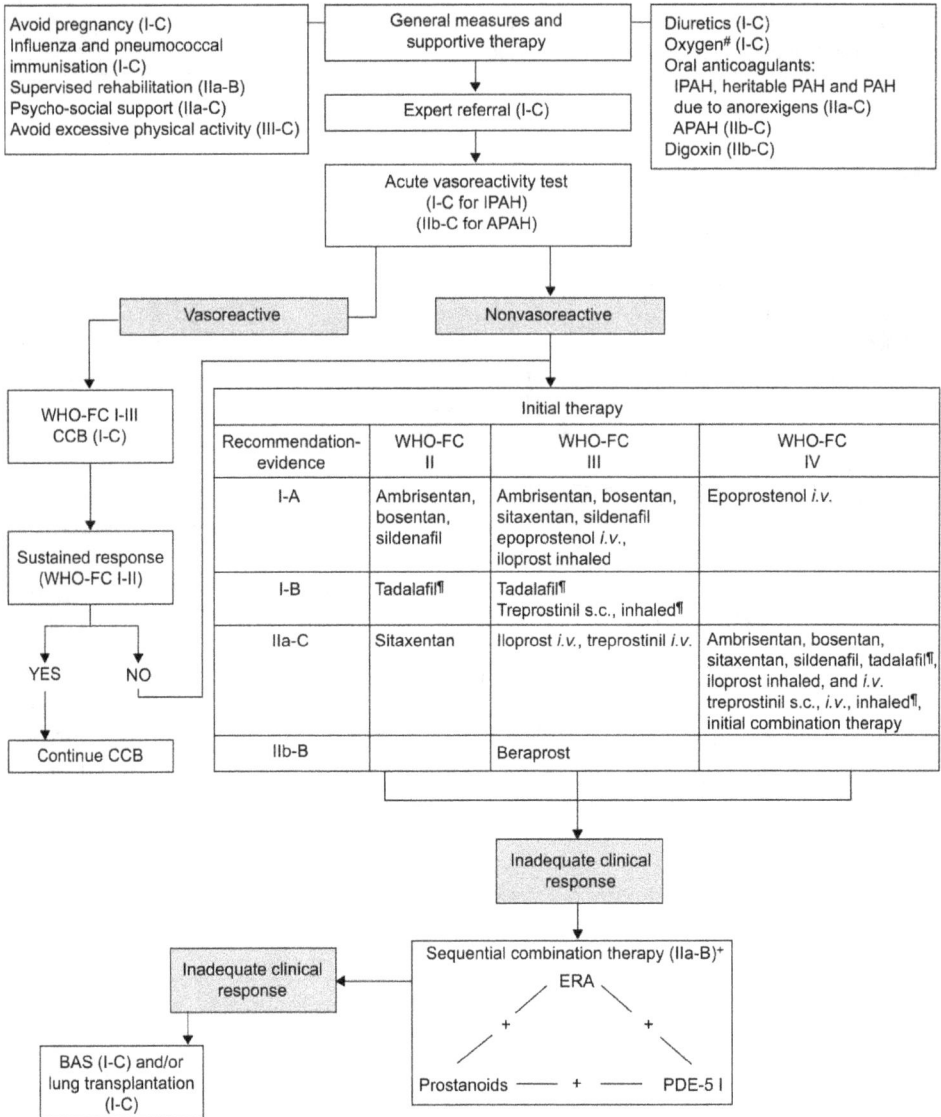

Fig. 2. Treatment algorithm for PAH-associated dyspnea
Evidence-based treatment algorithm for treatment of dyspnea caused by pulmonary arterial hypertension (group 1 patients only). APAH: associated pulmonary arterial hypertension; BAS: balloon atrial septostomy; CCB: calcium channel blocker; ERA: endothelin receptor antagonist; IPAH: idiopathic pulmonary arterial hypertension; PAH: pulmonary arterial hypertension; PDE-5 I: phosphodiesterase type-5 inhibitor; s.c.: subcutaneously; WHO-FC: World Health Organization functional class. #: to maintain arterial blood O_2 pressure >8 kPa (60 mmHg); ¶: under regulatory review in the European Union; +: IIa-C for WHO-FC II.

In summary, whether the response to monotherapy is sufficient or not can only be decided on an individual basis. Combination therapy is recommended for PAH patients not responding adequately to monotherapy and ideally should be instituted by experienced centres (Fig. 2).

5. Palliative and supportive treatments for residual dyspnea in treated progressive pulmonary hypertension

Since PAH is not a curable disease, many patients inevitably progress to WHO-FC IV with severe dyspnea. This necessitates additional palliative and supportive treatments. Exercise training, atrial septostomy and opioids are some of the interventions that may have a role in improving symptoms and exercise tolerance in patients with progressive PAH.

Exercise in the form of respiratory and physical training appears efficacious as part of the management of PAH. When superimposed on an optimal stable drug regimen, 15 weeks of respiratory and physical training led to an average increase of 111 m in 6MWT distance, in addition to improvements in other measures of exercise tolerance and quality of life (Mereles et al., 2006). This is a major benefit when put in the perspective of expensive PAH medications that may deliver more modest 20-40 m improvements in 6MWT distance.

Atrial septostomy performed by graded balloon dilatation may be suitable for selected patients with severe PAH. In patients with medically treated severe progressive PAH, atrial septostomy improved clinical symptoms and dyspnea, cardiac index, exercise endurance and systemic oxygen transport (Reichenberger et al., 2003; Sandoval et al., 1998).

Transplantation is an important option for selected PAH patients. Up to 25% of patients with PAH fail to improve on disease-specific therapy and the prognosis of patients who remain in WHO FC III or IV is poor. International guidelines to aid referral and listing have been published by the International Society for Heart and Lung Transplantation (Orens et al., 2006). Both heart–lung and double-lung transplantation have been performed for PAH and each centre has developed its own strategy for the choice of the type of transplantation in the individual patient. However, due to the shortage of donor organs, most patients are considered for double-lung transplantation. While right ventricular afterload is immediately reduced after double-lung transplantation, right ventricular systolic and left ventricular diastolic functions do not improve immediately and hemodynamic instability is a common problem in the early post-operative period. The overall 5-year survival following transplantation for PAH is 45–50%, with evidence of sustained improvement in dyspnea and quality of life (Trulock et al., 2006).

In parallel with attempts to treat the underlying pathology causing dyspnea, the sensation of breathlessness itself must be ameliorated. For many patients there comes a point when there are no further identifiable reversible components of PAH and the treatment focus needs to move to reducing the subjective sensation of breathlessness (Davis, 1994). Like pain, dyspnea has a sensory and an affective dimension. Therefore, treatment strategies in dyspnea should be similar to those used in pain. Recent neuroimaging studies suggest that neural pathways involved in pain and dyspnea sensation may be shared and, therefore, similar neurophysiological and psychological approaches used to understand and manage pain can be applied to dyspnea (Nishino, 2011). Previous randomised controlled trials have reported the effectiveness of sustained-release morphine in patients with refractory dyspnea, including those with severe COPD (Abernethy et al., 2003; Poole et al., 1998) and chronic heart failure (Johnson et al., 2002). Currently there is no data on use of opioids to relieve dyspnea in patients with progressive advanced PAH and clinical trials are on-going. Effective and predictive treatment of dyspnea remains elusive and a better understanding of the pathophysiology and neurophysiology of dyspnea may lead to more effective treatments.

6. Conclusion

Etiological diagnosis and assessment of pulmonary hypertension WHO functional class is critical for management. Despite recent advances in understanding and treatment of PAH it remains a progressive and incurable disease, with dyspnea and exercise intolerance being the major causes of distress to sufferers. More effective palliation of dyspnea in patients with PAH depends on better understanding of it's mechanisms. More randomised clinical trial evidence on combination and palliative treatments is needed to improve management of dyspnea in patients with advanced PAH.

7. Acknowledgement

Supported by a research grant from Foundation Daw Park Inc. and unrestricted educational grant from Actelion.

8. References

Abernethy, A.; Currow, D.; Frith, P.; Fazekas, B., McHugh, A. & Bui, C. (2003). Randomised, double blind, placebo controlled crossover trial of sustained release morphine for the management of refractory dyspnea. *British Medical Journal*, Vol.327, No.7417, (September 2003), pp. 523-528, ISSN 0959-8138

American Thoracic Society (2002). ATS Statement: Guidelines for the six minute walking test. *American Journal of Respiratory and Critical Care Medicine*, Vol.166, No.1, (July 2002); pp. 111-117, ISSN 1073-449X

Badesch, D.; Tapson, V.; McGoon, M.; Brundage, B.; Rubin, L.; Wigley, F.; Rich, S.; Barst, R.; Barrett, P.; Kral, K.; Jöbsis, M.; Loyd, J.; Murali, S.; Frost, A.; Girgis, R.; Bourge, R.; Ralph, D.; Elliott, C.; Hill, N.; Langleben, D.; Schilz, R.; McLaughlin, V.; Robbins, I.; Groves, B.; Shapiro, S. & Medsger, T. Jr. (2000) Continuous intravenous epoprostenol for pulmonary hypertension due to the scleroderma spectrum of disease. *Annals of Internal Medicine*, Vol.132, No.6, (March 2000); pp. 425-434, ISSN 1539-3704

Barst, R.; Galiè, N.; Naeije, R.; Simonneau, G.; Jeffs, R.; Arneson, C. & Rubin, L. (2006a). Long-term outcome in pulmonary arterial hypertension patients treated with subcutaneous treprostinil. *European Respiratory Journal*, Vol.28, No.6, (December 2006), pp. 1195-1203, ISSN 1399-3003

Barst, R.; Langleben, D.; Badesch, D.; Frost, A.; Lawrence, E.; Shapiro, S.; Naeije, R. & Galiè, N. (2006b). Treatment of pulmonary arterial hypertension with the selective endothelin-A receptor antagonist sitaxsentan. *Journal of the American College of Cardiology*, Vol.47, No.10, (May 2006), pp. 2049-2056, ISSN 0735-1097

Barst, R.; McGoon, M.; Torbicki, A.; Sitbon, O.; Krowka, M.; Olschewski, H. & Gaine, S. (2004). Diagnosis and differential assessment of pulmonary arterial hypertension. *Journal of the American College of Cardiology,* Vol.43, No.12 Supplement 1, (June 2004), pp. S40-S47, ISSN 0735-1097

Barst, R.; Rubin, L.; Walker, A.; Long, W.; McGoon, M.; Rich, S.; Badesch, D.; Groves, B.; Tapson, V.; Bourge, R.; Brundage, B.; Koerner, S.; Langleben, D.; Keller, C.; Murali, S.; Uretsky, B.; Clayton, L.; Pharm, D.; Jöbsis, M.; Blackburn, S. Jr.; Shortino, D. & Crow, J. for the Primary Pulmonary Hypertension Study Group (1996). A comparison of continuous intravenous epoprostenol (prostacyclin) with conventional therapy for primary pulmonary hypertension. *The New England Journal of Medicine,* Vol.334, No.5, (February 1996), pp. 296–302, ISSN 1533-4406

Benza, R; Barst, R.; Galiè, N.; Frost, A.; Girgis, R.; Highland, K.; Strange, C.; Black, C.; Badesch, D.; Rubin, L.; Fleming, T. & Naeije, R. (2008). Sitaxsentan for the treatment of pulmonary arterial hypertension: a 1-year, prospective, open-label observation of outcome and survival. *Chest,* Vol.134, No.4, (October 2008), pp. 775-782, ISSN 1931-3543

Chandra, S.; Shah, S.; Thenappan, T.; Archer, S.; Rich, S. & Gomberg-Maitland, M. (2010). Carbon monoxide diffusing capacity and mortality in pulmonary arterial hypertension. *The Journal of Heart and Lung Transplantation,* Vol.29, No.2, (February 2010), pp. 181-187, ISSN 1053-2498

Channick, R. ; Simonneau, G. ; Sitbon, O. ; Robbins, I. ; Frost, A. ; Tapson, V. ; Badesch, D. ; Roux, S. ; Rainisio, M. ; Bodin, F. & Rubin, L. (2001). Effects of the dual endothelin-receptor antagonist bosentan in patients with pulmonary hypertension: a randomised placebo-controlled study. *The Lancet,* Vol.358, No.9288, (October 2001), pp. 1119-1123, ISSN 1474-4465

D'Alonzo, G.; Barst, R.; Ayres, S.; Bergofsky, E.; Brundage, B.; Detre, K.; Fishman, A.; Goldring, R.; Groves, B.; Kernis, J.; Levy, P.; Pietra, G.; Reid, L.; Reeves, J.; Rich, S.; Vreim, C.; Williams, G. & Wu, M. (1991). Survival in patients with primary pulmonary hypertension. Results from a national prospective registry. *Annals of Internal Medicine,* Vol.115, No.5, (September 1991), pp. 343-349, ISSN 1539-3704

Davis, C. (1994). The therapeutics of dyspnea. *Cancer Surveys,* Vol.21 (1994), pp. 85-98, ISSN 0261-2429

Galié, N.; Badesch, D.; Oudiz, R.; Simonneau, G.; McGoon, M.; Keogh, A.; Frost, A.; Zwicke, D.; Naeije, R.; Shapiro, S.; Olschewski, H. & Rubin, L. (2005a). Ambrisentan therapy for pulmonary arterial hypertension. *Journal of the American College of Cardiology,* Vol.46, No.3, (August 2005), pp. 529-535, ISSN 0735-1097

Galiè, N.; Brundage, B.; Ghofrani, H.; Oudiz, R.; Simonneau, G.; Safdar, Z.; Shapiro, S.; White, R.; Chan, M.; Beardsworth, A.; Frumkin, L.; Barst, R. & Pulmonary Arterial Hypertension and Response to Tadalafil (PHIRST) Study Group. (2009a). Tadalafil therapy for pulmonary arterial hypertension. *Circulation,* Vol.119, No.22, (June 2009), pp. 2894-2903, ISSN 0009-7322

Galiè, N.; Ghofrani, H.; Torbicki, A.; Barst, R.; Rubin, L.; Badesch, D.; Fleming, T.; Parpia, T.; Burgess, G.; Branzi, A.; Grimminger, F.; Kurzyna, M.; Simonneau, G. & Sildenafil Use in Pulmonary Arterial Hypertension (SUPER) Study Group. (2005b). Sildenafil citrate therapy for pulmonary arterial hypertension. *The New England Journal of Medicine,* Vol.353, No.12, (November 2005), pp. 2148-2157, ISSN 1533-4406

Galiè, N.; Hoeper, M.; Humbert, M.; Torbicki, A.; Vachiery, J.; Barbera, J.; Beghetti, M.; Corris, P.; Gaine, S.; Gibbs, J.; Gomez-Sanchez, M.; Jondeau, G.; Klepetko, W.; Opitz, C.; Peacock, A.; Rubin, L.; Zellweger, M. & Simonneau, G. (2009b). Guidelines for the diagnosis and treatment of pulmonary hypertension. *European Respiratory Journal*, Vol.34, No.6, (December 2009), pp. 1219-1263, ISSN 1399-3003

Galiè, N.; Manes, A. & Branzi, A. (2002). The new clinical trials on pharmacological treatment in pulmonary arterial hypertension. *European Respiratory Journal*, Vol.20, No.4, (October 2002), pp. 1037-1049, ISSN 1399-3003

Galiè, N.; Rubin, L.; Hoeper, M.; Jansa, P.; Al-Hiti, H.; Meyer, G.; Chiossi, E.; Kusic-Pajic, A. & Simonneau, G. (2008). Treatment of patients with mildly symptomatic pulmonary arterial hypertension with bosentan (EARLY study): a double-blind, randomised controlled trial. *The Lancet*, Vol.371, No.9630, (June 2008), pp. 2093–2100, ISSN 1474-4465

Gomberg-Maitland, M.; Tapson, V.; Benza, R.; McLaughlin, V.; Krichman, A.; Widlitz, A. & Barst, R. (2005). Transition from intravenous epoprostenol to intravenous treprostinil in pulmonary hypertension. *American Journal of Respiratory and Critical Care Medicine*, Vol.172, No.12, (December 2005); pp. 1586-1589, ISSN 1073-449X

Hoeper, M.; Leuchte, H.; Halank, M.; Wilkens, H.; Meyer, F.; Seyfarth, H.; Wensel, R.; Ripken, F.; Bremer, H.; Kluge, S.; Hoeffken, G. & Behr, J. (2006). Combining inhaled iloprost with bosentan in patients with idiopathic pulmonary arterial hypertension. *European Respiratory Journal*, Vol.28, No.4, (October 2006), pp. 691-694, ISSN 1399-3003

Hoeper, M.; Schwarze, M.; Ehlerding, S.; Adler-Schuermeyer, A.; Spiekerkoetter, E.; Niedermeyer, J.; Hamm, M. & Fabel, H. (2000). Long-term treatment of primary pulmonary hypertension with aerosolized iloprost, a prostacyclin analogue. *The New England Journal of Medicine*, Vol.342, No.25, (June 2000), pp. 1866-1870, ISSN 1533-4406

Humbert, M.; Barst, R.; Robbins, I.; Channick, R.; Galiè, N.; Boonstra, A.; Rubin, L.; Horn, E.; Manes, A. & Simonneau, G. (2004a). Combination of bosentan with epoprostenol in pulmonary arterial hypertension: BREATHE-2. *European Respiratory Journal*, Vol.24, No.3, (September 2004), pp. 353-359, ISSN 1399-3003

Humbert, M.; Segal, E.; Kiely, D.; Carlsen, J.; Schwierin, B. & Hoeper, M. (2007). Results of European post-marketing surveillance of bosentan in pulmonary hypertension. *European Respiratory Journal*, Vol.30, No.2, (August 2007), pp. 338-344, ISSN 1399-3003

Humbert, M.; Sitbon, O. & Simonneau, G. (2004b). Treatment of pulmonary arterial hypertension. *The New England Journal of Medicine*, Vol.351, No.14, (September 2004), pp. 1425-1436, ISSN 1533-4406

Johnson, M.; McDonagh, T.; Harkness, A.; McKay, S. & Dargie, H. (2002). Morphine for the relief of breathlessness in patients with chronic heart failure – a pilot study. *European Journal of Heart Failure*, Vol.4, No.6, (December 2002), pp. 753-756, ISSN 1879-0844

Manning, H. & Schwartzstein, R. (1995). Pathophysiology of dyspnea. *The New England Journal of Medicine*, Vol.333, No.23, (December 1995), pp. 1547-1553, ISSN 1533-4406

McGoon, M.; Frost, A.; Oudiz, R.; Badesch, D.; Galiè, N.; Olschewski, H.; McLaughlin, V.; Gerber, M.; Dufton, C.; Despain, D. & Rubin, L. (2009). Ambrisentan therapy in patients with pulmonary arterial hypertension who discontinued bosentan or sitaxsentan due to liver function test abnormalities. *Chest*, Vol.135, No.1, (January 2009), pp. 122-129, ISSN 1931-3543

McLaughlin, V.; Benza, R.; Rubin, L.; Channick, R.; Voswinckel, R.; Tapson, V.; Robbins, I.; Olschewski, H.; Rubenfire, M. & Seeger, W. Addition of inhaled treprostinil to oral therapy for pulmonary arterial hypertension: a randomized controlled clinical trial. *Journal of the American College of Cardiology*, Vol.45, No.18, (May 2010), pp. 1915-1922, ISSN 0735-1097

McLaughlin, V.; Oudiz, R.; Frost, A.; Tapson, V; Murali, S.; Channick, R.; Badesch, D.; Barst, R.; Hsu, H. & Rubin, L. (2006). Randomized study of adding inhaled iloprost to existing bosentan in pulmonary arterial hypertension. *American Journal of Respiratory and Critical Care Medicine*, Vol.174, No.11, (December 2006); pp. 1257-1263, ISSN 1073-449X

McLaughlin, V.; Shillington, A. & Rich, S. (2002). Survival in primary pulmonary hypertension: the impact of epoprostenol therapy. *Circulation*, Vol.106, No.12, (September 2002), pp. 1477-1482, ISSN 0009-7322

McLaughlin, V.; Sitbon, O.; Badesch, D.; Barst, R.; Black, C.; Galiè, N.; Rainisio, M.; Simonneau, G. & Rubin, L. (2005). Survival with first-line bosentan in patients with primary pulmonary hypertension. *European Respiratory Journal*, Vol.25, No.2, (February 2005), pp. 244-249, ISSN 1399-3003

Mereles, D.; Ehlken, N.; Kreuscher, S.; Ghofrani, S.; Hoeper, M.; Halank, M.; Meyer, F.; Karger, G.; Buss, J.; Juenger, J.; Holzapfel, N.; Opitz, C.; Winkler, J.; Herth, F.; Wilkens, H.; Katus, H.; Olschewski, H. & Grünig, E. (2006). Exercise and respiratory training improve exercise capacity and quality of life in patients with severe chronic pulmonary hypertension. *Circulation*, Vol.114, No.14, (October 2006), pp. 1482-1489, ISSN 0009-7322

Myamoto, S.; Nagaya, N.; Satoh, T.; Kyotani, S.; Sakamaki, F.; Fujita, M.; Nakanishi, N. & Miyatake, K. (2000). Clinical correlates and prognostic significance of six-minute walk test in patients with primary pulmonary hypertension. Comparison with cardiopulmonary exercise testing. *Respiratory and Critical Care Medicine*, Vol.161, No.2 Pt 1, (February 2000), pp. 487-492, ISSN 1073-449X

Nishino T. (2011). Dyspnea: underlying mechanisms and treatment. *British Journal of Anaesthesia*, Vol.106, No.4, (February 2011), pp. 463-474. ISSN 1471-6771

O'Donnell, D.; Ora, J.; Webb, K.; Laveneziana, P. & Jensen, D. (2009). Mechanisms of activity-related dyspnea in pulmonary diseases. *Respiratory Physiology & Neurobiology*, Vol.167, No.1, (May 2009), pp. 116-132, ISSN 1569-9048

O'Callaghan, D. & Gaine, S. (2007). Combination therapy and new types of agents for pulmonary arterial hypertension. *Clinics in Chest Medicine*, Vol.28, No.1, (March 2007), pp.169-185, ISSN 0272-5231

Olschewski, H.; Simonneau, G.; Galiè, N.; Higenbottam, T.; Naeije, R.; Rubin, L.; Nikkho, S.; Speich, R.; Hoeper, M.; Behr, J.; Winkler, J.; Sitbon, O.; Popov, W.; Ghofrani, H.; Manes, A.; Kiely, D.; Ewert, R.; Meyer, A.; Corris, P.; Delcroix, M.; Gomez-Sanchez, M.; Siedentop, H.; Seeger, W. & Aerosolized Iloprost Randomized Study Group. (2002). Inhaled iloprost for severe pulmonary hypertension. *The New England Journal of Medicine*, Vol.347, No.5, (August 2002), pp. 322-329, ISSN 1533-4406

Orens, J.; Estenne, M.; Arcasoy, S.; Conte, J.; Corris, P.; Egan, J.; Egan, T.; Keshavjee, S.; Knoop, C.; Kotloff, R.; Martinez, F.; Nathan, S.; Palmer, S.; Patterson, A.; Singer, L.; Snell, G.; Studer, S.; Vachiery, J.; Glanville, A. & Pulmonary Scientific Council of the International Society for Heart and Lung Transplantation. (2006). International guidelines for the selection of lung transplant candidates: 2006 update–a consensus report from the Pulmonary Scientific Council of the International Society for Heart and Lung Transplantation. *The Journal of Heart and Lung Transplantation*, Vol.25, No. 7, (July 2006), pp. 745–755, ISSN 1053-2498

Paciocco, G.; Martinez, F.; Bossone, E.; Pielsticker, E.; Gillespie, B. & Rubenfire, M. (2001). Oxygen desaturation on the six-minute walk test and mortality in untreated primary pulmonary hypertension. *European Respiratory Journal*, Vol.17, No.4, (April 2001), pp. 647-652, ISSN 1399-3003

Palange, P.; Ward, S.; Carlsen, K.; Casaburi, R.; Gallagher, C.; Gosselink, R.; O'Donnell, D.; Puente-Maestu, L.; Schols, A.; Singh, S. & Whipp, B. (2007). Recommendations on the use of exercise testing in clinical practice. *European Respiratory Journal*, Vol.29, No.1, (January 2007), pp. 185-209, ISSN 1399-3003

Paul, G.; Gibbs, JS, Boobis, AR.; Abbas, A. & Wilkins, M. (2005). Bosentan decreases the plasma concentration of sildenafil when coprescribed in pulmonary hypertension. *British Journal of Clinical Pharmacology*, Vol.60, No.1, (July 2005), pp. 107–112, ISSN 1365-2125

Poole, P.; Veale, A. & Black, P. (1998). The effect of sustained-release morphine on breathlessness and quality of life in severe chronic obstruvtive pulmonary disease. *American Journal of Respiratory and Critical Care Medicine*, Vol.157, No.6 pt 1, (June 1998); pp. 1877-1880, ISSN 1073-449X

Provencher, S. ; Sitbon, O. ; Humbert, M. ; Cabrol, S. ; Jaïs, X. & Simonneau, G. (2006). Long-term outcome with first-line bosentan therapy in idiopathic pulmonary arterial hypertension. *European Heart Journal*, (March 2006), pp. 589-595, ISSN 1522-9645

Reichenberger, F.; Pepke-Zaba, J.; McNeil, K.; Parameshwar, J. & Shapiro, L. (2003). Atrial septostomy in the treatment of severe pulmonary arterial hypertension. *Thorax*, Vol.58, No.9, (September 2003), pp.797-800, ISSN 1468-3296

Rich S. & Brundage B. (1987). High-dose calcium channel-blocking therapy for primary pulmonary hypertension: evidence for long-term reduction in pulmonary arterial pressure and regression of right ventricular hypertrophy. *Circulation*, Vol.76, No.1, (July 1987), pp. 135-141, ISSN 0009-7322

Riley, M.; Pórszász, J.; Engelen, M.; Brundage, B. & Wasserman, K. (2000). Gas exchange responses to continuous incremental cycle ergometry exercise in primary pulmonary hypertension in humans. *European Journal of Applied Physiology*, Vol.83, No.1, (September 2000), pp. 63–70, ISSN 1439-6327

Rosenzweig, E. (2010). Tadalafil for the treatment of pulmonary arterial hypertension. *Expert Opinion on Pharmacotherapy*, Vol.11, No.1, (January 2010), pp. 127-132, ISSN 1744-7666

Rubin, L.; Badesch, D.; Barst, R.; Galiè, N.; Black, C.; Keogh, A.; Pulido, T.; Frost, A.; Roux, S.; Leconte, I.; Landzberg, M. & Simonneau, G. (2002). Bosentan therapy for pulmonary arterial hypertension. *The New England Journal of Medicine*, Vol.346, No.12, (March 2002), pp. 896-903, ISSN 1533-4406

Sandoval, J.; Gaspar, J.; Pulido, T.; Bautista, E.; Martínez-Guerra, M.; Zeballos, M.; Palomar, A. & Gómez, A. (1998). Graded balloon dilation atrial septostomy in severe primary pulmonary hypertension. *Journal of the American College of Cardiology*, Vol.32, No.2, (August 1998), pp. 297-304, ISSN 1558-3597

Simonneau, G.; Barst, R.; Galiè, N.; Naeije, R.; Rich, S.; Bourge, R.; Keogh, A.; Oudiz, R.; Frost, A.; Blackburn, S.; Crow, J.; Rubin, L. & Treprostinil Study Group. (2002). Continuous subcutaneous infusion of treprostinil, a prostacyclin analogue, in patients with pulmonary arterial hypertension: a double-blind, randomized, placebo-controlled trial. *American Journal of Respiratory and Critical Care Medicine*, Vol.165, No.6, (March 2002); pp. 800-804, ISSN 1073-449X

Simonneau, G.; Robbins, I.; Beghetti, M.; Channick, R.; Delcroix, M.; Denton, C.; Elliott, C.; Gaine, S.; Gladwin, M.; Jing, Z.; Krowka, M.; Langleben, D.; Nakanishi, N. & Souza, R. (2009). Updated clinical classification of pulmonary hypertension. *Journal of the American College of Cardiology*, Vol.54, No.1 suppl, (June 2009), pp. S43-S54, ISSN 1558-3597

Simonneau, G.; Rubin, L.; Galiè, N.; Barst, R.; Fleming, T.; Frost, A.; Engel, P.; Kramer, M.; Burgess, G.; Collings, L.; Cossons, N.; Sitbon, O.; Badesch, D. & the PACES Study Group. (2008). Addition of sildenafil to long-term intravenous epoprostenol therapy in patients with pulmonary arterial hypertension. *Annals of Internal Medicine*, Vol.149, No.8, (October 2008), pp. 521-530, ISSN 1539-3704

Sitbon, O.; Humbert, M.; Jaïs, X.; Ioos, V.; Hamid, A.; Provencher, S.; Garcia, G.; Parent, F.; Hervé, P. & Simonneau, G. (2005). Long-term response to calcium channel blockers in idiopathic pulmonary arterial hypertension. *Circulation*, Vol.111, No.23, (June 2005), pp. 3105-3011, ISSN 0009-7322

Sitbon, O.; Humbert, M.; Nunes, H.; Parent, F.; Garcia, G.; Hervé, P.; Rainisio, M. & Simonneau, G. (2002). Long-term intravenous epoprostenol infusion in primary pulmonary hypertension: prognostic factors and survival. *Journal of the American College of Cardiology*, Vol.40, No.4, (August 2002), pp. 780-788, ISSN 1558-3597

Steel, B. (1996). Timed walking tests of exercise capacity in chronic cardiopulmonary illness. *Journal of Cardiopulmonary Rehabilitation*, Vol.16, (1996), pp. 16:25-33, ISSN 0883-9212

Sun, X.; Hansen, J.; Oudiz, R. & Wasserman, K. (2002). Gas exchange detection of exercise-induced right-to-left shunt in patients with primary pulmonary hypertension. *Circulation*, Vol.105, No.1, (January 2002), pp. 54-60, ISSN 0009-7322

Tapson, V.; Gomberg-Maitland, M.; Mclaughlin, V.; Benza, R.; Widlitz, A.; Krichman, A. & Barst R. (2006). Safety and efficacy of intravenous treprostinil for pulmonary arterial hypertension: a prospective, multicenter, open-label 12-week trial. *Chest*, Vol.129, No.3, (March 2006), pp. 683-688, ISSN 1931-3543

Trulock, E.; Edwards, L.; Taylor, D.; Boucek, M.; Keck, B.; Hertz, M. & International Society for Heart and Lung Transplantation. (2006). Registry of the International Society for Heart and Lung Transplantation: twenty third official adult lung and heart lung transplantation report–2006. *The Journal of Heart and Lung Transplantation*, Vol.25, No. 8, (August 2006), pp. 880-892, ISSN 1053-2498

Valli, G.; Vizza, C.; Onorati, P.; Badagliacca, R.; Ciuffa, R.; Poscia, R.; Brandimarte, F.; Fedele, F.; Serra, P. & Palange, P. (2008). Pathophysiological adaptations to walking and cycling in primary pulmonary hypertension. *European Journal of Applied Physiology*, Vol.102, No.4, (March 2998), pp. 417-424, ISSN 1439-6327 von Romberg, E. (1892). Über Sklerose der Lungenarterie (in German). *Deutsches Archiv für Klinische Medizin,* Vol.48, (1891-1892) pp. 197–206.

Wensel, R.; Opitz, C.; Anker, S.; Winkler, J.; Höffken, G.; Kleber, F.; Sharma, R.; Hummel, M.; Hetzer, R. & Ewert, R. (2002). Assessment of survival in patients with Primary Pulmonary Hypertension. *Circulation,* Vol.106, No.3, (July 2002), pp. 319-324, ISSN 0009-7322

Yasunobu, Y.; Oudiz, R.; Sun, X.; Hansen, J. & Wasserman, K. (2005). End-tidal pCO_2 abnormality and exercise limitation in patients with primary pulmonary hypertension. *Chest,* Vol.127, No.5, (May 2005), pp. 1637-1646, ISSN 1931-3543

9

Assessment of Structural and Functional Pulmonary Vascular Disease in Patients with PAH

Juan Grignola[1], Enric Domingo[2,3],
Rio Aguilar-Torres[3,4] and Antonio Roman[5]
[1]Dept Pathophysiology, Hospital de Clínicas, Universidad de la República,
[2]Area del Cor, Hospital Universitari Vall d'Hebron
[3]Dept Physiology, Universitat Autonoma Barcelona
[4]Unit of Cardiac Image, Hospital Universitario Bellvitge
[5]Servei de Pneumologia i CIBERES, Hospital Universitari Vall d'Hebron
[1]Uruguay
[2,3,4,5]Spain

1. Introduction

Pulmonary arterial hypertension (PAH) is a life threatening disease characterized by a progressive increase in pulmonary blood pressure that often leads to right ventricular (RV) failure and death (McLaughlin et al., 2009). A review of the clinical trial data for the three classes of drugs approved for the treatment of PAH (prostanoids, endothelin antagonists, and phosphodiesterase-5 inhibitors) has shown that all agents have similar efficacy on the 6-min walking distance over 12 to 16 weeks, which was the primary endpoint in the randomized clinical trials. However, the improvement in the distance walked during the 6-min walking test in the patients receiving active therapy that led to drug approval ranged from 3 to 17% from baseline. With respect to hemodynamics (which provides direct information about the status of the pulmonary circulation) these treatments are unimpressive, producing only a minimal reduction in the pulmonary arterial (PA) pressure. Presently, it remains speculative how these different drugs act on the pulmonary vasculature of patients with PAH and little is known about their long-term efficacy (Rich, 2006). Likewise, recent metaanalysis reported that the pooled effect of all treatment strategies shows a significant reduction of 39% (2-62%, p=0.041) in all-cause mortality (Galié et al., 2009). The benefits were confined only to patients with advanced disease for only 16 weeks, regardless of which class of drug was used. However, the mechanism by which mortality decrease remains unknown because it was unrelated to a specific class of drug, the dose of the drug, or the effects of the drug on 6-minute walking distance or hemodynamics (Macchia et al., 2010).

The increase in pulmonary arterial pressure in patients with PAH is due to the combination of pulmonary vasoconstriction, pulmonary arterial wall remodeling and *in situ* thrombosis. The structural and functional changes in the pulmonary arteries of patients with idiopathic PAH (IPAH) (vascular remodeling) include wall thickening of all three layers of the blood vessel wall (adventitia, media and intima) and reduction of the arterial lumen. This is an important pathological feature of PAH which leads to increased steady and pulsatile components of the pulmonary vascular load. Several studies have shown that the proliferation of PA smooth muscle cells in PAH is enhanced, whereas apoptosis is depressed. Among the drugs currently used for the treatment of patients with PAH, it was demonstrated that prostacyclin analogues inhibit proliferation and promoting apoptosis to a greater extent in distal (< 1 mm external diameter) compared with proximal (> 8 mm external diameter) isolated human PA smooth muscle cells stimulating the cGMP pathway. These effects were potentiated by sildenafil in an independent cAMP pathway mechanism (Wharton et al., 2000, 2005). Recently, it was reported that imatinib (a tyrosine kinase inhibitor) also has anti-proliferative and pro-apoptotic effects on platelet-derived growth factor-stimulated PA smooth muscle cells from patients with IPAH (Nakamura et al., 2011). However, neither of the clinical trials characterize the direct effects of the treatments on the vasculature (*eg*, remodeling), until now. Direct measurement of PA structural/functional remodeling with new vascular imaging techniques such as cardiac magnetic resonance, intravascular ultrasound (IVUS) or optical coherence tomography (OCT) imaging needs to be investigated. Remarkable advances in these techniques provide an extraordinary opportunity to gain insight into histopathology that previously could only be obtained by open lung biopsy.

The aim of the present chapter is to evaluate the viscoelastic pulmonary artery properties (by IVUS) and PA fibrosis (by OCT) in patients with PAH and its relation to dynamic afterload. In addition, we also analyze acute vasoreactivity and its relationship with the viscoelastic properties of pulmonary artery vascular wall in patients with IPAH.

2. Physiological basis of normal local arterial viscoelastic properties

The viscoelastic properties of the great arteries determine their main functions: to conduct blood (conduction function) and to buffer the pulse pressure and flow generated by ventricular ejection (wall buffering function). In general, the elastic and viscous properties of the arterial wall have been characterized together as "viscoelasticity." Various studies have demonstrated that the elasticity and viscosity of the arterial wall play different roles in arterial function, and can also be independently affected by physiologic, pathologic or experimental conditions (Nichols & O'Rourke, 2005).

Elasticity depends strongly on pressure and therefore increases significantly during increased arterial pressure. Elastin, collagen, and vascular smooth muscle have different elastic moduli. They all start to stretch at different levels of arterial wall strain, thus the ratio of pressure to diameter is non-linear. At higher pressure, the recruitment of more rigid collagen fibers is greater, and elasticity increases. The degree of activation of vascular smooth muscle also affected arterial elasticity. Elastin and collagen keep the level of arterial stress stable, which allows cyclic elastic arterial stretching and recovery but prevents over-distension and arterial wall disruption. In contrast, vascular smooth muscle is a dynamic component whose elasticity depends not only on the distension pressure but also on its extent of activation. The elastic response of the artery is an important determinant of its conduction and buffering functions. An adequate elastic modulus allows systolic distension of the artery and the subsequent diastolic elastic recoil, which ensures the continuous anterograde blood flow. In addition, an adequate elastic modulus reduces the oscillations generated by the heart, ensuring a high mean arterial pressure and a low pulsatility.

Previous studies performed in systemic arteries and the PA showed that activation of vascular smooth muscle increases arterial wall elasticity as a function of deformation or diameter (isometric analysis), or decreases arterial stiffness as a function of strain or pressure (isobaric analysis). Our experimental data agree with these studies because elasticity, when measured at constant pressure, decreased with muscular activation (passive versus active PH) (Bia et al., 2005a).

Arterial wall viscosity has been associated mainly with energy loss during the cardiac cycle and might be directly associated with the amount and degree of activation of vascular smooth muscle. We have demonstrated that only the activation of vascular smooth muscle increased viscosity with respect to the control value in both PA and aorta. Moreover, viscosity was greater in the aorta than in the PA during control and hypertensive states (Bia et al., 2003). The viscosity of arterial tissue might be explained by one of two theories (Nichols & O'Rourke, 2005). The «passive» theory assumes that viscosity is a property of the constituents of the arterial wall (being vascular smooth muscle the most important). The «active» theory considers the mechanisms generating muscle contraction (activation) and myogenic response to stretching to be important. The viscous response of the arterial wall is independent of pressure and attenuates the highest frequency components of the incident waves of pressure and flow and the amplitude of the reflected waves that could trigger resonance phenomena in the system. A higher viscosity denotes a greater energy cost during the pulsatile expansion of the vessel in each cardiac cycle and is associated with a higher buffering function (Bia et al., 2005b).

Arterial wall buffering function could be defined by arterial wall viscosity/elasticity ratio. The arterial elasticity is highly dependent on blood pressure, and the viscosity values related to the amount of vascular smooth muscle and its degree of activation. Recently, in anesthetized animals, Bia et al found that the local wall buffering function of the ascending aorta and the main PA is similar despite their differences in elastic and viscous response. In both arteries, during active hypertension, the wall buffering function remained similar to the basal value, despite the increased pressure dependent upon the elastic modulus. This maintenance of the wall buffering function is due to the increase in the viscous modulus generated by the muscle activation (Bia et al., 2003).

3. Intravascular ultrasound (IVUS): A functional approach for the evaluation of pulmonary arterial wall viscoelasticity in PAH

In the clinical setting, the hemodynamic characterization of the pulmonary vascular tree and the response to vasoactive drugs is achieved by applying Poiseuille's law from pressure and cardiac output determinations during right heart catheterisation. However, these measurements have several limitations: a) they only assess the status of the stationary component of the pulmonary vasculature, neglecting the essentials of a pulsatile circulation; b) they correlate weakly with histological findings; and c) they do not have the ability to evaluate both structural and functional states of the PA wall (Saouti et al., 2010).

Resistance is only one component of afterload, and its calculations assume a constant blood flow, whereas compliance, capacitance and impedance are more useful to describe pulsatile flow. The PA stiffness assessment better reflects these latter components that could contribute to worsening right heart failure. Several studies have begun to measure and explore the clinical relevance of PA stiffness in PH.

PA stiffness is an important factor governing dynamic afterload. It has also been reported that proximal PA stiffness may increase early in the course of PH, suggesting a potential contributory role of PA stiffness in the development and progression of PH. The association between vascular stiffening and disease severity is believed to be due to several factors: a) stiffening reduces the windkessel effect of the elastic arteries, leading to greater flow inefficiency; b) stiffening increases RV afterload independent of pulmonary vascular resistance (PVR); and c) changes in the flow and pressure waveforms due to stiffening of the pulmonary circulation have been shown to stimulate cellular signaling pathways in distal vessels and the lungs that aggravate the existent vascular disease. Increased stiffness observed in PA hypertension may be secondary to elevated distending pressures or/and to structural changes of the PA wall. IVUS has been used for quantifying the pulsatility of PA (IVUSp) in IPAH (Berger et al., 2002; Rodés-Cabau et al., 2003). The arterial pulsatility depends on intraluminal pressure and on viscoelastic properties of the arterial wall, while stiffness depends on the extent of wall remodeling. The lack of correlation between IVUSp and usual hemodynamic variables in patients with IPAH suggests that wall remodeling may influence the functional properties of the arterial wall derived from IVUS. We have already experimentally demonstrated that only those indexes of wall stiffness that simultaneously consider changes of pressure and diameter of PA are correlated with the incremental elastic modulus (gold standard for the elastic properties of a vessel wall) (Bia et al., 2005a). It has been reported that a decreased pulsatility of both proximal (magnetic resonance imaging) (Gan et al., 2007; Sanz, Fernández-Friera & Moral, 2010) and distal (IVUS) (Rodés-Cabau et al., 2003) PA is related to increased long term mortality in patients with IPAH. However, because of the strong dependency of strain on underlying pressures, quantification of IVUSp alone is insufficient to fully characterize PA elastic properties, explaining the absence of its correlation with basic hemodynamic parameters (Rodés-Cabau et al., 2003; Grignola et al., 2010).

3.1 Estimation of local pulmonary arterial pulsatility and stiffness indexes by IVUS

We studied twenty five consecutive patients with IPAH who underwent cardiac catheterisation. Hemodynamic evaluation and IVUS imaging of the PA were performed during the same procedure according to a protocol previously reported. All patients underwent a routine right heart catheterisation and simultaneous IVUS in a supine position and breathing room air (Rodés-Cabau et al., 2003). A 7F Swan-Ganz catheter (Edwards Lifesciences, USA) was inserted into a brachial vein and a 5F end-hole catheter was inserted into the right radial artery to monitor systemic arterial pressure. Both catheters were connected to fluid-filled transducers which were positioned at the anterior axillary line level and zeroed at the atmospheric pressure. Right atrial pressure, PA pressure, pulmonary arterial occlusion pressure (PAOP) and systemic arterial pressure were measured. Cardiac output was estimated by the Fick method assuming basal oxygen consumption (125 ml O_2/min/m²) (Soto & Kleczka, 2008). Cardiac index was calculated by dividing the cardiac output by body surface area. After hemodynamic measurements were done, an Eagle Eye Gold catheter 20MHz, 3.5F (Volcano Corporation, USA) with an axial resolution of 200μm and a pullback of 0.5mm/s, was advanced over a 0.014" guidewire into the same PA branch using an exchange guidewire system and X-ray control (Fig. 1). This method guarantees that IVUS images and PA pressure are obtained from the same arterial segment in the pulmonary arterial tree. The images were obtained from the segmental PA of the inferior lobes (elastic PA between 2-4 mm) (Bressollette et al., 2001) and stored in digital format. The images were independently analyzed off-line by two observers blinded for clinical and hemodynamic findings (E.D., M.V.). The end-diastolic (minimal) and end-systolic (maximal) cross-sectional areas of the distal segment were measured (Fig. 2). Pulmonary vascular disease is diffuse but not uniform in the pulmonary tree. However, considering that Bresollette et al. have shown that structural abnormalities were significantly more severe in the lower lobes, it is possible that the pulmonary vascular disease process associated with PH begins in this region because of the higher hydrostatic pressure (Bresollette et al., 2001).

Steady (PVR) and pulsatile (pulmonary arterial capacitance, Cp) components of afterload were estimated. PVR and Cp were calculated as (mean PA pressure-PAOP)/cardiac output and the ratio between the stroke volume and the PA pulse pressure (SV/Pp), respectively. IVUSp was estimated as: ((systolic area-diastolic area)/diastolic area)) ×100; ((sA-dA)/dA) × 100 (Fig. 2).

PA stiffness indexes were assessed by arterial cross-sectional area and local Pp (Rodés-Cabau et al., 2003; Laurent et al., 2007; Grignola et al., 2010):

$$\text{Elastic modulus } (E_P)\text{: } dA \times Pp\,/(sA\text{-}dA) \tag{1}$$

$$\text{Cross-sectional distensibility } (D_{CS})\text{: IVUSp} \times Pp \tag{2}$$

$$\text{Local compliance } (C_L)\text{: } (sA\text{ - }dA)\,/\,Pp \tag{3}$$

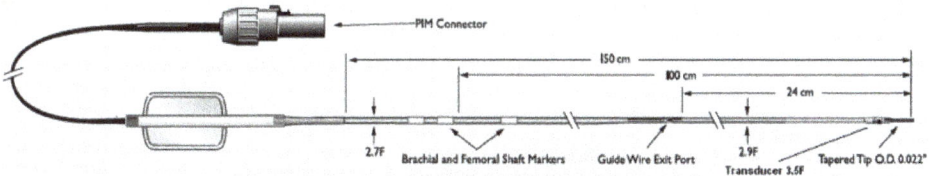

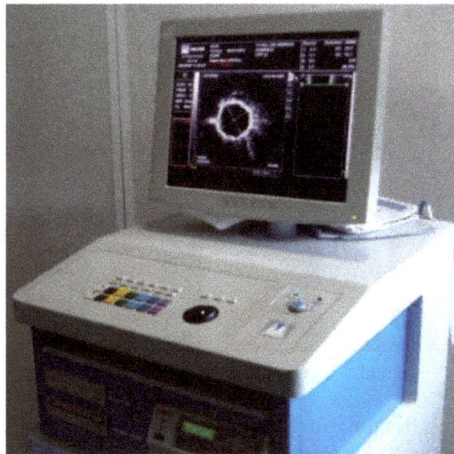

Fig. 1. Eagle Eye Gold imaging catheter (20 MHz) and console (Volcano Corporation).

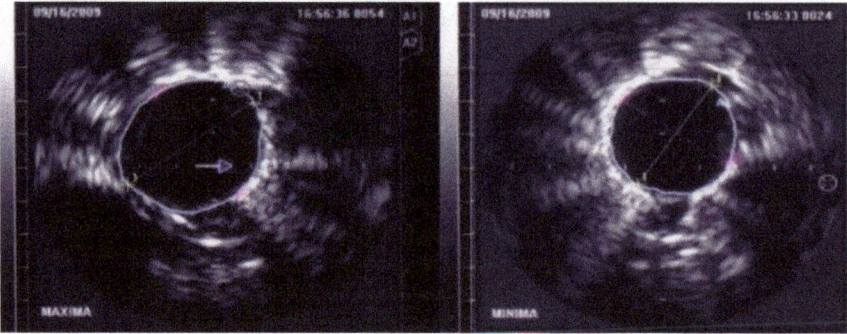

Fig. 2. Representative IVUS images of a patient with IPAH. Left side: systolic phase and right side: diastolic phase of the cardiac cycle. (IVUSp = 11.8-9.4/9.4 = 25.5%).

Figure 3 shows mean values of IVUSp and E_P in four groups of patients studied at our institution: ten control patients (with suspicion of PAH); a recent group of eighteen IPAH patients (2008-2009) split into two groups according to the median of E_P (group 1 ≤ 190 mmHg and group 2 > 190 mmHg) and a historical group of more severe IPAH patients (prior to 2003) (Rodés-Cabau et al., 2003; Domingo et al., 2011).

It can be seen that control group patients have a significantly lower E_P and higher IVUSp than IPAH patients. In according with our results, Berger et al. showed that arterial wall distensibility (the inverse of E_P) significantly decreased in children with advanced pulmonary vascular disease in comparison with normal subjects, corresponding with an average E_P of 182 mmHg versus 50 mmHg (Berger et al., 2001). However, they did not find differences in vascular pulsatility between patients with pulmonary vascular disease and control subjects.

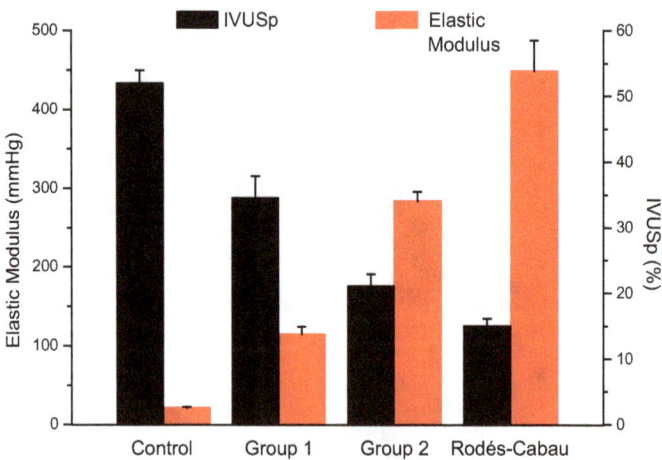

Fig. 3. Bar diagram showing the mean ± ES of elastic modulus and pulsatility (IVUSp) of control (n=10) and IPAH patients (Group 1, n=9; Group 2, n=10 and Rodés-Cabau, n=20).

We suggest that IVUSp and E_P are different qualitative indexes of the arterial wall viscoelastic properties. IVUSp is a normalized cross-sectional pulsatility that depends only on arterial cross-sectional signals (geometric related index) and E_P is a local PA stiffness index normalized by Pp.

We have previously shown that PA arterial wall indexes that depend only on arterial geometric signals (such as normalized cross-sectional pulsatility) do not follow the same patterns as the incremental elastic modulus (E_{INC}, gold standard of the elastic properties of a vessel wall) (Bia et al., 2005a). Only during vascular smooth muscle activation did arterial cross-sectional area and wall viscosity increase with regard to the passive situation and independent from the pulse pressure level, suggesting that absolute or normalized pulse cross-sectional area could be an indirect or qualitative marker of arterial wall viscosity status. In relation to this, the absence of a relation between IVUSp and hemodynamic variables suggests that changes in pulmonary vessel structure are responsible for functional alteration shown by ultrasound (Rodés-Cabau et al., 2003).

The incremental elastic modulus is commonly used in elasticity theory because it best defines the intrinsic properties (independently of size or geometry) of a given material (eg, the arterial wall). Consequently, it is considered the "gold standard" for the evaluation of the elastic response of a material. The requirement for the geometric characteristics of the arterial segment (thickness and diameter of the arterial wall) to be known makes this a difficult modulus to calculate in a clinical setting. The E_P allows calculation of the arterial rigidity in relation to the unit strain, and as such, is independent of the diameter or cross-sectional area. Its particular clinical usefulness comes from the fact that it is only necessary to know the maximum systolic and minimum diastolic values of the arterial pressure and cross-sectional signals in order to perform the calculation. However, since the calculation requires the use of the maximum and minimum values for pressure and cross-sectional in order to calculate the secant between these points, its values include both the elastic and viscous behavior of the arterial wall. Thus, due to the viscoelastic characteristic of the arterial wall, the maximum systolic diameter of the artery reached during arterial distension is highly dependent upon the level of arterial viscosity (Bia et al., 2005b).

Therefore, we can state that IVUSp is very dependent on wall viscosity and that E_P depends on the mechanical effect of PA pressure, the vascular smooth muscle tone variations, and the changes in the PA wall structure. So, as might be expected, control patients have the higher wall PA buffering function (higher IVUSp plus the lower E_P), and the group studied by Rodés-Cabau showed the worst PA buffering function (Fig. 3).

3.2 Correlation of local pulmonary arterial stiffness indexes with steady and pulsatile afterload

The arterial hydraulic load can be described completely by the so-called pulmonary arterial input impedance that accounts for the relationship between pulsatile pressure and flow. However, this description is not only difficult to derive but also complex to interpret (Nichols & O'Rourke, 2005). Therefore, several simplified descriptions of the arterial circulation have been proposed. One such description is the two-element Windkessel model which consists of physiologically easily interpretable parameters and describes the hemodynamics in terms of resistance and compliance. The resistance of the model is the

PVR. PVR is mainly located in the small arteries and arterioles, since resistance strongly depends on vessel diameter. The compliance of the model (Cp) is the storage capacity of all arteries and arterioles taken together. Cp is related to arterial wall elasticity and vessel size (i.e. radius and wall thickness). The compliance of the arterial tree allows the arteries to expand passively during systole and to recoil during diastole. This has two important effects: a) the compliant arteries are able to store the ejected blood-volume in systole and release this volume during diastole resulting in constant peripheral blood flow throughout the entire cardiac cycle and, b) the compliant arteries dampen/cushion the pressure so that pressure variations in the PA are smaller than in the ventricle. If we assume that the periphery is closed for a moment, the increase in pressure ($\Delta P = Pp$) resulting from a single stroke volume (SV) relates thus to compliance: $Cp = SV/Pp$, which overestimates the real compliance. Calculation of Cp is, in practice, more difficult because there is blood leaving the arterial system through the periphery (microcirculation) while cardiac ejection takes place. Although the pulse pressure method was shown to result in reliable data, the SV/Pp ratio is an acceptable method to derive compliance in vivo (Chemla et al., 1998; Stergiopulos, Segers & Westerhof, 1999).

Clinicians usually define RV afterload in terms of PVR and this measure is often used as a primary or secondary end-point in clinical studies. However, PVR only reflects the non-pulsatile (steady) component of blood flow, and neglects the important contribution of compliance. In recent years it has become clear that in PH not only the contribution of PVR is of importance but that the decrease in Cp plays an equally important role. Cp takes into account the pulsatile components of the arterial load and, therefore, is an important factor contributing to systolic and diastolic pressure. Besides, it was shown to be a prognosis factor for mortality (Mahapatra et al., 2006). It is noteworthy that the common PA and proximal left and right arteries together contribute only 15-20% of total Cp, suggesting that arterial compliance is distributed over the entire pulmonary arterial bed, like PVR (Saouti et al., 2010). On the contrary, in the systemic arterial tree the compliance is mainly located in the aorta (80% of total compliance in thoracic-abdominal aorta), and resistance is mainly located in arterioles. This distribution depends on the number of peripheral vessels, which is ≈ 8-10 times more in the pulmonary system than in the systemic tree (Saouti et al., 2010).

Cp quantifies total (rather than local) arterial compliance, given an average of what is happening in the whole arterial pulmonary tree without allowing the analysis of regional changes and to detect early-stage wall remodeling. As we previously mentioned, the simultaneous use of IVUS and conventional RHC allowed us to estimate local viscoelastic properties of the PA as a whole. A major advantage is that local arterial stiffness is directly determined from the change in pressure driving the change in volume, i.e. without using any model of the circulation. Both the change in pressure and size should be obtained from the same arterial segment. It has also been reported that proximal PA stiffness may increase early in the course of IPAH, suggesting a potential contributory role of PA stiffness in the development and progression of PAH (Sanz et al., 2009).

In spite of IPAH patients with higher wall stiffness (group 2 and Rodés-Cabau group) showing lower IVUSp are associated with decreased Cp and increased PVR, neither Cp nor PVR correlated with IVUSp (Fig. 4). On the contrary, the three local PA stiffness indexes (normalized by pulse pressure) correlated significantly with global capacitance and resistance properties of the pulmonary arterial tree (Fig. 5) (Grignola et al., 2010).

As mentioned before, the assessment of PA stiffness indexes requires the use of the maximum and minimum values for pressure and cross-sectional area including both the elastic and viscous behavior of the PA arterial wall.

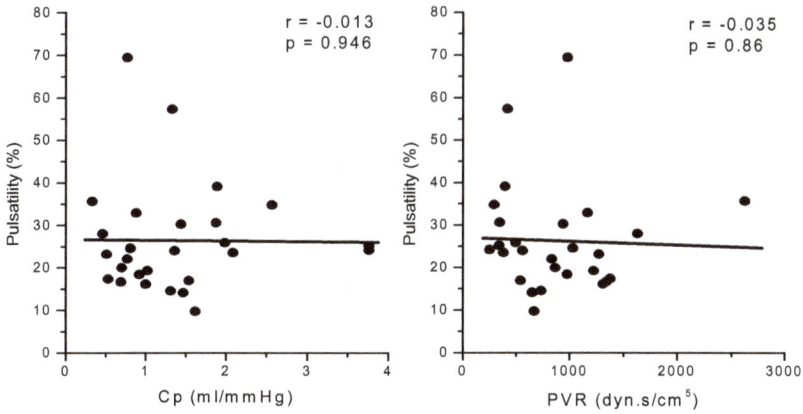

Fig. 4. Absence of correlation between pulsatility (IVUSp) and pulsatile (Cp, capacitance index) and steady (PVR, pulmonary vascular resistance) pulmonary afterload components.

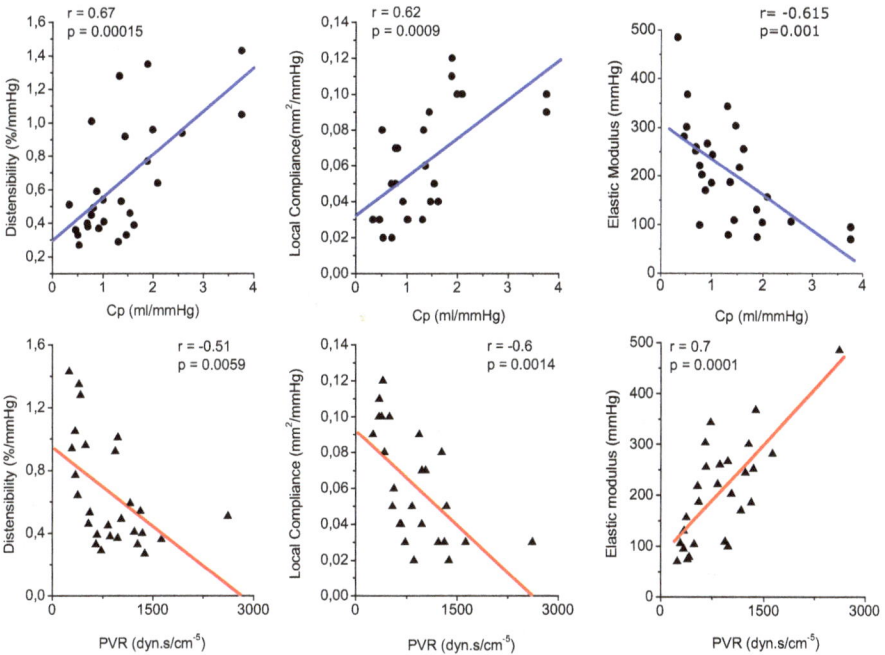

Fig. 5. Correlations between local PA stiffness indexes normalized by pulse pressure and pulsatile (Cp, capacitance index) and steady (PVR, pulmonary vascular resistance) pulmonary afterload (n=25).

By contrast, IVUSp is only an indirect marker of arterial wall viscosity status, explaining the absence of correlation between IVUSp and afterload parameters.

Recent studies showed that PVR and Cp are inversely related by a hyperbola, and in combination describe the RV afterload better than either PVR or Cp separately (Lankhaar et al., 2006, 2008). In other words, the product i.e. the RC-time, in the pulmonary circulation remains the same in healthy subjects and in patients with IPAH and chronic thromboembolic pulmonary hypertension, and even after treatment (Saouti et al., 2010).

Figure 6 shows that in the early stage of PAH a small increase in PVR will be accompanied by a relatively large drop in Cp (patient A). However, in later stages when the vascular disease progresses, the increase in PVR will continue but the drop in Cp will be limited as the vascular wall stiffness will reach a maximum (patient B).

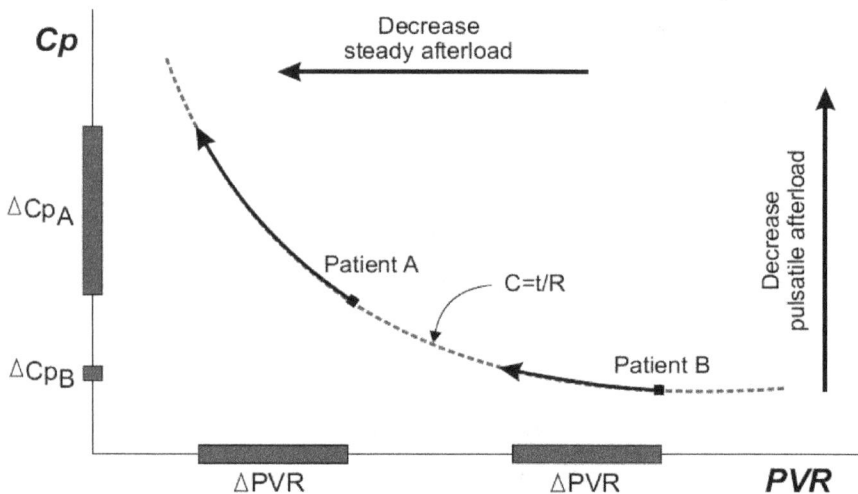

Fig. 6. Inverse hyperbolic relationship between pulmonary arterial compliance (Cp) and pulmonary vascular resistance (PVR). Δ: change.

Finally, compliance in the pulmonary arterial system is distributed over the entire arterial system and stands at the basis of the constancy of the RC time. Applying this RC approach, we can see that patients with an E_P lower than the median (group 1, $E_P < 190$ mmHg) are distributed in the upper left of the hyperbola and that patients of group 2 ($E_P \geq 190$ mmHg) hold the bottom right of the RC curve (Fig. 7A). On the contrary, splitting the patients according to the median of the IVUSp (23%) does not reveal any specific distribution along the RC curve (Fig. 7B). We can affirm that patients with lesser changes in pulmonary vascular bed ($E_P < 190$ mmHg) are characterized by the fact that a small change of PVR leads to a considerable change in Cp and can, therefore, be better detected by a change in compliance than a change in PVR and viceversa.

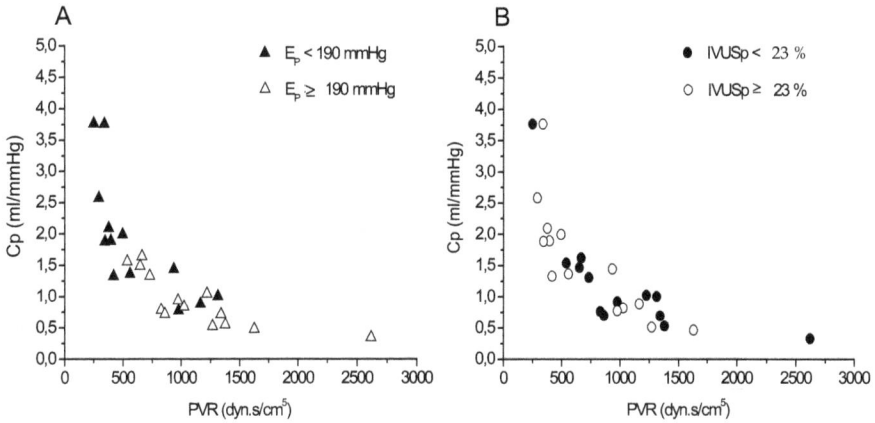

Fig. 7. RC curve of patients with IPAH. The population was split into two groups according to the median of E_P and IVUSp.

3.3 Correlation of local pulmonary arterial elastic modulus with acute vasoreactivity

Detection of acute pulmonary vasoreactivity is important for the evaluation of patients with PAH in different scenarios (Tonelli, Alnuaimat & Mubarak, 2010). However, the clinical relevance of acute vasoreactivity testing in PAH for identifying patients with a marked vasoreactive component, who may thus benefit from chronic calcium channel blocker therapy, has been established only in IPAH (Ghofrani, Wilkins & Rich, 2008). The criteria for identifying responder and non-responder patients in IPAH have been changed in the last twenty years (Tonelli, Alnuamat & Mubarak, 2010). Nowadays, according to the retrospective study of Sitbon et al., a positive response is defined as a decrease in mean PA pressure (Pm) > 10 mmHg, reaching an absolute Pm < 40 mmHg with an unchanged or increased cardiac output (Sitbon et al., 2005). However, the acute response to a vasodilator agent is not an all-or-nothing phenomenon, since different degrees of vasoreactivity are present in all patients with PAH, even in those defined as non-responders by the revised current criteria (Vieira Costa et al., 2005). Pathophysiologically, the different criteria used throughout time to define a positive response may identify patients with different degrees of vascular remodeling. It has been suggested that the currently used criteria of acute responder might identify those patients with a predominant vasoconstriction, a better hemodynamic profile and less remodeling of the vascular wall (Vieira Costa et al., 2005). Recently, Jardim et al. have proposed PA distensibility ≥ 10% (magnetic resonance imaging) as a noninvasive surrogate response marker to the acute vasodilator test in patients with PAH (Jardim et al., 2007).

However, one aspect that has not been evaluated to date is the relationship between pulmonary arterial wall stiffness, real absolute vasodilatation, and vasoreactivity response (in terms of conventional vasoreactivity criteria) during the acute vasoreactivity testing. Hemodynamic evaluation and IVUS imaging of the PA were performed in the same procedure according to a protocol previously reported (Rodés-Cabau et al., 2003; Grignola et al., 2011). Table 1 describes the baseline clinical and hemodynamic characteristics of the 19 IPAH patients enrolled in the study.

Variables	Value
Demographic variables	
Age, years	52 ± 15
Gender, M / F	6 / 13
Functional status	
NYHA class I-II / III-IV	12 / 7
6MWD, m	386 ± 105
Hemodynamic measurements	
CI, l/m/m²	2.4 ± 0.8
SVI ml/m²	30 ± 10
Pm, mmHg	47 ± 18
Pp, mmHg	47 ± 20
RAP, mmHg	8.2 ± 4.8
PVRi, WU.m²	21 ± 12
PAOP, mmHg	10 ± 3
SvO₂, %	64 ± 7

Table 1. Clinical and hemodynamic data of the patients with IPAH (n=19). (CI: cardiac index; PAOP: pulmonary arterial occlusion pressure; Pm and Pp: mean and pulse arterial pulmonary pressures; PVRi: pulmonary vascular resistance index; RAP: mean right atrial pressure; SVI: stroke volume index; SvO₂: mixed venous oxygen saturation; 6MWD: six-minute walking distance).

Acute vasoreactivity testing was performed after baseline measurements, using intravenous epoprostenol. The infusion of epoprostenol was started at a dose of 2 ng/kg/min, and increased progressively (2 ng/kg/min every 10 to 15 min) until a positive response was obtained or until side effects occurred (Grignola et al., 2011). Both the pressure and cross-sectional area changes of PA were obtained during two stable hemodynamic states: baseline and epoprostenol infusion. The population was split into two groups according to the presence of real absolute vasodilatation (delta dA ≥ 10%) (Jardim et al, 2007). The mean dose of epoprostenol was similar in both groups (11 ± 2 ng/kg/min in the vasodilator group and 10 ± 1.2 ng/kg/min in the non-vasodilator group) (Table 2).

Both groups showed a significant heart rate increase and mean aortic pressure decrease ($p<0.05$). PAOP did not change during epoprostenol infusion. Among patients who showed a real vasodilatation (delta dA ≥ 10%), 5 of the 6 had an elastic modulus below the median value (190 mmHg), and presented baseline lower elastic modulus and higher IVUSp. On the other hand, among the patients who did not present a vasodilatation, 9 of 13 had an elastic modulus above the median value. A ROC curve showed that the presence of PA stiffness below the median value was able to differentiate patients with an acute vasodilator response, with 83% sensitivity (95% confidence interval of 54-113%) and 70% specificity

(95% confidence interval of 44-94%). The area under the ROC curve was found to be 0.81 (95% confidence interval 0.58-1.04; $p<0.05$). We choose this cut-off value for E_P since it corresponds to the maximum Youden's index ($J=0.53$). However, no significant relationship has been found between baseline PA wall stiffness and vasodilator response and the decrease in Pm and/or in PVRi during acute vasoreactivity testing.

	All patients (n=19)		Vasodilator group (n=6)		Non-vasodilator group (n=13)	
	Basal	Epo	Basal	Epo	Basal	Epo
CI, $l/m/m^2$	2.3 ± 0.6	2.7 ± 1.3†	2.7 ± 1.0	3.3 ± 1.2†	2.3 ± 0.6‡	2.5 ± 0.9
SVI ml/m^2	30 ± 10	33 ± 15	30 ± 14	42 ± 16†	30 ± 8‡	28 ± 7
Pm, mmHg	50 ± 18	47 ± 18	49 ± 17	48 ± 20	46 ± 16	42 ± 14
Pp, mmHg	50 ± 20	31 ± 12†	50 ± 18	46 ± 20	44 ± 16	41 ± 16
PVRi, Wu.m^2	21 ± 12	15 ± 9†	24 ± 17	17 ± 11†	19 ± 10	15 ± 7
Cp, ml/mmHg	1.38 ± 1	2.1 ± 1.1†	1.4 ± 0.9	1.8 ± 1.2†	1.3 ± 0.8	1.4 ± 0.7
IVUSp, %	27.8 ± 12.9	23.8 ± 10.5†	35.6 ± 17	26.5 ± 15†	24.0 ± 8.4‡	22.1 ± 6.5
E_P, mmHg	195 ± 97	220 ± 124	173 ± 85	244 ± 110	224 ± 81	206 ± 87
dArea, mm^2	11.7 ± 7.6	10.3 ± 7.2	11.3 ± 10.8	12.4 ± 11.6	12.0 ± 6.0	9.1 ± 2.6
sArea, mm^2	15.1 ± 10	12.7 ± 9	15.2 ± 14.5	15.5 ± 14.5	15.0 ± 8.0	11.0 ± 3.4
ΔArea, mm^2	3.3 ± 2.7	2.3 ± 2.1†	4.0 ± 3.9	3.3 ± 3.3	3.0 ± 2.1	1.9 ± 1.1

Table 2. Hemodynamic and IVUS data before (baseline) and after acute vasoreactivity testing (Epo) of both groups. (CI: cardiac index; Cp: pulmonary capacitance index; dArea and sArea: diastolic and systolic lumen area; E_P: elastic modulus; IVUSp: pulmonary arterial pulsatility; Pm and Pp: mean and pulse arterial pulmonary pressures; PVRi: pulmonary vascular resistance index; SVI: stroke volume index. †$p<0.05$ Basal vs. Epo; ‡$p<0.05$ between basal conditions of two groups).

The similar baseline Pm and Pp between both groups allows to state that the acute real vasodilator response is the direct consequence of better preserved viscoelastic wall properties of PAs. No significant relationship has been found between PA wall stiffness and vasodilator response and the decrease in Pm and/or in PVRi during acute vasoreactivity testing. This is not consistent with the hypothesis that a favorable vasoreactive response is related to a less advanced stage of the pulmonary vascular disease (Raffy et al., 1996). Therefore, the acute vasodilatation responder patient may not always be the acute vasoreactive responder patient (current criteria).

The analysis of IVUSp and E_P during the acute vasoreactivity testing showed that the patients with a vasodilator response had an isobaric (similar Pm) worsening of IVUSp ($p<0.05$) and of E_P ($p=0.08$). This is in agreement with Cholley et al. who reported that the isobaric relaxation of vascular wall smooth muscle produces a paradoxical increase in aortic stiffness with a concomitant increase in the incremental elastic modulus (Cholley et al., 2001). In other words, PA vasodilation by itself may cause the vessel to become stiffer since it is operating at a higher internal diameter. This fact would cause a redistribution of parietal stress into the different components of the PA wall, recruiting collagen fibers with higher stiffness, lower viscosity and lower wall buffering function, producing deterioration of IVUSp and E_P. This paradoxical response may also explain the lack of correlation between baseline E_P and hemodynamic vasoreactivity during epoprostenol infusion.

In our cohort, the patients who showed a real absolute pulmonary artery vasodilation during acute vasoreactivity testing, had an isobaric response (absence of changes in Pm) with a concomitant stroke volume index increase (40%), Cp increase (29%) and PVRi decrease (30%). The patients with a positive vasoreactive response according to current criteria do not necessarily have a real absolute vasodilatation on IVUS (Grignola et al., 2011). As proposed by Raffy et al., acute positive vasoreactive response to epoprostenol could be used identify a particular subgroup in the IPAH population that is characterized by a spontaneously slower evolution and hence a better prognosis (Raffy et al., 1996). The absence of IVUSp and E_P worsening during short-term response to epoprostenol in the non-vasodilator and higher remodeling group of IPAH patients could support the greater benefit of epoprostenol in patients with worse functional class. Future studies should analyse whether absolute vasodilatation during acute vasodilator challenge is the most useful criterion to determine responders to calcium channel blocking therapy. We firmly believe that the study of local stiffness indexes of distal PA in IPAH may be useful for analyzing direct and long term effects of specific drugs designed for IPAH treatment on the remodeling process of the pulmonary arterial vascular tree (Rich, 2009; Rich et al., 2010).

4. Optical Coherence Tomography (OCT): A structural approach for the evaluation of pulmonary arterial wall in PAH

Optical Coherence Tomography (OCT) has emerged in recent years as one of the most promising intravascular imaging modalities, capable of providing cross-sectional images of tissue with a homoaxial resolution of 10 μm and a lateral resolution of 20 μm, which is ≈ 10 times higher than that of any available imaging modality (Table 3).

The principle of OCT is analogous to pulse-echo ultrasound imaging: however, light is used rather than sound to create the image. Whereas US produces images from the backscattered sound "echoes", OCT uses infrared light waves that reflected off the internal microstructure within the biological tissues due to their differing optical indices. The use of light provides significantly higher spatial resolution than that of any ultrasound technique. However, this is at the expense of a reduced penetration depth and the need to create a blood-free environment for imaging. In small arteries (diameter lesser than 2-3 mm), blood (namely red blood cells) represents a non-transparent tissue causing multiple scattering and substantial signal attenuation. As a consequence, blood must be displaced during OCT imaging, with the need for balloon occlusion and intra-arterial flush (Pratty et al., 2010).

OCT utilizes a near-infrared light emitted by a super-luminescent diode in combination with advanced fibre-optics to create a dataset of the artery studied. Both the bandwidth of the infrared light used and the wave velocity are orders of magnitude higher than in medical ultrasound. The resulting resolution depends primarily on the ratio of these parameters, and is one order of magnitude larger than that of IVUS (Table 3).

	TD-OCT	IVUS
Energy source	Near-infrared light	Ultrasound (20-45 MHz)
Wave-length, μm	1.3	35 - 80
Resolution, μ	15-20 (axial); 20-40 (lateral)	100-200 (axial); 200-300 (lateral)
Probe size (μ)	400	1100
Frame rate, frames/s	15-20	30
Tissue penetration, mm	1-2.5	10
Pull-back rate, mm/s	1-3	0.5-1, up to 40
Max scan diameter, mm	7	15

Table 3. Physical characteristics of time-domain optical coherence tomography vs. IVUS.

Analogous to ultrasound imaging, the echo time delay of the emitted light is used to generate spatial image information and the intensity of the received (reflected or scattered) light is translated into a (false) colour scale. As the speed of light is much faster than that of sound, an interferometer is required to measure the backscattered light (Regar et al., 2003; Farooq et al., 2009; Pratty et al., 2010). OCT produces accurate images of the arterial lumen and the lumen-vessel wall interface. Normal arteries show a clear demarcation between tunica intima (highly reflective), tunica media (poorly reflective) and tunica adventitia (highly reflective) by OCT (Regar et al., 2003) (Fig. 8). Lipid and necrotic tissue are visualized as poorly reflective structures, while fibrous tissue shows a highly reflective, uniform pattern within the artery wall.

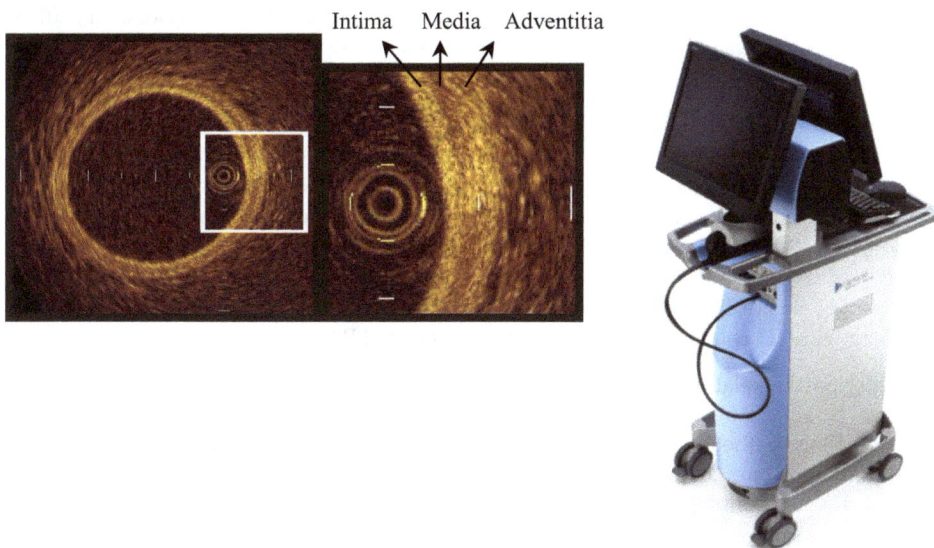

Fig. 8. Left and middle: *in vivo* OCT image of a normal artery with the different layers. Right: Time-Domain OCT system (Lightlab Imaging, Westford, MA, USA).

Second-generation OCT systems have now been developed that potentially overcome many of the practical limitations of the TD-OCT scanners. This technology utilizes a detection method termed Fourier or frequency-domain detection, which allows high-speed data acquisition and real-time imaging. Using guide catheter flush without balloon occlusion, imaging at ≥ 100 frames per second with a pull-back rate of up to 20 mm/second has been achieved, in contrast to 5.6 frames/second for the TD-OCT system. This development has led to faster image acquisition speeds, with greater penetration depth and without loss of vital detail or resolution, and represents a great advance on current conventional OCT systems (Raffel et al., 2008; Gonzalo et al., 2010).

4.1 Estimation of local pulmonary fibrosis by OCT

Although the focus in understanding the mechanism of PAH has been on the small PA (< 500 μ), there is evidence that changes in impedance, resulting from stiffening of the more proximal conduit PAs, may also be a critical determinant not only of the pressure but of the ability of the right ventricle to function (Rabinovitch, 2008).

In Heath and Edwards' histopathological classification, structural changes in the PAs include the progressive intimal fibrosis from the smaller muscular PA to the medium-sized PA (Heath & Edwards, 1958). In spite of similar clinical and hemodynamic profiles, patients differed considerably with respect to the nature of their pulmonary vascular obstructive lesions. Palevsky et al showed that an intimal area of more than 18% of the vascular cross-sectional area had an 85% predictive value for identifying patients with a poor outcome during 36 months of follow-up (Palevsky et al., 1989). Therefore, accurate detection and quantification of intimal fibrosis would be important in the assessment of PA remodeling, irreversibility and prognosis of the disease. Besides, it has recently been shown that collagen content is important in extralobar PA stiffening caused by chronic hypoxia (Ooi et al., 2010). Finally, there is evidence that conduit PA stiffness is a strong predictor of mortality in PAH (Mahapatra et al., 2006; Gan et al., 2007).

According to our knowledge, there is scarce and poorly analyzed literature on the use of OCT in PAH. Tatebe et al reported the potential usefulness of OCT as a novel diagnostic tool for the differential diagnosis of distal type chronic thromboembolic PH from PAH (Tatebe et al., 2010). They showed that PA > 1 mm in diameter had no obstruction in the control of PAH subjects, although the media of the arteries appeared to be thickened in PAH subjects compared with controls. Finally, Hou et al. reported the OCT findings of one case of severe IPAH (Hou et al., 2010). They showed that the intima was more than twice the thickness in this patient with PH compared with a patient with normal PA pressure.

We quantified the relative PA wall fibrosis (%Fib) by OCT in patients with stable IPAH (Domingo et al., 2010). After hemodynamic and IVUS measurements, a Helios coaxial occlusion balloon catheter (LightLab Imaging Inc, Westford MA, USA) was advanced over a 0,014" guidewire into the same pulmonary artery branch, using an exchange guidewire system and X-ray control. This method guarantees that IVUS, OCT and PA pressure are obtained at the same level of the studied PA branch. The Helios is situated in the distal part of the vessel. The guidewire is replaced by an ImageWire 2000 OCT imaging catheter (LightLab Imaging Inc, Westford MA, USA). While maintaining the ImageWire in its place, the balloon is retracted to the proximal part of the branch. To prevent blood from entering the region of interest, the balloon is inflated to 0.6 atm. Total occlusion is verified angiographically with a contrast injection. When occlusion is achieved, a manual continuous flush with saline is initiated for blood clearing. According to the study from Yabushita et al., fibrosis is represented by OCT as intimal thickening with a bright and homogeneous signal (Yabushita et al., 2002). In the same image the inner lumen area and the area limited by the outer boundary of fibrosis are measured. Subtraction of these two areas represents fibrosis area. Percentage of fibrosis is calculated as the ratio between the fibrosis/lumen cross-sectional areas (%Fib):

$$\%Fib = (area\ of\ Fib/PA\ cross\ sectional\ area) \times 100 \qquad (4)$$

A typical OCT image of a distal PA in a patient with IPAH is shown in Fig. 9. External and internal markers outline the area of fibrosis and the ratio between the fibrosis area and the external cross-sectional area estimates the percentage of wall fibrosis.

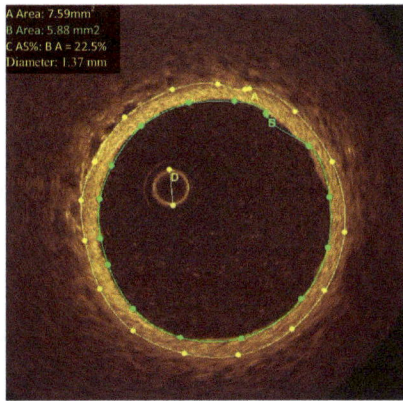

Fig. 9. In vivo OCT image of a distal pulmonary artery in a patient with IPAH. Calculation of the fibrosis of the arterial wall.

The mean OCT %Fib was 23 ± 7, with an IVUSp of $33 \pm 21\%$ and an E_P of 185 ± 107 mmHg.

4.2 Correlation of local pulmonary fibrosis with steady and pulsatile afterload

Histopathology of PAH is founded on structural modifications of the vascular wall of small PA characterized by thickening of all its layers. These changes include vascular wall proliferation, fibrosis and vessel obstruction (Sakao, Tatsumi & Voekel, 2010).

In a model of chronic hypoxia PH, pulmonary vascular remodeling increases conduit PA stiffness. Vascular collagen accumulation is a major cause of extralobar PA stiffening in hypoxia PH. On the contrary, no significant change in elastin wall content has been observed (Ooi et al., 2010). In accordance with this, we found higher OCT %Fib in PA (1.5 to 2 mm of diameter) of patients with IPAH with respect to control patients (23 ± 7 vs. $1.4 \pm 1.3\%$). Patients with a higher wall fibrosis showed higher steady (PVR increase) and pulsatile (Cp decrease) components of PA afterload. OCT %Fib was better correlated with capacitance ($r = -0.47$; $p = 0.04$), than with PVR ($r = 0.44$; $p = 0.06$) (Domingo et al., 2010). Although wall fibrosis is associated with an increase in E_P, the absence of correlation between structural (OCT fibrosis) and functional (IVUSp; E_P) wall remodeling, reveals the complex interaction between the different PA wall components in the remodeling process. The increased E_P not only depends on the extent of wall fibrosis. Vasoconstriction, change in elastin wall content, transmural PA pressure and wall geometrical factors (thickness/radius ratio) also influence E_P. Neither IVUS %Fib nor pulsatility was correlated with PA afterload.

5. Conclusion

PAH is a rare and severe condition characterized by vascular proliferation and remodeling of the small PA wall, resulting in a progressive increase in pulmonary vascular impedance and ultimately right ventricular failure and death. Both PA elastic modulus assessed by IVUS and wall percentage of fibrosis assessed by OCT correlated with the severity of PA dynamic afterload (global capacitance and resistance properties of the pulmonary arterial tree). Patients with a higher degree of remodeling had a worse clinical and hemodynamic profile. The severity of remodeling of elastic distal PA did not correlate with the acute response of mean PA pressure and/or PVRi to epoprostenol during the acute vasoreactivity test.

We suggest the potential usefulness of IVUS and OCT as novel diagnostic tools for evaluation of PA wall functional and structural remodeling in patients with PAH group I, during acute vasoreactivity testing, along the disease process, and as a marker of treatment response, complementary to clinical and hemodynamic evaluation. It is possible that the current criteria for an acute positive pulmonary vasoreactivity test (decrease in Pm > 10 mmHg, reaching an absolute Pm < 40 mmHg with an unchanged or increased cardiac output) would not necessarily identify patients with lower vascular remodeling. This fact would explain the long-term clinical benefit of calcium blockers in only 50% of patients considered hemodynamic responders in the acute vasoreactivity testing.

6. Acknowledgements

To Manuel Vázquez (RN) for his technical assistance. This work was partially supported by a financial grant from Glaxo Smith Kline. Juan C Grignola is supported by CSIC (Comisión Sectorial de Investigación Científica) and ANII (Agencia Nacional de Investigación e Innovación).

7. References

Berger, R.M.F., Cromme-Dijkhuis, A.H., Hop, W.C.J., Kruit, M.N. & Hess, J. (2002). Pulmonary arterial wall distensibility assessed by intravascular ultrasound in children with congenital heart disease. *Chest* Vol. 122, pp. 549-557, ISSN 0012-3692.

Bia, D., Armentano, R.L., Grignola, J.C., Craiem, D., Zócalo, Y., Ginés, F. & Levenson, J. (2003). The vascular smooth muscle of great arteries: local control site of arterial buffering function? *Revista Española de Cardiología* Vol. 56, pp. 1202-1209, ISSN 0300-8932.

Bia, D., Barra, J.G., Grignola, J.C., Ginés, F. & Armentano, R.L. (2005a). Pulmonary artery smooth muscle activation attenuates arterial dysfunction during acute pulmonary hypertension. *Journal of Applied Physiology* Vol. 98, pp. 605-613, ISSN 1439-6327.

Bia, D., Aguirre, I., Zócalo, Y., Devera, L., Cabrera Fischer, E. & Armentano, R.L. (2005b). Regional differences in viscosity, elasticity, and wall buffering function in systemic arteries: pulse wave analysis of the arterial pressure-diameter relationship. *Revista Española de Cardiología* Vol. 58, pp. 167-174 ISSN 0300-8932.

Bressollette, E., Dupuis, J., Bonan, R., Doucet, S., Cernacek, P. & Tardif, J.C. (2001). Intravascular ultrasound assessment of pulmonary vascular disease in patients with pulmonary hypertension. *Chest* Vol. 120, pp. 809-815, ISSN 0012-3692.

Chemla, D., Hébert, J.L., Coirault, C., Zamani, K., Suard, I., Colin, P. & Lecarpentier, Y. (1998). Total arterial compliance estimated by stroke volume-to-aortic pulse pressure ratio in humans. *American Journal of Physiology* Vol. 274, pp. 500-505, ISSN 0363-6143.

Cholley, B.P., Lang, R.M., Korcarz, C.E. & Shroff, S.G. (2001). Smooth muscle relaxation and local hydraulic impedance properties of the aorta. *Journal of Applied Physiology* Vol. 90, pp. 2427-2438, ISSN 1439-6327.

Domingo, E., Grignola, J.C., Aguilar, R., Lopez-Messeguer, M., Vazquez, M. & Roman, A. (2010). Pulmonary artery fibrosis by optical coherence tomography is correlated with pulmonary dynamic afterload in pulmonary arterial hypertension *European Heart Journal* Vol. 31(Suppl1), 750, P4459, ISSN 1520-765X.

Domingo, E., Grignola, J.C., Aguilar, R., Vázquez, M., López-Messeguer, M., Bravo, C. & Roman, A. (2011). Correlation between local pulmonary stiffness and the acute vasoreactivity test in pulmonary arterial hypertension. *American Journal of Respiratory and Critical Care Medicine* Vol. 183, A5745, ISSN 1073-449X.

Farooq, U.M., Khasnis, A., Majid, A. & Kassab, M.Y. (2009). The role of optical coherence tomography in vascular medicine. *Vascular Medicine* Vol. 14, pp. 63-71, ISSN 1538-5744.

Galié, N., Manes, A., Negro, L., Palazzini, M., Bacchi-Reggiani, M.L. & Branzi, A. (2009). A meta-analysis of randomized controlled trials in pulmonary arterial hypertension. *European Heart Journal* Vol. 30, pp. 394-403, ISSN 1520-765X.

Gan, C.T., Lankhaar, J.W., Westerhof, N., Marcus, T., Becker, A., Twisk, J.W.R., Boonstra, A., Postmus, P.E. & Vonk-Noordegraf, A. (2007). Noninvasively assessed pulmonary artery stiffness predicts mortality in pulmonary arterial hypertension. *Chest* Vol. 132, pp. 1906-1912, ISSN 0012-3692.

Ghofrani, H.A., Wilkins, M.W. & Rich, S. (2008). Uncertainties in the diagnosis and treatment of pulmonary arterial hypertension. *Circulation* Vol. 118, pp. 1195-1201, ISSN 0009-7322.

Gonzalo, N., Tearney, G.J., Serruys, P.W., van Soest, G., Okamura, T., García-García, H.M., van Geuns, R.J., van der Ent, M., Ligthart, J., Bouma, B.E. & Regar, E. (2010). Second-generation optical coherence tomography in clinical practice. High-speed data acquisition is highly reproducible in patients undergoing percutaneous coronary intervention. *Revista Española de Cardiología* Vol. 63, pp. 893-903, ISSN 0300-8932.

Grignola, J.C., Domingo, E., Bravo, C., Aguilar, R., López-Messeguer, M., Vázquez, M. & Roman, A. (2010). Local pulmonary artery stiffness indexes are correlated with steady and pulsatile components of right ventricular afterload in pulmonary arterial hypertension. *Journal of the American College of Cardiology* Vol. 55(Suppl1): A367, ISSN 0735-1097.

Grignola, J.C., Domingo, E., Aguilar, R., Vázquez, M., López-Messeguer, M., Bravo, C. & Roman, A. (2011). Acute absolute vasodilatation is associated with lower vascular wall stiffness in pulmonary arterial hypertension. *International Journal of Cardiology*, doi:10.1016/j.ijcard.2011.07.020, ISSN 0167-5273.

Heath, D., & Edwards, J.E. (1958). The pathology of hypertensive pulmonary disease: A description of six grades of structural changes in the pulmonary arteries with special reference to congenital cardiac septal defects. *Circulation* Vol. 18, pp. 533-547, ISSN 0009-7322.

Hou, J., Qi, H., Zhang, M., Meng, L., Han, Z., Yu, B. & Jang, K. (2010). Pulmonary vascular changes in pulmonary hypertension: optical coherence tomography findings. *Circulation: Cardiovacular Imaging* Vol. 3, pp. 344-345, ISSN 1941-9651.

Jardim, C., Rochitte, C.E., Humbert, M., Rubenfeld, G., Jasinowodolinski, D., Carvalho, C.R.R. & Souza, R. (2007). Pulmonary artery distensibility in pulmonary arterial hypertension: an MRI pilot study. *European Respiratory Journal* Vol. 29, pp. 476-481, ISSN 0903-1936.

Lankhaar, J.W., Westerhof, N., Faes, T.J., Marques, K.M., Marcus, J.T., Postmus, P.E. & Vonk-Noordegraaf, A. (2006). Quantification of right ventricular afterload in patients with and without pulmonary hypertension. *American Journal of Physiology* Vol. 291, pp. H1731-H1737, ISSN 0363-6143.

Lankhaar, J.W., Westerhof, N., Faes, T.J., Tji-Joong Gan, C., Marques, K.M., Boonstra, A., van den Berg, F.G., Postmus, P.E. & Vonk-Nordegraaf, A. (2008). Pulmonary vascular resistance and compliance stay inversely related during treatment of pulmonary hypertension. *European Heart Journal* Vol. 29, pp. 168-1695, ISSN 1520-765X.

Laurent, S., Cockroft, J., Van Bortel, L., Boutouyrie, P., Gianattasio, C., Hayoz, D., Pannier, B., Vlachopoulos, Ch., Wilkinson, I. & Struijker-Boudier, H. (2006). Expert consensus document of arterial stiffness: methodological issues and clinical applications. *European Heart Journal* Vol. 27, pp. 2588-2605, ISSN 1520-765X.

Macchia, A., Marchioli, R., Tognoni, G., Scarano, M., Marfisi, R.M., Tavazzi, L. & Rich, S. (2010). Systematic review of trials using vasodilators in pulmonary arterial hypertension: why a new approach is needed. *American Heart Journal* Vol. 159, pp. 245-257, ISSN 0363-6135.

Mahapatra, S., Nishimura, R.A., Sorajja, P., Cha, S. & McGoon, M.D. (2006). Relationship of pulmonary arterial capacitance and mortality in idiopathic pulmonary arterial hypertension. *Journal of the American College of Cardiology* Vol. 47, pp. 799-803, ISSN 0735-1097.

McLaughlin, V.V., Archer, S.L., Badesch, D.B., Barst, R.J., Farber, H.W., Lindner, J.R., Mathier, M.A., McGoon, M.D., Park, M.H., Rosenson, R.S., Rubin, L.J., Tapson, V.F. & Varga, J. (2009). ACCF/AHA expert consensus document on pulmonary hypertension. *Circulation* Vol. 119, pp. 2250-2294, ISSN 0009-7322.

Nakamura, K., Akagi, S., Ogawa, A., Kusano, K.F., Matsubara, H., Miura, D., Fuke, S., Nishii, N., Nagasea, N., Kohno, K., Morita, H., Oto, T., Yamanaka, T., Otsuka, F., Miura, A., Yutani, Ch., Ohe, T. & Ito, H. (2011). Pro-apoptotic effects of imatinib on PDGF-stimulated pulmonary artery smooth muscle cells from patients with idiopathic pulmonary arterial hypertension. *International Journal of Cardiology*, doi:10.1016/ j.ijcard.2011.02.024, ISSN 0167-5273.

Nichols W.W. & O'Rourke M.F. (2005). *McDonald's Blood Flow in Arteries: Theoretical Experimental and Clinical Principles.* ISBN 0 340 80941 8 London, UK. Hodder Arnold.

Ooi, C.Y., Wang, Z., Tabima, D.M., Eickhoff, J.C. & Chesler, N.C. (2010). The role of collagen in extralobar pulmonary artery stiffening in response to hypoxia induced pulmonary hypertension. *American Journal of Physiology* Vol. 299, pp. H1823-1831, ISSN 0363-6143.

Palevsky, H.I., Schloo, B.L., Pietra, G.G., Weber, K.T., Janicki, J.S., Rubin, E. & Fishman, A.P. (1989). Primary pulmonary hypertension: Vascular structure, morphometry and responsiveness to vasodilator agents. *Circulation* Vol. 80, pp. 1207-21, ISSN 0009-7322.

Pratty, F., Regar, E., Mintz, G.S., Arbustini, E., DiMario, C., Jang, I-K., Akasaka, T., Costa, M., Guagliumi, G., Grube, E., Ozaki, Y., Pinto, F. & Serruys, P.W.J. (2010). Expert review document on methodology, terminology, and clinical applications of optical coherence tomography. *European Heart Journal* Vol. 31, pp. 401–415, ISSN 1520-765X.

Raffel, O.C., Akasaka, T. & Jang I-K. (2008). Cardiac optical coherence tomography. *Heart* Vol. 94, pp. 1200-1210, ISSN 1355-6037.

Raffy; O., Azarian, R., Brenot, F., Parent, F., Sitbon, O., Petitpretz, P., Hervé, P., Duroux, P., Dinh-Xuan, A.T. & Simonneau G. (1996). Clinical significance of pulmonary vasodilator response during short-term infusion of prostacyclin in primary pulmonary hypertension. *Circulation* Vol. 93, pp. 484-488, ISSN 0009-7322.

Rabinovitch, M. (2008). Molecular pathogenesis of pulmonary arterial hypertension. *Journal of Clinical Investigation* Vol. 118, pp. 2372–2379, ISSN 0021-9738.

Regar, E., Schaar, J.A., Mont, E., Virmani, R. & Serruys, P.W.J. (2003). Optical coherence tomography. *Cardiovascular Radiation Medicine* Vol. 4, pp. 198-204, ISSN 1522-1865.

Rich, S. (2006). The current treatment of pulmonary arterial hypertension. Time to redefine success. *Chest* Vol. 130, pp. 1198-1202, ISSN 0012-3692.

Rich, S. (2009). The effects of vasodilators in pulmonary hypertension. Pulmonary vascular or peripheral vascular?. *Circulation Heart Failure* Vol. 2, pp. 145-150, ISSN 1941-3289.

Rich, S., Pogoriler, J., Husain, A.N., Toth, P.T., Gomberg-Maitland, M. & Archer, S.L. (2010). Long-term effects of epoprostenol on pulmonary vasculature in idiopathic pulmonary arterial hypertension. *Chest* Vol. 138, pp. 1234-1239, ISSN 0012-3692.

Rodés-Cabau, J., Domingo, E., Roman, A., Majo, J., Lara, B., Padilla, F., Anívarro, I., Angel, J., Tardif, J.C. & Soler-Soler, J. (2003). Intravascular ultrasound of the elastic pulmonary arteries: a new approach for the evaluation of primary pulmonary hypertension. *Heart* Vol. 89, pp. 311-315, ISSN 1355-6037.

Sakao, S., Tatsumi, K. & Voelkel, N.F. (2010). Reversible or irreversible remodeling in pulmonary arterial hypertension. *American Journal of Respiratory Cell and Molecular Biology* Vol. 43, pp. 629-634, ISSN 1044-1549.

Sanz, J., Kariisa, M., Dellegrottaglie, S., Prat-González, S., Garcia, M.J., Fuster, V. & Rajagopalan, S. (2009). Evaluation of pulmonary artery stiffness in pulmonary hypertension with cardiac magnetic resonance. *Journal of the American College of Cardiology: Cardiovascular Imaging* Vol. 2, pp. 286-295, ISSN 1936-878X.

Sanz, J., Fernández-Friera, L. & Moral, S. (2010). Imaging techniques and the evaluation of the right and the pulmonary circulation. *Revista Española de Cardiología* Vol. 63, pp. 209-223, ISSN 0300-8932.

Saouti, N., Westerhof, N., Postmus, P.E., Vonk-Noordegraaf., A.V. (2010). The arterial load in pulmonary hypertension. *European Respiratory Review* Vol. 19, pp. 197-203, ISSN 0905-9180.

Sitbon, O., Humbert, M., Jais, X., Ioos, V., Hamid, A.M., Provencher, S. Garcia, G., Parent, F., Hervé, P. & Simonneau G. (2005). Long-term response to calcium channel blockers in idiopathic pulmonary arterial hypertension. *Circulation* Vol. 111, pp. 3105-3111, ISSN 0009-7322.

Soto, F.J. & Kleczka, J.F. (2008). Cardiopulmonary hemodynamics in pulmonary hypertension: pressure tracings, waveforms and more. *Advances in Pulmonary Hypertension* Vol. 7, pp. 386-393, ISSN 1933-088X.

Stergiopulos, N, Segers, P, & Westerhof, N. (1999). Use of pulse pressure method for estimating total arterial compliance in vivo. *American Journal of Physiology* Vol. 276, pp. 424-428, ISSN 0363-6143.

Tatebe, S., Yoshihiro, F., Koichiro, S., Makoto, N., Saori, M., Kimio, S., Oikawa, M & Shimokawa, H. (2010). Optical coherence tomography as a novel diagnostic tool for distal type chronic thromboembolic pulmonary hypertension. *Circulation Journal* Vol. 74, pp. 1742-44, 1346-9843, ISSN 1346-9843.

Tonelli, A.R., Alnuaimat, H. & Mubarak, K. (2010). Pulmonary vasodilator testing and use of calcium channel blockers in pulmonary arterial hypertension. *Respiratory Medicine* Vol. 104, pp. 481-496, ISSN 0954-6111.

Vieira Costa, E.L., Jardim, C., Bassin Bogossian, H., Passos Amato, M.B., Ribeiro Carvalho, C., & Souza, R. (2005). Acute vasodilator test in pulmonary arterial hypertension: evaluation of two response criteria. *Vascular Pharmacology* Vol. 43, pp. 143-147, ISSN 1537-1891.

Wharton, J., Davie, N., Upton, P.D., Yacoub, M.H., Polak, J.M. & Morrell, N.W. (2000). Prostacyclin analogues differentially inhibit growth of distal and proximal human pulmonary artery smooth muscle cells. *Circulation* Vol. 102, pp. 3130-36, ISSN 0009-7322.

Wharton, J., Strange, J.W., Møller, G.M.O; Growcott, E.J., Ren, X., Franklyn, A.P., Phillips, S.C. & Wilkins M.R. (2005). Antiproliferative effects of phosphodiesterase type 5 inhibition in human pulmonary artery cells. *American Journal of Respiratory and Critical Care Medicine* Vol. 127, pp. 105-113, ISSN 1073-449X.

Yabushita, H., Bouma, B.E., Houser, S.L., Aretz, H.T., Jang, I.K., Schlendorf, K.H., Kauffman, C.R., Shishkov, M., Kang, D.H., Halpern, E.F. & Tearney, GJ. (2002). Characterization of human atherosclerosis by optical coherence tomography. *Circulation* Vol. 106, pp. 1640-1645, ISSN 0009-7322.

10

Echocardiography in Pulmonary Hypertension

Chin-Chang Cheng and Chien-Wei Hsu
Kaohsiung Veterans General Hospital
Taiwan

1. Introduction

The gold standard for diagnosis and confirmation of PH is right heart catheterization. But right heart catheterization is an invasive procedure, and it associated with morbidity (1.1%) and mortality (0.55%)(Hoeper et al. 2006). Although right heart catheterization is the method to measure pulmonary arterial pressures, it is not suitable in daily practice to screen the possible candidates of PH. Echocardiography is an widely available non-invasive tool, and it can offer the information on the structures of hearts and the estimated pressure profiles of cardiovascular system. Therefore, echocardiography plays an important role in diagnosis and monitoring treatment effects.

The classification of pulmonary hypertension (PH) includes 5 groups: 1) pulmonary arterial hypertension (PAH); 2) pulmonary hypertension owing to left heart disease; 3) pulmonary hypertension due to lung disease; 4) chronic thromboembolic pulmonary hypertension; 5) miscellaneous.(Simonneau et al. 2009) In the clinical situation, while suspecting a patient with PH, it plays an important role in screening the patients with suspected PH, ruling in or out PH due to left heart disease, and evaluating the presence of congenital heart disease. If the patient is diagnosed as PAH, echocardiography can afford the semi-quantitative methods to evaluate the effects of treatment.

2. Echocardiography in diagnosis of PH

2.1 Structures of heart

Conventional echocardiography can provide the two-dimensional images to evaluate the structural abnormalities of heart. Group 2 PH account for the most cases of PH (Oudiz 2007), therefore examination of the function and structure of left heart is the first thing to do in diagnosis of PH. Congenital heart disease is another common cause of PH, and it usually can be corrected by surgery. Therefore, it is important in evaluating the gross anatomy of left heart, the systolic function of left ventricle, mitral valve and aortic valve disorders, the diastolic dysfunction of left heart, and the congenital heart defects. The detail evaluation of structural evaluation of heart is beyond the scope of this book. In the beginner of PH, who is not the cardiologist, cardiovascular consultant is necessary. But diastolic dysfunction is usually overlooked in the clinical practice. The possible clue of isolated diastolic dysfunction of left heart is dilated left atrium. If this sign is present and the pulmonary capillary wedge pressure is less than 15 mmHg during right heart catheterization, saline replacement during right heart catheterization may uncover the occult diastolic dysfunction.(Hoeper et al. 2009). It not uncommon that congenital heart disease cannot be diagnosed by transthoracic echocardiography due to limited windows, transesophageal echocardiography is a necessary tool in this situation, especially in atrial septal defect and pulmonary vein stenosis.

Because of chronic right ventricular (RV) pressure overload, most patients present with enlarged right-side chambers, RV hypertrophy, and reduced global RV systolic function.(Bossone et al. 1999) The hallmark of RV pressure overload is systolic flattening of the interventricular septum with D-shape of left ventricle (Figure 1A), with reduced diastolic and systolic left ventricular volumes, but preserved global left ventricular systolic function. The eccentric index of left ventricle, which measured at papillary muscle level of mitral valve in paraternal short-axis view, is less than 1. (Figure 1A) Pericardial effusions have also been described in PAH patients, and this sign represents higher right atrial pressures, higher pulmonary arterial pressures and poor prognosis. (Park et al. 1989) (Figure 1B)

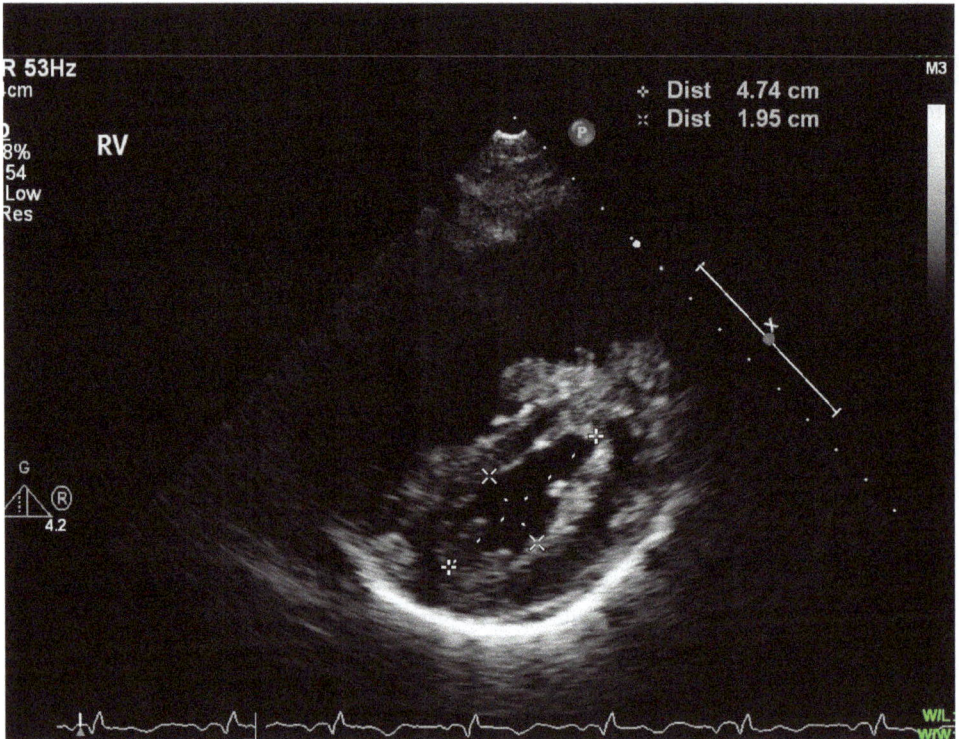

Fig. 1. Echocardiographic parasternal short-axis view. The interventricular septum is flattened due to pressure overload of the right ventricle.

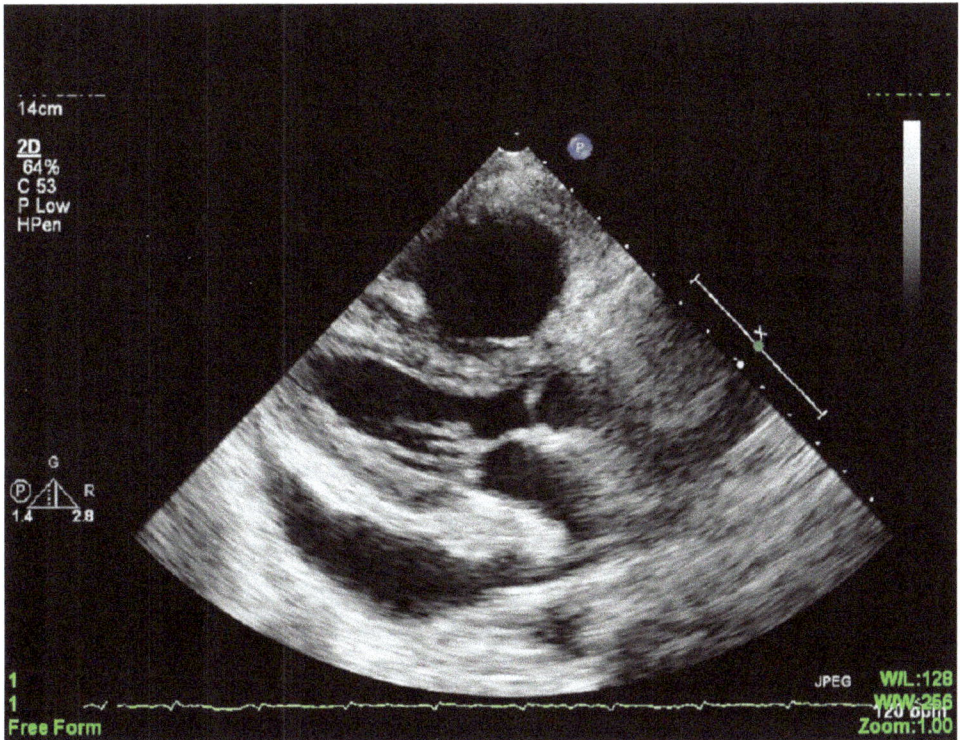

Fig. 2. Presence of pericardial effusion in a patient with severe pulmonary arterial hypertension.

2.2 Hemodynamics

As mentioned before, right heart catheterization is the gold standard in diagnosis of PH, but non-invasive Doppler echocardiography can also afford estimates of hemodynamic parameters, such as pulmonary arterial pressure, cardiac output, pulmonary vascular resistance and pulmonary capillary wedge pressures. Therefore, it is a good screening tool in patients with PH.

2.2.1 Pulmonary arterial pressures

The hemodynamic criterion of pulmonary hypertension is mean pulmonary arterial pressure greater than 25 mmHg by right heart catheterization. Pulmonary arterial pressures can also be measured semi-quantitatively by echocardiography. For calculating pulmonary arterial systolic pressures, the first step is to estimate right atrial pressure (RAP), which is evaluate by examining the diameter of inferior vena cava. IVC diameter < 2.1 cm that collapses >50% with a sniff suggests normal RA pressure of 3 mm Hg (range, 0-5 mm Hg), whereas IVC diameter > 2.1 cm that collapses < 50% with a sniff suggests high RA pressure of 15 mm Hg (range, 10-20 mm Hg). In scenarios in which IVC diameter and collapse do not fit this paradigm, an intermediate value of 8 mm Hg (range, 5-10 mm Hg) may be used. (Table 1) (Rudski et al.

2010) The second step is search the presence of tricuspid regurgitation (TR). When TR is present, measurement of the peak TR velocity (V_{TR}) should be performed. Because velocity measurements are angle dependent, it is recommended to obtain TR signals from several windows and to use the signal with the highest velocity. The third step is calculating pulmonary arterial systolic pressure (PASP) by the following equation:

$$PASP = RAP + V_{TR}^2 \quad \text{(Figure 3)}$$

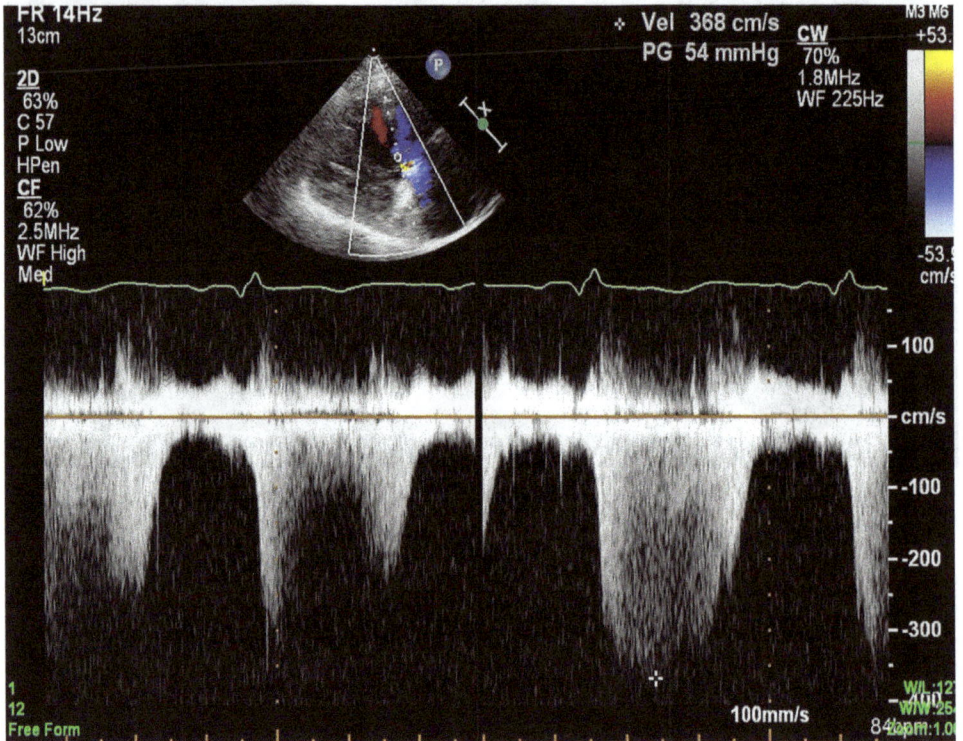

Fig. 3. A 51-year-old female, with a history of systemic lupus erythematousus and pulmonary arterial hypertension, had an estimated tricuspid regurgitation pressure gradient of 54mmHg. After adding estimated right atrial pressure, pulmonary artrerial systolic pressure would be obtained.

But the accuracy of the estimated PASP depends on recording a clear envelope of the TR velocity by continuous-wave Doppler tracing. If the signal of TR is not clear or incomplete, underestimation of peak velocity of TR will occurs.

Estimation of pulmonary arterial diastolic pressure (PADP) is similar to that of PASP, and the velocity used in estimated PADP is the pulmonary regurgitation (PR) velocity at end-diastole. The formula to calculate PADP is as following:

$$PADP = RAP + V_{end\text{-}diastole\ PR}^2 \quad (Figure\ 4)$$

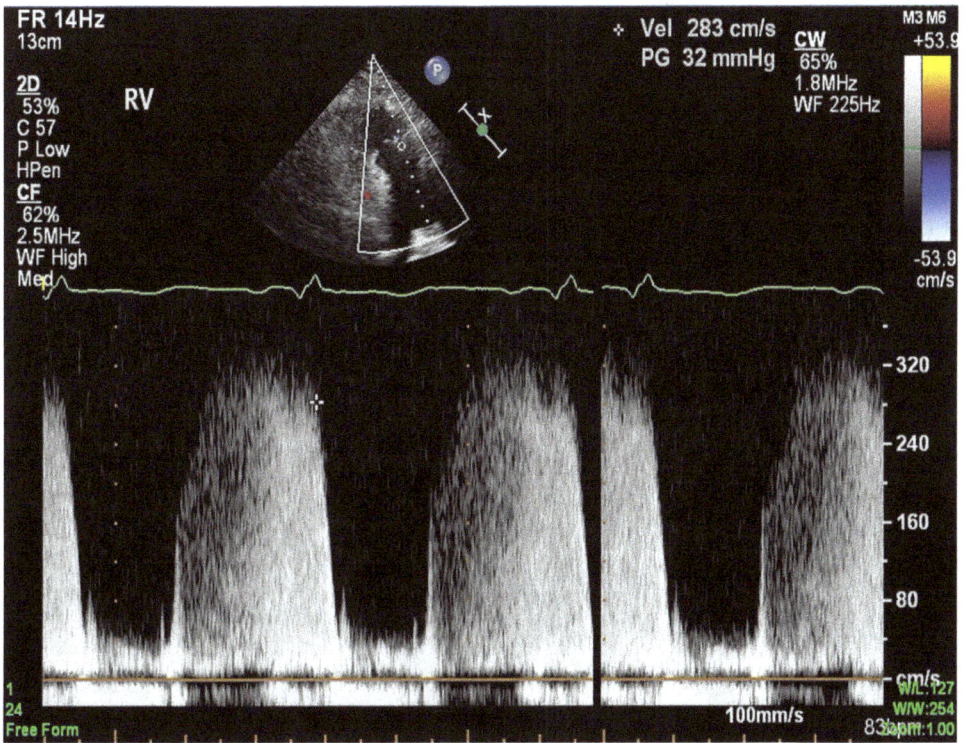

Fig. 4. A 51-year-old female, with a history of systemic lupus erythematousus and pulmonary arterial hypertension, had an estimated pulmonary regurgitation pressure gradient of 32mmHg. After adding estimated right atrial pressure, pulmonary artrerial diastolic pressure would be obtained.

After obtaining PASP and PADP, the mean PA pressure (MPAP) can be obtained as following:

$$MPAP = PADP + 1/3\ (PASP\text{-}PADP) \quad (Figure\ 3)$$

RAP (mmHg)	Normal (0-5)	Intermediate (5-10)		High (15)
IVC diameter (mm)	< 21	<21	>21	>21
Collapse with sniff	>50%	<50%	>50%	<50%
Secondary indices of elevated RAP				Restrictive filling Tricuspid E/E' > 6 Diastolic flow predominance in hepatic vein (systolic filling fraction < 55%)

Table 1. Estimation of right atrial pressure (RAP) on the basis of IVC diameter and collapse (Rudski et al. 2010)

2.2.2 Cardiac output

Cardiac output is related to the symptoms and prognosis of PH. Cardiac output can also be calculated by echocardiography. Before calculating cardiac output, the presumption is absence of intra-cardiac or great vessel shunt, and the cardiac output can be measured from left ventricular outflow tract (LVOT) or right ventricular outflow tract. In daily practice, measurements of diameters and velocity time integral of left ventricular outflow tract is a routine practice in our echocardiographic laboratory. Therefore, application of pulse-wave Doppler over LVOT, a clear envelope of LVOT flow (VTI_{LVOT}) can be acquired. The diameter of LVOT (D_{LVOT}) can be measured at parasternal long-axis view. The cardiac output can be calculated as the following equation:

$$\text{Cardiac output} = 0.785 * D_{LVOT}{}^2 * VTI_{LVOT} * \text{heart rate} / 1000 \qquad \text{(Figure 5)}$$
$$*1000 \text{ is for conversion of units}$$

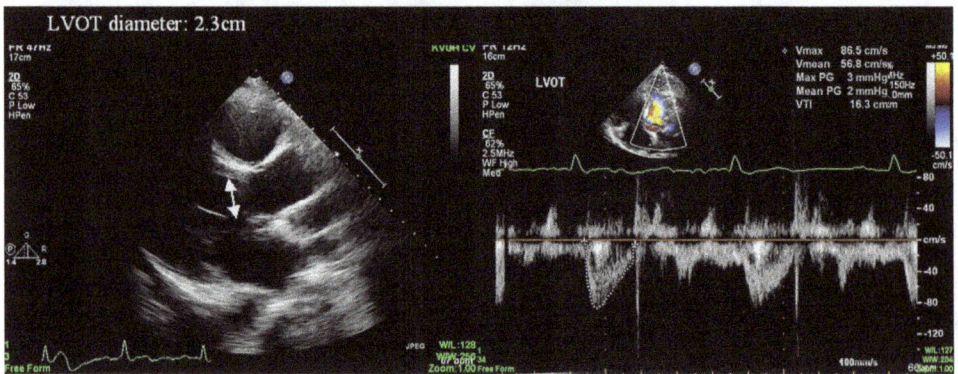

Fig. 5. A 34-year-old male with thalassemia and chronic hemolytic anemia related pulmonary hypertension. (VTI_{LVOT}: 16.3cm/s, D_{LVOT}: 2.3cm, Cardiac output= $0.785 * 2.3^2 * 16.3 * 66 / 1000 = 4.4$L/min)

3. Echocardiography in evaluation of right heart function

Right ventricular function is a prognostic factor of PH. However, because of complex geometry of right ventricle, it is difficulty to evaluate right ventricular function. In current era, more studies demonstrated the clinical utility and value of right ventricular myocardial performance index, tricuspid annular plane systolic excursion (TAPSE), right ventricular fractional area changes and Sm of the tricuspid annulus.

3.1 Right ventricular myocardial performance index (RVMPI)

RVMPI is an index of global RV function, and it is calculated by summation of isovolumic contraction time (IVCT) and isovolumic relaxation time (IVRT) and divided by ejection time (ET). (Figure 6)

$$RVMPI = \frac{IVCT + IVRT}{ET}$$

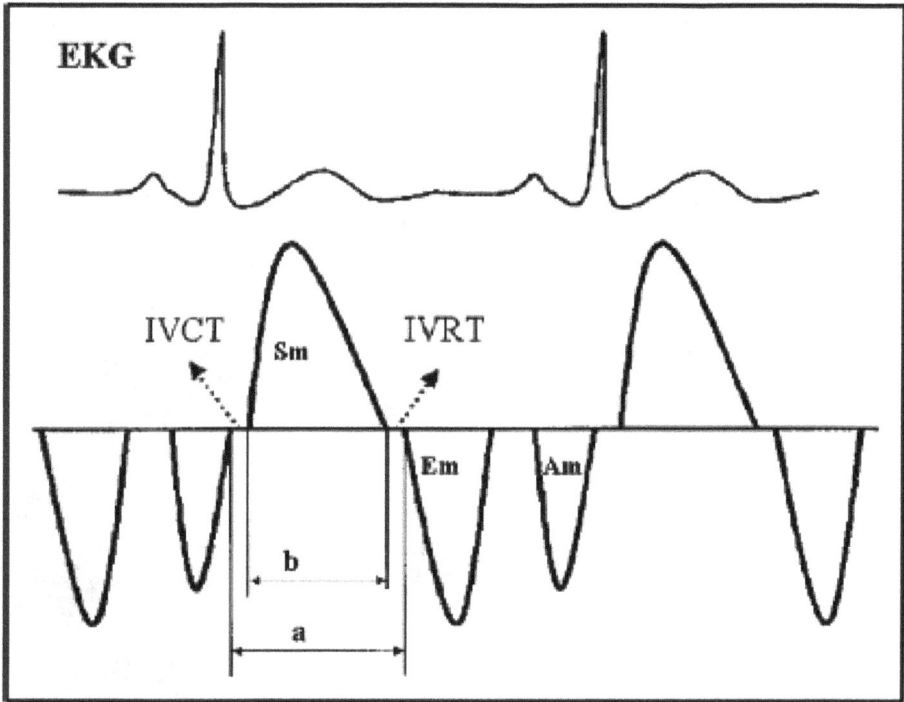

Fig. 6. Myocardial TDI includes all 3 phases. The MPI was calculated as (a-b)/b. a: the time interval from the onset of isovolumic contraction to the end of isovolumic relaxation; Am: late diastolic wave; b = ventricular ejection time; Em: early diastolic wave; EKG: electrocardiogram; IVCT : isovolumic contraction time; IVRT: isovolumic relaxation time; Sm: the wave for the systolic phase.

It can be obtained by flow-Doppler and tissue Doppler technique. By using flow-Doppler technique, pulse-wave Doppler tracings are obtained from tricuspid valve and right ventricular outflow tract. By using tissue-Doppler technique, IVCT, IVRT and ET are obtained from the lateral tricuspid annulus. (Figure 6) RVMPI > 0.40 by flow-Doppler technique and > 0.55 by tissue-Doppler technique indicate RV systolic dysfunction. (Rudski et al. 2010)

3.2 Tricuspid annulus plane systolic excursion (TAPSE)

Although the morphology of RV is complex, contraction of the longitudinal fibers of RV cause most of RV systolic function and measurement of RV longitudinal motion can represent RV systolic function. TAPSE is an easy and convenient way to evaluate the RV longitudinal motion. In apical four-chamber view, the cursor line is placed across the lateral tricuspid annulus, and M-mode imaging of the cursor line reveals the longitudinal motion of lateral tricuspid annulus. TAPSE is the distance, which tricuspid annulus moves from the end-diastole phase to the end-systolic phase, and it represents the RV systolic function. When TAPSE < 16mm, RV systolic dysfunction may be present. (Figure 7)

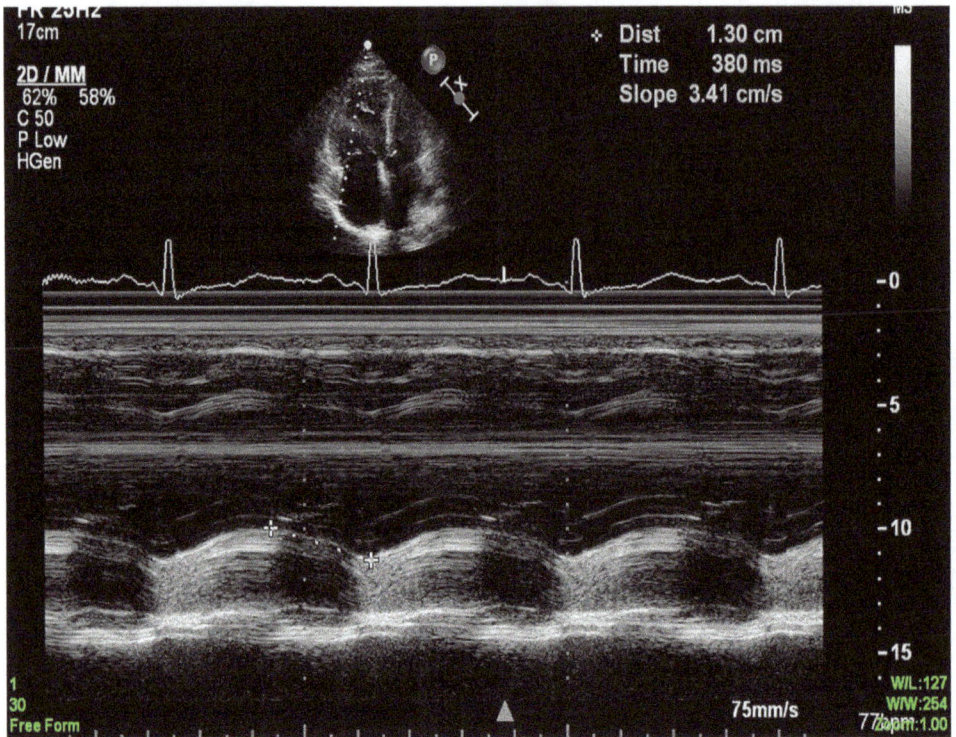

Fig. 7. A 35-year-old female with a history of idiopathic pulmonary arterial hypertension, with low TAPSE (13mm), which indicates poor RV systolic function

3.3 Right ventricular fractional area change (RVFAC)

RVFAC, which resembles left ventricular ejectional fraction, provides an estimate of RV systolic function. To obtain RVFAC, clear RV morphology and endocardial border should be clear at apical four-chamber views. RV end-diastolic and end-systolic areas (RVEDA & RVESA) are obtained after tracing RV area.

$$RVFAC = \frac{RVEDA - RVESA}{RVEDA} \times 100\%$$

RVFAC > 40% is normal. RVFAC <35% indicates RV systolic dysfunction. It is important to make sure that the entire right ventricle is in the view, including the apex and the lateral wall in both systole and diastole. Care must be taken to exclude trabeculations while tracing the RV area.

3.4 Peak Sm of lateral tricuspid annulus

Although tissue Doppler imaging detects regional myocardium function, pulmonary hypertension causes global RV change and lateral tricuspid annulus function can represent global RV function. Peak Sm of lateral tricuspid annulus is obtained by tissue-Doppler technique at end-expiration period. Peak Sm> 10 cm/s is normal, and peak Sm< 10cm/s represents depressed RV systolic function. (Figure 8)

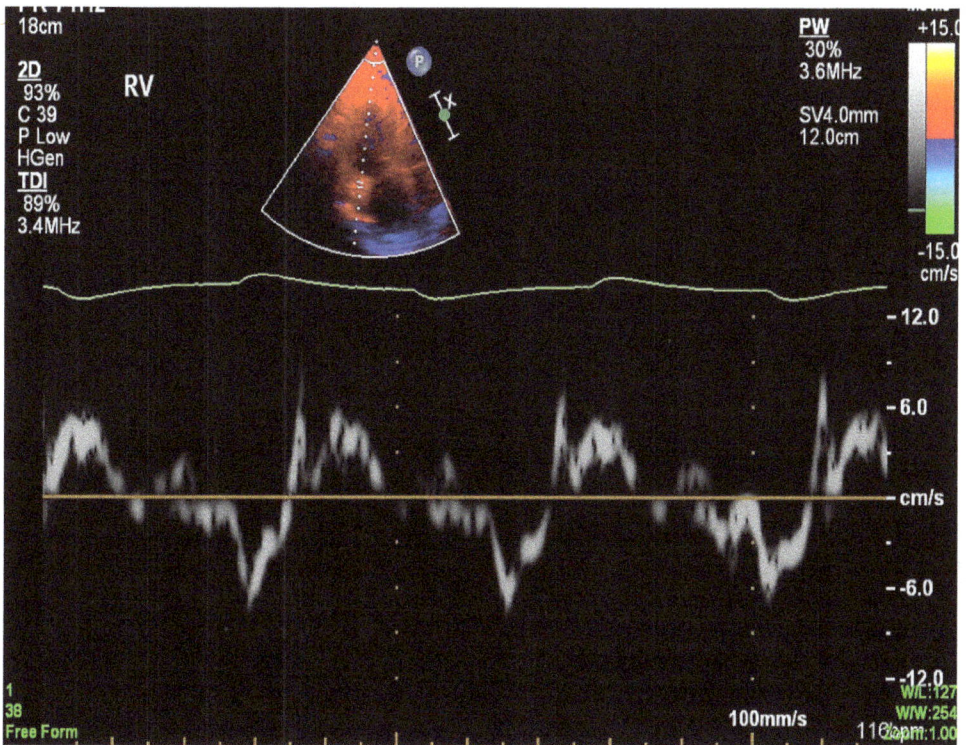

Fig. 8. A 45-year-old female with systemic lupus erythematosus and pulmonary arterial hypertension, had a low peak Sm (6.0cm/s) at lateral tricuspid annulus, which indicates poor RV systolic function.

4. Conclusion

Echocardiography is a useful tool in diagnosis of PH, evaluating the left heart disease, and estimation of pulmonary arterial hemodynamics. After diagnosis of PH is established, TAPSE, peak Sm velocity and RVMPI are simple methods to monitor treatment effects.

5. References

Bossone, E., T. H. Duong-Wagner, G. Paciocco, H. Oral, M. Ricciardi, D. S. Bach, M. Rubenfire & W. F. Armstrong (1999) Echocardiographic features of primary pulmonary hypertension. *Journal of the American Society of Echocardiography : official publication of the American Society of Echocardiography*, 12, 655-662.

Hoeper, M. M., J. A. Barbera, R. N. Channick, P. M. Hassoun, I. M. Lang, A. Manes, F. J. Martinez, R. Naeije, H. Olschewski, J. Pepke-Zaba, M. M. Redfield, I. M. Robbins, R. Souza, A. Torbicki & M. McGoon (2009) Diagnosis, assessment, and treatment of non-pulmonary arterial hypertension pulmonary hypertension. *Journal of the American College of Cardiology*, 54, S85-96.

Hoeper, M. M., S. H. Lee, R. Voswinckel, M. Palazzini, X. Jais, A. Marinelli, R. J. Barst, H. A. Ghofrani, Z.-C. Jing, C. Opitz, H.-J. Seyfarth, M. Halank, V. McLaughlin, R. J. Oudiz, R. Ewert, H. Wilkens, S. Kluge, H.-C. Bremer, E. Baroke & L. J. Rubin (2006) Complications of right heart catheterization procedures in patients with pulmonary hypertension in experienced centers. *Journal of the American College of Cardiology*, 48, 2546-2552.

Oudiz, R. J. (2007) Pulmonary Hypertension Associated with Left-Sided Heart Disease. *Clinics in chest medicine*, 28, 233-241.

Park, B., H. C. Dittrich, R. Polikar, L. Olson & P. Nicod (1989) Echocardiographic evidence of pericardial effusion in severe chronic pulmonary hypertension. *The American journal of cardiology*, 63, 143-145.

Rudski, L. G., W. W. Lai, J. Afilalo, L. Hua, M. D. Handschumacher, K. Chandrasekaran, S. D. Solomon, E. K. Louie & N. B. Schiller (2010) Guidelines for the echocardiographic assessment of the right heart in adults: a report from the American Society of Echocardiography endorsed by the European Association of Echocardiography, a registered branch of the European Society of Cardiology, and the Canadian Society of Echocardiography. *Journal of the American Society of Echocardiography : official publication of the American Society of Echocardiography*, 23, 685-713; quiz 786-8.

Simonneau, G., I. M. Robbins, M. Beghetti, R. N. Channick, M. Delcroix, C. P. Denton, C. G. Elliott, S. P. Gaine, M. T. Gladwin, Z.-C. Jing, M. J. Krowka, D. Langleben, N. Nakanishi & R. Souza (2009) Updated clinical classification of pulmonary hypertension. *Journal of the American College of Cardiology*, 54, S43-54.

Part 4

Several Clinical Forms of Pulmonary Hypertension

11

Pulmonary Hypertension in Systemic Sclerosis

Muhammad Ishaq Ghauri[1],
Jibran Sualeh Muhammad[2] and Kamran Hameed[3]
[1]Department of Medicine, Jinnah Medical College Hospital
[2]Department of Biological and Biomedical Sciences, Aga Khan University
[3]Department of Medicine, Ziauddin Medical University, Karachi,
Pakistan

1. Introduction

Pulmonary complications of systemic sclerosis (SSc) are both frequent and the leading cause of SSc-related death (Steen & Medsger, 2007; Ferri *et al.*, 2002). The most common pulmonary manifestations of SSc are the following:

- Pulmonary arterial hypertension (PAH)
- Interstitial lung disease (ILD)
- Pulmonary hypertension (PH) due to ILD
- A combination of ILD and PAH

2. Classification

The World Health Organization (WHO) classifies patients with pulmonary hypertension into five groups, as shown in the table (table 1) (Simonneau *et al.*, 2009).

1. Pulmonary arterial hypertension (PAH)
1.1. Idiopathic PAH
1.2. Heritable
1.2.1. BMPR2
1.2.2. ALK1, endoglin (with or without hereditary hemorrhagic telangiectasia)
1.2.3. Unknown
1.3. Drug- and toxin-induced
1.4. Associated with
1.4.1. Connective tissue diseases
1.4.2. HIV infection
1.4.3. Portal hypertension
1.4.4. Congenital heart diseases
1.4.5. Schistosomiasis
1.4.6. Chronic hemolytic anemia
1.5 Persistent pulmonary hypertension of the newborn

1'. Pulmonary veno-occlusive disease (PVOD) and/or pulmonary capillary hemangiomatosis (PCH)
2. Pulmonary hypertension owing to left heart disease
2.1. Systolic dysfunction
2.2. Diastolic dysfunction
2.3. Valvular disease
3. Pulmonary hypertension owing to lung diseases and/or hypoxia
3.1. Chronic obstructive pulmonary disease
3.2. Interstitial lung disease
3.3. Other pulmonary diseases with mixed restrictive and obstructive pattern
3.4. Sleep-disordered breathing
3.5. Alveolar hypoventilation disorders
3.6. Chronic exposure to high altitude
3.7. Developmental abnormalities
4. Chronic thromboembolic pulmonary hypertension (CTEPH)
5. Pulmonary hypertension with unclear multifactorial mechanisms
5.1. Hematologic disorders: myeloproliferative disorders, splenectomy
5.2. Systemic disorders: sarcoidosis, pulmonary Langerhans cell histiocytosis: lymphangioleiomyomatosis, neurofibromatosis, vasculitis
5.3. Metabolic disorders: glycogen storage disease, Gaucher disease, thyroid disorders
5.4. Others: tumoral obstruction, fibrosing mediastinitis, chronic renal failure on dialysis

ALK1: activin receptor-like kinase type 1; BMPR2: bone morphogenetic protein receptor type 2; HIV: human immunodeficiency virus.

Table 1.

Patients in the first group are considered to have pulmonary arterial hypertension (PAH). In contrast, patients in the remaining four groups are considered to have pulmonary hypertension (PH):

- Group 2 PH consists of patients who have pulmonary venous hypertension, which is usually due to left heart disease
- Group 3 PH includes patients who have PH due to lung disease and/or chronic hypoxemia (ie, interstitial lung disease, chronic obstructive airways disease, and obstructive sleep apnea)
- Group 4 PH consists of patients with chronic thromboembolic pulmonary hypertension
- Group 5 PH includes patients whose PH is of uncertain cause and likely multifactorial

When all five groups are described collectively, the term PH is used.

Systemic sclerosis (SSc) is unique among the different forms of PH because it can be associated with group 1 PAH or group 3 PH. In addition, patients with SSc frequently have diastolic dysfunction and group 2 PH. As a result, the precise classification of the type of PH can be challenging in patients with SSc. Group 1 PAH is the focus of this review.

3. Definition

Systemic sclerosis (SSc)-associated pulmonary arterial hypertension (PAH) is defined as a mean pulmonary artery pressure greater than 25 mmHg at rest (measured by right heart catheterization) with a wedge pressure less than or equal to 15 mmHg in a patient who has systemic sclerosis without significant coexisting interstitial lung disease and chronic hypoxemia. (Badesch *et al.*, 2009)

4. Risk factors

It is important to recognize patients who are at increased risk for developing systemic sclerosis (SSc)-associated pulmonary arterial hypertension (PAH). Vigilant monitoring and early detection facilitates the timely initiation of therapy, which improves symptoms and may prolong survival.

The following risk factors for PAH have been identified in patients with SSc:

- Long-standing limited cutaneous SSc with a positive anti-centromere antibody. The total burden of cutaneous telangiectasias correlates positively with the risk of PAH. (Shah *et al.*, 2010)
- Patients with diffuse cutaneous SSc tend to develop PAH less commonly; however, those with a nucleolar pattern of anti-nuclear antibody (ANA) are at increased risk. (Steen, 2005)
- Progressive decrease of the diffusion capacity (DLCO) over serial measurements. This was demonstrated by a case control study of 212 patients with limited cutaneous SSc (Steen & Medsger, 2003). Patients with PAH were matched to patients without PAH according to age, gender, extent of skin involvement, and disease duration. The mean DLCO was 52 percent of predicted five years before PAH developed. A linear decline of 50 percent was found over a 10 to 15 year period among patients who developed PAH. In contrast, the DLCO remained unchanged in patients who did not develop PAH.
- Exercise-induced PH on right heart catheterization. Nearly 20 percent of patients with SSc and exercise-induced PH may progress to PAH, according to an observational study. (Steen *et al.*, 2008; Condliffe *et al.*, 2009)

In contrast to these risk factors, patients with Scl 70 autoantibodies are more likely to have PH associated with interstitial lung disease (group 3 PH). Patients with SSc who have anti-RNA polymerase III autoantibodies characteristically have extensive skin involvement and increased risk for scleroderma renal crisis, but uncommonly develop PAH. (Steen, 2005)

5. Screening

Patients with systemic sclerosis (SSc) who have never been diagnosed with pulmonary vascular disease have been screened for pulmonary arterial hypertension (PAH) in numerous observational studies. Doppler echocardiography was the most common screening method, but exercise echocardiography and diagnostic algorithms were also used:

- Doppler echocardiography — In a study that included 669 patients with SSc or mixed connective tissue disease, 13 percent had an elevated right ventricular systolic pressure (an indicator of PAH). In another study of 227 patients with SSc, serial Doppler echocardiograms found a high tricuspid gradient (also an indicator of PAH) in 11 percent of patients during the initial echocardiogram and 17 percent during a subsequent echocardiogram. (Wigley *et al.*, 2005; Hesselstrand *et al.*, 2005)

- Exercise echocardiography — A study of 54 patients with SSc found that 44 percent had an abnormal response to exercise (defined as a ≥20 mmHg increase of the estimated pulmonary arterial systolic pressure during exercise, as measured echocardiographically) (Steen *et al.*, 2008). Right heart catheterization confirmed the presence of resting or exercise induced PAH in 81 percent of these patients. Thus, resting PAH was identified in nearly 36 percent of the study population. Of note, the abnormal response to exercise strongly correlated with a very low diffusion capacity (DLCO) and a high forced vital capacity to DLCO ratio (FVC/DLCO).
- Diagnostic algorithms — A study of 709 patients who had SSc identified PAH in 8 percent of the patients using an algorithm that included Doppler echocardiography and right heart catheterization. (Hachulla *et al.*, 2005)

Taken together, the studies have estimated that the prevalence of PAH is 8 to 37 percent among patients with SSc who have never been diagnosed with pulmonary vascular disease range (Steen *et al.*, 2008; Wigley *et al.*, 2005; Hesselstrand *et al.*, 2005; Hachulla *et al.*, 2005). This high prevalence, combined with the high mortality rate of SSc-associated PAH and the availability of therapies that improve symptoms and may prolong survival, has been used as an argument to screen patients who have SSc for PAH.

These factors must be weighed against the potential pitfalls of screening, which include the impact of false positive and false negative results. False positive results may lead to unnecessary right heart catheterization and related complications, as well as unnecessary patient anxiety. False negative results may lead to false reassurance and decreased vigilance in the clinical assessment of symptoms and signs of PAH, ultimately delaying diagnosis and therapy. False positive and false negative results are most common among patients who have interstitial lung disease. (Arcasoy *et al.*, 2003)

All patients with SSc should be evaluated regularly and thoroughly for symptoms and/or signs of PAH, as well as having regular pulmonary function tests (PFTs) to look for changes in the diffusion capacity (DLCO).

The diagnostic evaluation of suspected SSc-associated PAH is the same as that for other types of PAH, which is discussed in detail elsewhere. Suspected SSc-associated PAH should not be treated without first performing a right heart catheterization.

6. Prognosis

Pulmonary arterial hypertension (PAH) is an independent risk factor for mortality among patients with systemic sclerosis (SSc) (Hachulla *et al.*, 2009). The severity of the PAH and the presence of coexisting interstitial lung disease (ILD) directly correlate with mortality (Condliffe *et al.*, 2009; MacGregor *et al.*, 2001; Mukerjee *et al.*, 2003; Mathai *et al.*, 2009):

- A prospective cohort study of 794 patients with SSc found a prevalence of PAH of 12 percent, which was confirmed by right heart catheterization (Mukerjee *et al.*, 2003). The two year mortality rates among patients with mean pulmonary artery pressures of <32 mmHg and >45 mmHg were 22 and 61 percent, respectively. A high right atrial pressure (indicative of right ventricular failure) was the strongest hemodynamic predictor of mortality.

- A prospective cohort study of 59 patients with SSc and pulmonary hypertension (confirmed by right heart catheterization) compared patients with coexisting ILD to patients without ILD. Survival was significantly worse among patients with coexisting ILD (46 versus 79 percent). Most deaths among the patients with ILD are due to respiratory failure, whereas most deaths among patients without ILD are due to right heart failure. (Mathai *et al.*, 2009)

Progression of SSc-associated PAH is not inevitable. In one observational study of patients with SSc, 30 percent of those who had an estimated pulmonary artery pressure of >30 mmHg on an echocardiogram were found to have an estimated pulmonary artery pressure <30 mmHg two years later.

The prognosis for patients with SSc-associated PAH is worse than that for patients with idiopathic pulmonary arterial hypertension (IPAH). This was suggested by a retrospective cohort study of 91 patients that found that patients with SSc-associated PAH had one-, two-, and three-year survival rates of 87, 64, and 64 percent, respectively. In contrast, patients with IPAH had one-, two-, and three-year survival rates of 91, 88, and 78 percent, respectively. Patients with SSc-associated PAH also had higher serum levels of N-terminal brain natriuretic peptide (NT-BNP) than patients with IPAH. NT-BNP is an index of cardiac strain. (Fisher *et al.*, 2006; Mathai *et al.*, 2010)

Survival among patients with SSc-associated PAH appears to have improved modestly over the past decade. This is most likely the consequence of earlier diagnosis and more effective supportive and directed therapies. A prospective cohort study of 92 patients with SSc-associated PAH (confirmed by right heart catheterization) compared the survival of patients prior to 2002 with that of patients in the current treatment era (Williams *et al.*, 2006). Two year survival was significantly better in the current era (71 versus 47 percent). Therapy generally consisted of diuretics, digoxin, oxygen, warfarin, and prostanoids prior to 2002, but the endothelin-1 antagonists became the most frequently used first-line therapy during the current era.

Despite its improvement, the mortality rate of SSc-associated PAH remains unacceptably high, particularly when associated with ILD.

7. Treatment

PRIMARY THERAPY – Primary therapy of pulmonary hypertension refers to treatment that is directed at the underlying cause. In the case of systemic sclerosis (SSc)-associated pulmonary arterial hypertension (PAH), primary therapy refers to treatment of the SSc.

There are no established, disease-modifying therapies for SSc. However, there are effective treatments for many of its organ-based complications. The indications for the treatment of these complications are reviewed separately.

DIRECTED THERAPY – Directed therapy targets the pulmonary arterial hypertension (PAH), rather than the cause of the PAH. It is administered by clinicians with expertise in the evaluation and management of patients with pulmonary hypertension. Most aspects of directed therapy for patients with systemic sclerosis (SSc)-associated PAH are identical to those for patients with other types of PAH:

- Directed therapy is indicated for patients whose PAH is symptomatic, defined as a World Health Organization (WHO) functional class of II, III, or IV (table 1).
- Right heart catheterization is performed prior to the initiation of directed therapy in order to confirm the PAH and assess its severity.
- Classes of drugs approved for directed therapy include endothelin-1 antagonists, phosphodiesterase type 5 inhibitors, and prostanoids. (Hassoun, 2009)
- The preferred agent depends upon the severity of functional limitation, clinician preference, and patient preference.

The clinical outcomes of directed therapy in patients with SSc-associated PAH are the focus of this section. An important caveat to consider when appraising the evidence is that most trials used the six-minute walk test (6MWT) as the primary outcome. While this may be a reasonable surrogate outcome for patients with idiopathic pulmonary arterial hypertension (IPAH), it has not been validated as a reliable tool for evaluating the severity of pulmonary hypertension and the response to therapy in patients with SSC-associated PAH. (Impens *et al.*, 2008; Kowal-Bielecka *et al.*, 2010)

Endothelin-1 receptor antagonists — Endothelin-1 receptor antagonists can be either non-selective, blocking signaling mediated by type A and type B endothelin-1 receptors, or selective, blocking signaling mediated by only type A endothelin-1 receptors.

Nonselective — Bosentan is a non-selective endothelin-1 receptor antagonist. The following evidence suggests that bosentan is beneficial in SSc-associated PAH, although the response may be less than that in IPAH:

- The multicenter BREATHE-1 trial randomly assigned 213 patients with PAH (approximately 30 percent of whom had SSc- or systemic lupus erythematosus [SLE]-associated PAH) to receive bosentan or placebo (Rubin *et al.*, 2002). The patients with SSc- or SLE-associated PAH who received bosentan had an increase in their 6MWT of 3 m, while those who received placebo had a decrease of 40 m (mean difference 43 m). In comparison, patients with IPAH who received bosentan had an increase in their 6MWT of 46 m, while those who received placebo had a decrease of 5 m (mean difference 51 m). Patients with SSc- or SLE-associated PAH who received bosentan also had delayed progression to clinical worsening compared those treated with placebo. So, it is clearly seen that bosentan prevented deterioration of the 6MWT in the scleroderma subgroup.
- In a study of 53 patients who had PAH associated with either SSc- or scleroderma spectrum disorder, bosentan therapy was associated with a 48-week survival of 92 percent (Denton *et al.*, 2008). This exceeds that of historical controls, which had estimated two year survival rates of only 50 percent. (Koh *et al.*, 1996; Kawut *et al.*, 2003)

Selective — Ambrisentan and sitaxsentan are selective type A endothelin-1 receptor antagonists. Ambrisentan is available in the United States. Sitaxsentan is not yet available in the United States, but is available in Europe. The evidence suggests that both are beneficial in patients with SSc-associated PAH, although the response may be less than that in IPAH:

- The multicenter ARIES-1 and ARIES-2 trials randomly assigned 394 patients with PAH to receive either ambrisentan or placebo (Galiè *et al.*, 2008). The 6MWT improved among all patients at 12 weeks, including patients with SSc- or connective tissue disease-associated PAH. However, those with SSc- or connective tissue disease-associated PAH had a more modest response (mean difference 15 to 23 m) when compared to patients with IPAH (mean difference 50 to 60 m).

- A post hoc subgroup analysis compared sitaxsentan to placebo in 42 patients with connective tissue disease-associated PAH, using data from an earlier randomized trial (Girgis *et al.*, 2007; Barst *et al.*, 2004). The subgroup analysis found that the sitaxsentan group had an increase in their 6MWT of 20 m, while the placebo group had a decrease of 38 m (mean difference 58 m). Patients with SSc who received sitaxsentan also had a delay in clinical worsening.

The poor therapeutic response of SSc-associated PAH, compared with other types of PAH, may reflect the multisystemic nature of SSc, the frequent involvement of the heart and lungs, and/or differences in vascular pathogenesis.

Phosphodiesterase type 5 inhibitors – The phosphodiesterase type 5 (PDE-5) inhibitors reduce the catabolism of cGMP, enhancing the pulmonary vasodilatation induced by endogenous nitric oxide. Sildenafil and tadalafil are the PDE-5 inhibitors that have been approved for the treatment of PAH.

- Sildenafil – The effects of sildenafil were demonstrated by the multicenter SUPER-1 trial, which compared three doses of sildenafil (20, 40, or 80 mg three times daily for 12 weeks) to placebo in 278 patients with symptomatic PAH (Galiè *et al.*, 2005). A subgroup analysis of 84 patients with SSc- or connective tissue disease-associated PAH detected improvement in the 6MWT, New York Heart Association (NYHA) functional class, pulmonary artery pressure, and pulmonary vascular resistance among those treated with sildenafil at a dose of 20 mg three times daily (Badesch *et al.*, 2007). There was no dose-response gradient in this group (different than patients with IPAH). The long-term effectiveness of sildenafil in SSc-associated PAH has not been reported.
- Tadalafil – Tadalafil has the advantage of being administered once daily. However, its efficacy in the treatment of connective tissue disease-associated PAH has not been evaluated.

Prostanoids – The prostanoids were the first agents shown to improve symptoms, functional ability, and hemodynamic parameters of patients with SSc-associated PAH (Badesch *et al.*, 2000). Formulations include epoprostenol, treprostinil, and iloprost.

Epoprostenol – The following studies illustrate the short-term and long-term efficacy of epoprostenol:

- The short-term efficacy of continuous intravenous epoprostenol in SSc-associated PAH was demonstrated by a randomized trial of 111 patients. The mean pulmonary artery pressure decreased 10 percent among patients treated with epoprostenol, compared to an increase of 2 percent among those who received placebo. In addition, epoprostenol therapy decreased pulmonary vascular resistance, increased cardiac output, and improved the functional class.
- The long-term benefits of continuous intravenous epoprostenol in SSc-associated PAH are uncertain due to methodological limitations of the relevant studies. An analysis of data from the original epoprostenol trial and its open-label extension study found one-, two-, three-, and four-year survival rates of 71, 52, 48, and 48 percent, respectively, among patients with SSc-associated PAH (Badesch *et al.*, 2009). These survival rates are better than those of historical controls.

Treprostinil — Treprostinil is a stable prostacyclin analogue that can be administered by either continuous intravenous infusion or subcutaneous infusion using a portable microinfusion pump (similar to an insulin pump). Inhaled treprostinil has been developed, which can be administered by only four inhalations daily. (Voswinckel *et al.*, 2009)

In a randomized trial that compared subcutaneous treprostinil to placebo, a subgroup analysis of 90 patients with SSc- or connective tissue disease-associated PAH found that treprostinil was associated with improved dyspnea, cardiac index, and pulmonary vascular resistance (Oudiz *et al.*, 2004). The treprostinil group also had an improved 6MWT, but the effect was modest (mean difference 25 m).

Iloprost — An inhaler that produces aerosol particles small enough to ensure alveolar deposition delivers Iloprost. The usual formulation requires as many as nine daily doses because of its relatively short duration of action, with each dose requiring 10 to 15 minutes. A newer, more concentrated formulation still requires 6 to 9 inhalations daily, but each dose requires less time.

The effect of iloprost was demonstrated by an open-label, uncontrolled trial of five patients with SSc-associated PAH (Launay *et al.*, 2001). Iloprost therapy was associated with an increased 6MWT (85 m) at six months.

SUPPORTIVE THERAPY — Supportive therapy targets the sequelae of the pulmonary arterial hypertension (PAH) and should be considered in all patients who have systemic sclerosis (SSc)-associated PAH. It includes supplemental oxygen for patients with resting or exercise hypoxemia and diuretics for patients with fluid retention.

SSc-associated PAH is not one of the widely accepted indications for anticoagulation. However, anticoagulation may be considered on a case-by-case basis after carefully weighing the potential benefits of fewer potential thromboembolic complications against the risk of bleeding.

LUNG TRANSPLANTATION — Lung transplantation remains an option for suitable operative candidates who have severe symptoms due to systemic sclerosis (SSc)-associated pulmonary arterial hypertension (PAH) and have failed to respond to intravenous epoprostenol, either alone or in combination with other agents.

The morbidity and mortality of lung transplantation in patients with SSc-associated PAH does not appear to be significantly different from that of patients undergoing lung transplantation for idiopathic pulmonary fibrosis. This was illustrated by a retrospective study of 14 patients with SSc-associated PAH who had undergone lung transplantation (Schachna *et al.*, 2006). The two-year survival rate was 64 percent.

8. References

Arcasoy SM, Christie JD, Ferrari VA, et al. Echocardiographic assessment of pulmonary hypertension in patients with advanced lung disease. Am J Respir Crit Care Med 2003; 167:735.

Badesch DB, Tapson VF, McGoon MD, et al. Continuous intravenous epoprostenol for pulmonary hypertension due to the scleroderma spectrum of disease. A randomized, controlled trial. Ann Intern Med 2000; 132:425.

Badesch DB, Hill NS, Burgess G, et al. Sildenafil for pulmonary arterial hypertension associated with connective tissue disease. J Rheumatol 2007; 34:2417.

Badesch DB, Champion HC, Sanchez MA, et al. Diagnosis and assessment of pulmonary arterial hypertension. J Am Coll Cardiol 2009; 54:S55.

Badesch DB, McGoon MD, Barst RJ, et al. Longterm survival among patients with scleroderma-associated pulmonary arterial hypertension treated with intravenous epoprostenol. J Rheumatol 2009; 36:2244.

Barst RJ, Langleben D, Frost A, et al. Sitaxsentan therapy for pulmonary arterial hypertension. Am J Respir Crit Care Med 2004; 169:441.

Condliffe R, Kiely DG, Peacock AJ, et al. Connective tissue disease-associated pulmonary arterial hypertension in the modern treatment era. Am J Respir Crit Care Med 2009; 179:151.

Denton CP, Pope JE, Peter HH, et al. Long-term effects of bosentan on quality of life, survival, safety and tolerability in pulmonary arterial hypertension related to connective tissue diseases. Ann Rheum Dis 2008; 67:1222.

Ferri C, Valentini G, Cozzi F, et al. Systemic sclerosis: demographic, clinical, and serologic features and survival in 1,012 Italian patients. Medicine (Baltimore) 2002; 81:139.

Fisher MR, Mathai SC, Champion HC, et al. Clinical differences between idiopathic and scleroderma-related pulmonary hypertension. Arthritis Rheum 2006; 54:3043.

Galiè N, Ghofrani HA, Torbicki A, et al. Sildenafil citrate therapy for pulmonary arterial hypertension. N Engl J Med 2005; 353:2148.

Galiè N, Olschewski H, Oudiz RJ, et al. Ambrisentan for the treatment of pulmonary arterial hypertension: results of the ambrisentan in pulmonary arterial hypertension, randomized, double-blind, placebo-controlled, multicenter, efficacy (ARIES) study 1 and 2. Circulation 2008; 117:3010.

Girgis RE, Frost AE, Hill NS, et al. Selective endothelin A receptor antagonism with sitaxsentan for pulmonary arterial hypertension associated with connective tissue disease. Ann Rheum Dis 2007; 66:1467.

Hachulla E, Gressin V, Guillevin L, et al. Early detection of pulmonary arterial hypertension in systemic sclerosis: a French nationwide prospective multicenter study. Arthritis Rheum 2005; 52:3792.

Hachulla E, Carpentier P, Gressin V, et al. Risk factors for death and the 3-year survival of patients with systemic sclerosis: the French ItinérAIR-Sclérodermie study. Rheumatology (Oxford) 2009; 48:304.

Hassoun PM. Therapies for scleroderma-related pulmonary arterial hypertension. Expert Rev Respir Med 2009; 3:187.

Hesselstrand R, Ekman R, Eskilsson J, et al. Screening for pulmonary hypertension in systemic sclerosis: the longitudinal development of tricuspid gradient in 227 consecutive patients, 1992-2001. Rheumatology (Oxford) 2005; 44:366.

Impens AJ, Wangkaew S, Seibold JR. The 6-minute walk test in scleroderma--how measuring everything measures nothing. Rheumatology (Oxford) 2008; 47 Suppl 5:v68.

Kawut SM, Taichman DB, Archer-Chicko CL, et al. Hemodynamics and survival in patients with pulmonary arterial hypertension related to systemic sclerosis. Chest 2003; 123:344.

Koh ET, Lee P, Gladman DD, Abu-Shakra M. Pulmonary hypertension in systemic sclerosis: an analysis of 17 patients. Br J Rheumatol 1996; 35:989.

Kowal-Bielecka O, Avouac J, Pittrow D, et al. Echocardiography as an outcome measure in scleroderma-related pulmonary arterial hypertension: a systematic literature analysis by the EPOSS group. J Rheumatol 2010; 37:105.

Launay D, Hachulla E, Hatron PY, et al. Aerosolized iloprost in CREST syndrome related pulmonary hypertension. J Rheumatol 2001; 28:2252.

MacGregor AJ, Canavan R, Knight C, et al. Pulmonary hypertension in systemic sclerosis: risk factors for progression and consequences for survival. Rheumatology (Oxford) 2001; 40:453.

Mathai SC, Hummers LK, Champion HC, et al. Survival in pulmonary hypertension associated with the scleroderma spectrum of diseases: impact of interstitial lung disease. Arthritis Rheum 2009; 60:569.

Mathai SC, Bueso M, Hummers LK, et al. Disproportionate elevation of N-terminal pro-brain natriuretic peptide in scleroderma-related pulmonary hypertension. Eur Respir J 2010; 35:95.

Mukerjee D, St George D, Coleiro B, et al. Prevalence and outcome in systemic sclerosis associated pulmonary arterial hypertension: application of a registry approach. Ann Rheum Dis 2003; 62:1088.

Oudiz RJ, Schilz RJ, Barst RJ, et al. Treprostinil, a prostacyclin analogue, in pulmonary arterial hypertension associated with connective tissue disease. Chest 2004; 126:420.

Rubin LJ, Badesch DB, Barst RJ, et al. Bosentan therapy for pulmonary arterial hypertension. N Engl J Med 2002; 346:896.

Schachna L, Medsger TA Jr, Dauber JH, et al. Lung transplantation in scleroderma compared with idiopathic pulmonary fibrosis and idiopathic pulmonary arterial hypertension. Arthritis Rheum 2006; 54:3954.

Shah AA, Wigley FM, Hummers LK. Telangiectases in scleroderma: a potential clinical marker of pulmonary arterial hypertension. J Rheumatol 2010; 37:98.

Simonneau G, Robbins IM, Beghetti M, et al. Updated clinical classification of pulmonary hypertension. J Am Coll Cardiol 2009; 54:S43.

Steen V, Medsger TA Jr. Predictors of isolated pulmonary hypertension in patients with systemic sclerosis and limited cutaneous involvement. Arthritis Rheum 2003; 48:516.

Steen VD. Autoantibodies in systemic sclerosis. Semin Arthritis Rheum 2005; 35:35.

Steen VD, Medsger TA. Changes in causes of death in systemic sclerosis, 1972-2002. Ann Rheum Dis 2007; 66:940.

Steen V, Chou M, Shanmugam V, et al. Exercise-induced pulmonary arterial hypertension in patients with systemic sclerosis. Chest 2008; 134:146.

Voswinckel R, Reichenberger F, Gall H, et al. Metered dose inhaler delivery of treprostinil for the treatment of pulmonary hypertension. Pulm Pharmacol Ther 2009; 22:50.

Wigley FM, Lima JA, Mayes M, et al. The prevalence of undiagnosed pulmonary arterial hypertension in subjects with connective tissue disease at the secondary health care level of community-based rheumatologists (the UNCOVER study). Arthritis Rheum 2005; 52:2125.

Williams MH, Das C, Handler CE, et al. Systemic sclerosis associated pulmonary hypertension: improved survival in the current era. Heart 2006; 92:926.

12

Sarcoidosis Associated Pulmonary Hypertension

Veronica Palmero, Phillip Factor and Roxana Sulica
Albert Einstein College of Medicine, Beth Israel Medical Center, New York
United States of America

1. Introduction

Pulmonary hypertension (PH) is a serious complication of sarcoidosis, a multi-systemic inflammatory disease characterized by the presence of widespread non-caseating granulomas. When PH develops in patients with sarcoidosis, it is associated with increased morbidity and mortality.

Sarcoidosis-associated pulmonary hypertension (SAPH) is most commonly seen in patients with advanced pulmonary sarcoidosis as a result of pulmonary fibrosis and chronic hypoxemia. However, the presence of PH in individuals with extra-pulmonary sarcoidosis and normal pulmonary physiology suggests that SAPH may be due to other mechanisms. Appropriate understanding of this disease and its complex pathophysiology is essential for early recognition and therapy.

2. Definition

SAPH is defined as mean pulmonary artery pressure (mPAP) above 25 mm Hg at rest with a pulmonary artery occlusion pressure (PAOP) or left ventricular end-diastolic pressure (LVEDP) less than 15 mmHg, in patients with sarcoidosis, diagnosed by clinical, radiological and histological criteria, in the absence of other risk factors for pulmonary hypertension. (Badesch et al., 2009) Because of the complex pathogenetic mechanisms of SAPH, it is classified under group 5 (i.e. Pulmonary Hypertension with Unclear Multifactorial Mechanisms) of the Updated Clinical Classification of Pulmonary Hypertension (Dana Point, 2008). (Simonneau et al., 2009)

3. Epidemiology

The prevalence of SAPH in general sarcoidosis population is 5% to 28% and varies with geographical location, clinical characteristics and diagnostic method. (Palmero & Sulica, 2010)

In case series of unselected sarcoidosis patients, the prevalence of SAPH is as low as 5-15%. If only dyspneic patients are considered, SAPH frequency can be as high as 60%. (Baughman et al., 2011) The prevalence of SAPH has been reported to be 73.8% in patients being evaluated for lung transplantation, with severe PH (mPAP >40 mm Hg) present in 36% of patients. (Shorr et al., 2005) SAPH is more prevalent in patients with advanced radiographic stage, but can develop in the absence of parenchymal lung abnormalities. In one cohort of 54 patients with sarcoidosis and elevated pulmonary pressures by echocardiography, 60% of the patients had radiographic stage IV disease, while 10% had radiologically normal lung parenchyma (stages 0 and I). (Sulica et al., 2005) When right heart catheterization (RHC) was used to measure mPAP, pulmonary hypertension was found in 31.8% of 22 patients without lung fibrosis. (Nunes et al., 2006)

4. Pathophysiology

Multiple mechanisms have been proposed to explain the development of pulmonary hypertension in patients with sarcoidosis. Pulmonary fibrosis with destruction of the pulmonary vascular bed and chronic hypoxemia is a major cause of increased pulmonary artery pressures in advanced pulmonary sarcoidosis. Since SAPH may develop in the absence of pulmonary fibrosis, alternative pathogenic mechanisms have been proposed and include elevated levels of endothelin-1 (ET-1), decreased nitric oxide synthesis, structural abnormalities such as granulomatous vasculitis, pulmonary veno-occlusive disease, external compression of the pulmonary vessels by enlarged mediastinal lymph nodes, hypoxia-induced vasoconstriction, and pulmonary vascular remodeling. In addition, a significant percent (i.e. approximately 30%) of patients with sarcoidosis have elevated pulmonary artery pressures due to left heart disease. (Baughman et al., 2010).

Presence of multiple mechanisms of increased pulmonary pressures in sarcoidosis underscores the importance of different management and therapeutic options in SAPH.

4.1 Nitric oxide

The synthesis and release of nitric oxide (NO) from the endothelial cells and other sources is a key element in the maintenance of the low pulmonary artery vasomotor tone characteristic of the normal pulmonary circulation. (Sterling & Creager, 1999) Decreased production of NO has been associated with the development of various forms of pulmonary hypertension. There is indirect evidence that a NO-dependent mechanism is operative in certain cases of SAPH. Inhaled NO administration acutely reduces the pulmonary vascular resistance (PVR) up to 20% in patients with SAPH, even in the presence of significant parenchymal lung disease. Although PVR reduction was not maintained over time, specific treatment targeting NO production might still be beneficial. (Preston et al., 2001)

4.2 Endothelin-1

Endothelin-1 (ET-1) is a peptide synthesized by the vascular endothelium with potent vasoconstrictor, pro-inflammatory and proliferative properties. This peptide has been found to contribute to increased pulmonary arterial tone and smooth-muscle proliferation in patients with pulmonary arterial hypertension. (Giaid et al., 1993) Similarly, elevated levels of ET-1 in plasma, bronchio-alveolar lavage and urine have been found in SAPH. Moreover, ET-1 levels decrease with clinical remission of sarcoidosis. (Letizia et al, 2001; Reichenberger et al., 2001; Sofia et al., 1995; Terashita et al., 2006) These findings suggest an important role for ET-1 in the pathogenesis of sarcoidosis and PH and raise the possibility of use of endothelin receptor antagonists in patients with SAPH.

4.3 Granulomatous vasculitis

Sarcoidosis is characterized by the presence of generalized granulomatous inflammation in organs and tissues, including the pulmonary vascular wall. This includes inflammation and necrosis of the vessel wall with destruction of the elastic media of small and medium-sized vessels, with subsequent vascular remodeling and occlusive narrowing of the vascular lumen. These changes are reflected hemodynamically in elevated pulmonary vascular resistance and pulmonary hypertension. (Takemura et al., 1991, 1992)

Granulomatous angiitis has been found in 69-100% of lung biopsies from patients with sarcoidosis, with a predilection for venous structures, although arterial involvement has been reported as well. (Rosen et al., 1977)

4.4 Pulmonary veno-occlusive disease (PVOD)

PVOD is an occlusive venopathy characterized by extensive and diffuse fibrosis of the intima of the venules and small intralobular veins. Recanalization occurs over time, resulting in chronic hemosiderosis and calcium deposition in the elastic laminae, altering the normal hemodynamics. These changes have been found in explanted lung specimens of patients with sarcoidosis, suggesting an association of a PVOD-like disease with the development of pulmonary hypertension in sarcoidosis. (Nunes et al., 2006) Typical radiologic findings of PVOD, such as ground glass opacities and inter-lobular septal edema, have been frequently found in patients with SAPH, suggesting that PVOD accounts for some of the PVR increase seen in SAPH. (Handa et al., 2006; Nunes et al., 2006)

4.5 Extrinsic compression of pulmonary vasculature

Extrinsic compression of the pulmonary vasculature by enlarged lymph nodes may be associated with significant increases in PVR and mPAP if the vascular lumen is reduced more than 50%. Nunes et al. described extrinsic compression of large pulmonary arteries by lymphadenopathy in 21.4% of patients with sarcoidosis that developed pulmonary hypertension. It was typically attributed to bilateral mediastinal and hilar lymph node involvement. Sarcoidosis-associated mediastinal fibrosis can also contribute to external compression of the pulmonary vasculature. The diagnostic method of choice in cases of extrinsic pulmonary artery compression is pulmonary angiography, which demonstrates extrinsic pulmonary artery stenosis without intraluminal obstruction. (Damuth et al., 1980; Nunes et al., 2006; Wescott & DeGraff, 1973)

4.6 Hypoxia-induced vasoconstriction

Chronic hypoxemia and resulting pulmonary vascular remodeling are implicated in the pathogenesis of pulmonary hypertension in chronic parenchymal lung disease. Correction of **hypoxemia** with supplemental oxygen has been shown to ameliorate the progression of **pulmonary hypertension** in patients with COPD. It is reasonable to extrapolate that patients with sarcoidosis and impaired pulmonary function, destruction of the lung parenchyma and hypoxemia are at similar risk for pulmonary hypertension by the same mechanisms.

4.7 Pulmonary hypertension due to left heart disease

Cardiac factors, either direct granulomatous myocardial involvement or left ventricular diastolic dysfunction with impaired relaxation have also been linked with increased pulmonary artery pressures in patients with sarcoidosis. In these circumstances, pulmonary hypertension is postcapillary in nature (i.e. pulmonary venous hypertension). This mechanism implies a different prognosis and requires different management strategies from precapillary SAPH treatment. (Baughman et al., 2006, 2010)

5. Clinical presentation

Persistent or progressive dyspnea on exertion in excess to that expected from the parenchymal lung involvement is the sentinel symptom of SAPH. (Handa et al., 2006; Nunes et al., 2006; Sulica et al., 2005) Similarly, appearance or worsening of dyspnea in a patient with stable or improved pulmonary function or despite optimization of immunosuppressive therapy may suggest SAPH. (Baughman et al., 2010) Other symptoms such as cough, chest pain, palpitations, and pre-syncope or syncope are suggestive, but not specific of SAPH. Less than 10% of patients with SAPH are asymptomatic. SAPH should be considered in patients presenting with syncope, although this symptom could also represent sarcoid cardiac involvement. (Sulica et al., 2005) Specific signs of pulmonary hypertension, such as a loud pulmonary component of the second heart sound, tricuspid or pulmonary regurgitant murmurs, and right-sided gallop may be present in SAPH. Signs of right ventricular failure, like lower extremity edema, right ventricular heave, and elevated jugular venous pressure, are present in 21% of the patients with SAPH. (Sulica et al., 2005) Hypoxemia and decreased functional status, measured by the 6-minute-walk distance, exercise desaturation and decreased distance-saturation product (DSP), tend to be more pronounced in patients with SAPH compared to sarcoidosis patients without PH. (Alhamad et al., 2010; Baughman et al., 2007; Bourbonnais & Samavati, 2008)

6. Diagnosis

Initial diagnosis of SAPH is based on a high index of suspicion. If pulmonary hypertension is clinically suspected in patients with sarcoidosis, a comprehensive series of diagnostic tests should be performed to confirm the diagnosis and to exclude other causes of pulmonary hypertension. A 2- dimensional echocardiography is an appropriate initial step to screen for SAPH. Basic evaluation includes an electrocardiogram and laboratory tests, such as liver function tests, HIV testing, and markers of connective tissue disease. Ventilation-perfusion scan should be performed to rule out chronic thrombo-embolic pulmonary hypertension as an alternative explanation for pulmonary hypertension in these patients. Pulmonary function tests and tests of exercise capacity (such as the 6-minute-walk test or cardio-pulmonary exercise testing) are recommended to gauge baseline functional status of the SAPH patient.

The gold standard for diagnosis of SAPH is right heart catheterization (RHC), although there are no published guidelines for which patients should undergo RHC in this patient population. Given the high prevalence of pulmonary venous hypertension in patients with sarcoidosis, RHC is the only reliable diagnostic method to differentiate precapillary SAPH from postcapillary PVH.

We recommend that RHC be performed in all patients in whom SAPH is suspected, particularly if initiation of PH therapy is contemplated.

6.1 Pulmonary Function Tests (PFTs)

Compared to patients with sarcoidosis without PH, patients who develop SAPH tend to demonstrate more pulmonary functional abnormalities and a more pronounced reduction in the diffusing capacity of the lung for carbon monoxide (DLCO).

Forced vital capacity% (FVC %), forced expiratory volume in 1 second % (FEV_1 %), mid-expiratory flow (FEF $_{25-75}$), DLCO %, and total lung capacity % (TLC %) have been reported to be significantly lower in patients with sarcoidosis and PH when compared with patients without PH. (Baughman et al., 2007; Bourbonnais & Samavati, 2008; Handa et al., 2006; Sulica et al., 2005)

A very common finding in patients with PH is the presence of a disproportionate decrease in the diffusing capacity of the lung for carbon monoxide to the degree of pulmonary impairment and restriction, similar to PAH associated with scleroderma.

Decreases in DLCO% below 50% in the absence of radiographic pulmonary fibrosis and below 30% in patients with stage 4 CXR may signify the development of SAPH. (Sulica et al., 2005)

6.2 Six Minute Walk Test (6MWT)

The six minute walk test is an inexpensive, simple and reproducible test used to assess the functional status of patients with pulmonary, cardiac and pulmonary vascular disease. Six minute walk distance is reduced in the majority of patients with sarcoidosis, and this reduction is even more pronounced in patients with SAPH, when compared with sarcoidosis patients without PH. (Baughman et al., 2007, Bourbonnais & Samavati, 2008) In a prospective study of 142 patients with sarcoidosis, the median 6MWD walked by SAPH patients was 280 m, which was significantly lower compared to the median distance of 411 m, walked by the patients without documented PH. (Baughman et al., 2007)

In addition, compared to patients without PH, during a 6MWT, SAPH patients demonstrate more significant degree of oxygen desaturation, increased Borg Dyspnea Score and a lower distance saturation product (DSP, defined as the product between the distance walked and the lowest oxygen saturation achieved during the 6MWT). (Alhamad et al., 2010; Baughman et al., 2007; Bourbonnais & Samavati, 2008) We recommend using the 6MWT at initial evaluation and periodically thereafter to monitor disease progression and response to therapy. However, it is important to recognize that, as opposed to patients with non-sarcoid pulmonary arterial hypertension (PAH), the clinical significance of the 6MWT results is more complex in SAPH patients. In these patients, other factors besides the presence of pulmonary vascular disease determine the 6MWD, such as the degree of desaturation with exercise, lung functional parameters (FVC), and self reported respiratory health. (Baughman et al., 2007)

6.3 Radiology

As mentioned above, SAPH is more frequently encountered in patients with advanced radiographic stage and pulmonary fibrosis. The role of high resolution chest tomography (HRCT) in diagnosing SAPH is unclear. Compared to controls with sarcoidosis but no PH, Nunes et al noted a more frequent occurrence of ground glass attenuation in patients with SAPH without fibrosis, and significantly higher frequency of septal lines in patients with SAPH and pulmonary fibrosis. Conversely, Handa et al were unable to correlate the presence of lymph node enlargement, lung opacities and thickening of bronchovascular bundles on HRCT with SAPH.

Thus, pending additional results, at this time it is reasonable to conclude that tomographic imaging studies are usually not helpful in predicting the presence of SAPH. (Handa et al., 2006; Nunes et al., 2006)

6.4 Echocardiography

Transthoracic echocardiography (TTE) is a noninvasive screening method commonly used to test for the presence of pulmonary hypertension in sarcoidosis. It is also helpful to detect other cardiac abnormalities, such as left heart disease, presence of shunts or pericardial effusion, and particularly to evaluate the right heart, anatomically and functionally. Echocardiography may be used to estimate the right ventricular systolic pressure (RVSP) from the tricuspid regurgitation jet velocity. Arcasoy et al reviewed 374 patients with advanced lung disease and found that RVSP could be estimated in only 44% of the subjects due to the lack of tricuspid regurgitant jet in the majority of patients. (Arcasoy et al., 2003). For the patients in whom RVSP estimation was feasible, even though there was a good correlation with RHC-determined RVSP (r= 0.69, p<0.0001), the agreement was very poor. Notably, echocardiographically estimated RVSP differed from RHC measured RVSP by more than 10 mmHg in 52% of cases. This study suggests that echocardiography may be a useful screening tool for pulmonary hypertension, but may not be accurate enough for quantification of pulmonary artery pressures. As such, echocardiography cannot substitute right heart catheterization for the accurate diagnosis of SAPH.

6.5 Right Heart Catheterization (RHC)

RHC is the gold standard for diagnosis of SAPH and for determining the degree of right ventricular dysfunction. In a single-center series, 53 patients with sarcoidosis and persistent dyspnea despite systemic immunosuppressive therapy underwent right heart catheterization. Notably, TTE was unable to detect RVSP in 30% of these patients and 24% of the patients with elevated RVSP on TTE had PCWP greater than 20 mmHg. This study underscores the importance of RHC in precisely identifying and categorizing PH in sarcoidosis. (Baughman et al., 2006) In a subsequent study, Baughman and colleagues performed RHC in 130 patients with sarcoidosis and unexplained dyspnea. They found that 70 patients (53.8%) had PH. Of these, 20 patients (15.4 %) had postcapillary, pulmonary venous hypertension (PH with left ventricular disease), while 50 patients (38.5 %) had precapillary PH, with normal left-sided filling pressures. Importantly, the presence of PH was associated with a higher risk for death; patients with precapillary PH and post-capillary PH had hazard ratios for death of 10.39 and 3.14 respectively. (Baughman et al., 2010) In conclusion, RHC is of paramount importance in the diagnosis of SAPH, not only for establishing an accurate diagnosis, evaluation of the right ventricular function and ruling out pulmonary venous hypertension, but also for valuable prognostic information.

7. Treatment

There are no specific therapies or treatment guidelines currently available for the management of PH in association with sarcoidosis. The current management of these patients is based on PAH therapeutic options and from observational studies.

7.1 Corticosteroids and immunosuppressive therapy

Corticosteroids and other immunosuppressive agents have been long used for the treatment of sarcoidosis, but they do not have an established role in the treatment of SAPH. Gluskowski et al used RHC to study 22 patients with pulmonary sarcoidosis and radiographic stage 2 and 3 disease that were treated with corticosteroids for 12 months.

Radiological regression was seen in 91% of the patients. At baseline, 75% of the evaluated patients had elevated PAP with exercise and 16% had elevated PAP at rest. They found that half of the patients in each group had markedly reduced mPAP after treatment, but were unable to correlate corticosteroid treatment with changes in lung function, radiographic changes or mPAP decrease. (Gluskowski et al., 1990) A possible explanation for the lack of uniform hemodynamic response to corticosteroids in this study is that, in patients without a hemodynamic response, healing of the intravascular granulomas with fibrosis resulted in further narrowing of the pulmonary vessels and permanently increased pulmonary vascular resistance.

Nunes and colleagues found an even lower response to corticosteroids. They retrospectively studied 10 patients with SAPH treated with corticosteroids (oral prednisone 0.5 to 1 mg/kg/day). These patients were evaluated at 3 and 6 months by Doppler echocardiography. In 3 of the 10 patients without evidence of pulmonary fibrosis they noted a decrease of more than 20% from baseline in RVSP by echocardiography. None of the patients with stage IV chest radiograph showed significant hemodynamic response to corticosteroids. (Nunes et al., 2006)

7.2 Specific pulmonary hypertension therapy

7.2.1 Prostacyclins

Intravenous epoprostenol is a prostaglandin with potent vasodilatory activity and inhibitory effect on platelet aggregation used for the treatment of PAH. Fisher et al evaluated the long-term effect of intravenous epoprostenol in 8 patients with moderate to severe PH (mean PVR > 1,176 dynes s cm^{-5}) and WHO functional class III and IV symptoms. Majority of the patients showed evidence of pulmonary fibrosis, had restrictive physiology, decreased DLCO% and required supplemental oxygen. One of the 8 patients died from right heart failure prior to RHC. An acute vasodilator trial with intravenous epoprostenol was done in 7 of the 8 patients. Six of the 7 patients demonstrated acute vasoreactivity defined as a 25% or more decrease in the PVR in response to maximally tolerated dose of epoprostenol. These 6 patients were started on intravenous epoprostenol, but one died from cardiac arrest within hours of initiation. Five patients were followed for an average of 29 months while receiving intravenous epoprostenol (mean dose 55.6 ng/kg/min) and all showed functional improvement by 1 or 2 WHO classes. This limited evidence suggests that PAH therapies may be beneficial for SAPH patients. (Fisher et al., 2006)

Inhaled iloprost, a prostacyclin analogue, has been administered as monotherapy to 22 patients with SAPH in an open label prospective study. Fifteen patients completed 16 weeks of iloprost administration, most common causes of discontinuation being cough and lack of compliance with 6-9 daily inhalations. Six patients showed hemodynamic improvement, with a more than 20% decrease in PVR. The 6MWD increased by more than 30 m in 3 patients. Quality of life, as measured by the Saint George Respiratory Questionnaire, also improved in 7 of the SAPH patients who completed the study. (Baughman et al., 2009)

7.2.2 Phosphodiesterase inhibitors

Selective inhibitors of cGMP-specific phosphodiesterase type 5 (PDE5) increase local NO in the pulmonary vasculature, thereby promoting vasodilation and are currently approved for the treatment of PAH. Only limited data is available for their use in SAPH. A small, single center retrospective study evaluated 25 patients with end-stage pulmonary sarcoidosis referred for transplantation. Twelve patients were treated with sildenafil for 1-12 months. Although there was no significant impact on the 6MWD, a significant reduction in mPAP (average mPAP for the group decreased from 48 mmHg to 39 mmHg), PVR (average PVR decreased from 10.7 to 5.6 Wood units), and an increase in the cardiac index from 2.3 to 2.9 L/min/m²) was noted. (Milman et al., 2008)

7.2.3 Endothelin receptor blockers

Endothelin-1 receptor blockers are used in PAH to reverse the endothelin system activation, which results in deleterious vasoconstriction and cardiac and vascular remodeling. Increased levels of endothelin-1 have been found in patients with sarcoidosis that have developed PH, suggesting this might be a contributing mechanism to the development of SAPH. Published experience with endothelin receptor blockers in SAPH is limited to a few retrospective case series and one prospective study.

Baughman and colleagues evaluated 53 patients with sarcoidosis and persistent dyspnea and assessed their pulmonary pressures by RHC. Out of those, 5 patients with SAPH were treated with bosentan for 4 months, with a decrease in mPAP from 50 mmHg to 35 mmHg at follow-up. (Baughman et al., 2006; 2007)

We have reported a retrospective case series of 40 patients with SAPH who received bosentan and were followed for an average of 38 months. These patients demonstrated a significant reduction in their mean PAP and PVRI at follow-up RHC. (P=0.0048 and P=0.017, respectively). We also observed an increase in the 6MWD of 74.6 m (p=0.0013) and less dyspnea. (Palmero & Sulica, 2011)

Judson and colleagues enrolled 21 SAPH patients in a proof of concept prospective study designed to investigate the effect of ambrisentan therapy over 6 months. Ten patients completed the study. There were no significant changes in the 6MWD, gas exchanges or hemodynamic variables. However, there was a significant improvement in the WHO functional class and quality of life assessed by the Sarcoidosis Health Questionnaire. (Judson et al., 2011)

7.2.4 Two-center experience

Barnett et al evaluated 22 patients with SAPH treated with specific PAH therapeutic agents. These patients had moderate restrictive pulmonary dysfunction, severely decreased DLCO, radiologic stage IV disease (68%), and a mean PAP of 46 mm Hg. Following treatment with different PH agents (sildenafil, bosentan, and intravenous epoprostenol), there were improvements in WHO functional class, 6MWD (p=0.032), mean PAP (p=0.008) and PVR (p=0.011). Transplant free survival rates at 1 and 3 years were reported as 90% and 74%, respectively, and no serious adverse events were attributed to the any of the drugs. (Barnett et al., 2009)

All these findings suggest a potential benefit from specific PAH therapeutic agents in selected patients with SAPH. However, large multicenter trials are required prior to recommending their use as standard of care in patients with SAPH.

8. Prognosis

The development of PH reduces life expectancy in patients with sarcoidosis. Certain risk factors have been associated with worse outcomes and increased mortality. These factors include the presence of hypoxemia, mPAP above 35 mmHg, a cardiac index below $2 L/min/m^2$, and high right atrial pressure ≥ 15 Hg. (Arcasoy et al., 2001; Shorr et al., 2002)

9. Conclusion

SAPH is common in advanced sarcoidosis, although it can be found in earlier stages of the disease as well. Presence of SAPH is usually associated with increased or unexplained dyspnea, decreased functional status, increased oxygen requirements, and lower survival rates. When clinically suspected, appropriate diagnostic tests, particularly echocardiography and right heart catheterization, should be promptly performed. There is a variable and inconsistent response to the available therapeutic agents in small series of patients with SAPH. Further studies are necessary to better understand this disease and to define more effective therapeutic strategies.

10. References

Alhamad EH, Ahmad Shaik S, Idrees MM, et al. Outcome measures of the 6 minute walk test: relationships with physiologic and computed tomography findings in patients with sarcoidosis. Pulmonary Medicine 2010, 10: 42.

Arcasoy S, Christie J, Pochettino A, et al. Characteristics and outcomes of patients with sarcoidosis listed for lung transplantation. Chest 2001; 120:873.

Arcasoy S, Christie J, Ferrari V, et al. Echocardiographic assessment of pulmonary hypertension in patients with advanced lung disease. Am J Respir Crit Care Med 2003; 167: 735.

Badesch DB, Hunter CC, Gomez Sanchez Miguel Angel et al, Diagnosis and Assessment of Pulmonary Arterial Hypertension. J Am Coll Cardiol 2009; 54: S55-66.

Barnett C, Bonura E, Nathan S, et al. treatment of sarcoidosis-associated pulmonary hypertension. Chest 2009; 135:1455.

Baughman RP, Engel PJ, Meyer CA et al. Pulmonary hypertension in sarcoidosis. Sarcoidosis Vasc Diffuse Lung Dis 2006; 23:108.

Baughman R, Sparkman B, Lower E. Six-Minute Walk Test and Health Status Assessment in Sarcoidosis. Chest 2007; 132:207.

Baughman, RP. Pulmonary hypertension associated with sarcoidosis. Arthritis Research & Therapy 2007; 9:S2.

Baughman RP, Judson MA, Lower EE, et al. Inhaled iloprost for sarcoidosis-associated pulmonary hypertension. Sarcoidosis Vasculitis and Diffuse Lung Diseases 2009; 26; 110-120.

Baughman RP, Engel PJ, Taylor L et al. Survival in Sarcoidosis-Associated Pulmonary Hypertension. The Importance of Hemodynamic Evaluation. Chest 2010 ; 138 (5) : 1078-1085.

Baughman RP, Culver DA, and Judson MA. A Concise Review of Pulmonary Sarcoidosis. Am J Respir Crit Care Med 183: 573-581, 2011

Bourbonnais JM and Samavati L. Clinical predictors of pulmonary hypertension in sarcoidosis. Eur Respir J 2008 ; 32 : 296-302.

Damuth T, Bower J, Cho K, et al. Major pulmonary artery stenosis causing pulmonary hypertension in sarcoidois. Chest 1980; 78:888.

Fisher K, Serlin D, Wilson K et al. Sarcoidosis-associated pulmonary hypertension. Chest 2006; 130:1481.

Giaid A, Yanagisawa M, Langleben D, et al. Expression of endothelin-1 in the lung of patients with pulmonary hypertension. N Engl J Med 1993; 328:1732.

Gluskowski J, Hawrylkiewicz I, Zych D, et al. Effect of corticosteroid treatment on pulmonary haemodynamics in patients with sarcoidosis. Eur Respir J 1990; 3: 403.

Handa T, Nagai S, Miki S, et al. Incidence of pulmonary hypertension and its clinical relevance in patients with sarcoidosis. Chest 2006; 129:1246.

Judson MA, Kwon S, Highland KB, et al. The assessment of three health-related quality of life measurements assessed in an ambrisentan trial for sarcoidosis-associated pulmonary hypertension. Sarcoidosis Vasculitis and Diffuse Lung Diseases 2011; 28 (Suppl N:1); 20, E8.

Letizia C, Danese A, Reale M, et al. Plasma levels of endothelin-1 increase in patients with sarcoidosis and fall after disease remission. Panminerva Med 2001; 43:257.

Milman N, Burton C, Iversen M, et al. Pulmonary hypertension in end-stage pulmonary sarcoidosis: therapeutic effects of sildenafil?. J Heart Lung Transplant 2008; 27:329.

Nunes H, Humbert M, Capron F, et al. Pulmonary hypertension associated with sarcoidosis: mechanisms, haemodynamics and prognosis. Thorax 2006; 61:68.

Palmero V, Sulica R. Sarcoidosis-Associated Pulmonary Hypertension: Assessment and Management. Sem Resp Crit Care Med. 2010;31:494-500.

Palmero V, Sulica R. Bosentan for the Treatment of Sarcoidosis-Associated Pulmonary Hypertension. Am. J. Respir. Crit. Care Med., May 2011; 183: A5889.

Preston I, Klinger J, Landzberg M, et al. Vasoresponsiveness of Sarcoidosis-associated pulmonary hypertension. Chest 2001; 120:866.

Reichenberger F, Schauer J, Kellner k, et al. Different expression of endothelin in the bronchoalveolar lavage in patients with pulmonary Disease. Lung 2001; 179:163.

Rosen Y, Moon S, Huang C, et al. Granulomatous pulmonary angiitis in sarcoidosis. Arch Pathol Lab Med 1977; 101:170.

Shorr A, Davies D, Nathan S. Outcomes for patients with sarcoidosis awaiting lung transplantation. Chest 2002; 122:233.

Shorr AF, Helman DL, Davies DB, et al. Pulmonary hypertension in advanced sarcoidosis: epidemiology and clinical characteristics. Eur Respir J 2005; 25:783.

Simonneau G, Robbins IM, Beghetti M, et al. Clinical classification of pulmonary hypertension. J Am Coll Cardiol 2009; 54: S43-54.

Sofia M, Mormile M, Faraone S, et al: Endothelin-1 excretion in urine in active pulmonary sarcoidosis and in other interstitial lung diseases. Sarcoidosis 1995; 12:118.

Sterling R, Creager M. Nitric oxide and pulmonary hypertension. Coron Artery Dis 1999; 10:287.

Sulica R, Teirstein AS, Kakarla S, et al. Distinctive clinical, radiographic and functional characteristic of patients with sarcoidosis-related pulmonary hypertension. Chest 2005; 128:1483.

Takemura T, Matsui Y, Oritsu M, et al. Pulmonary vascular involvement in sarcoidosis: granulomatous angiitis and microangiopathy in transbronchial lung biopsies. Virchows Arch A Pathol Anat Histopathol 1991; 418:281.

Takemura T, Matsui Y, Saiki S, et al. Pulmonary vascular involvement in sarcoidosis: a report of 40 autopsy cases. Hum Pathol 1992; 23:1216.

Terashita K, Kato S, Sata M, et al. Increased endotelin-1 levels in BAL fluid in patients with pulmonary sarcoidosis. Respirology 2006 ; 11 : 145-151

Wescott J, DeGraff A. Sarcoidosis, hilar adenopathy and pulmonary artery narrowing. Radiology 1973; 108:585.

13

Clinical Syndromes and Associations with Persistent Pulmonary Hypertension of the Newborn

Jae H. Kim and Anup Katheria
Division of Neonatal-Perinatal Medicine, Department of Pediatrics
University of California San Diego
United States of America

1. Introduction

Persistent pulmonary hypertension of the newborn (PPHN) occurs when the normal cardiopulmonary transition fails to occur. In term infants, PPHN is thought to occur in 2 per 1000 infants, and in approximately 10 percent of infants with respiratory failure. PPHN is a significant source of morbidity and mortality in this population. Early identification of infants with PPHN is difficult because it is the failure of the newborn to lower its pulmonary pressure and vascular resistance over time that must occur in order to make the diagnosis. However, it is imperative for the clinician to identify the newborn with clinical features that may be associated with PPHN since making the clinical diagnosis of a genetic syndrome or association can considerably alter the overall prognosis of the infant.

The transitional period from fetus to newborn is marked by changes in blood flow that are necessary for the newborn to adapt to an extrauterine environment. During fetal circulation, blood flows across the fetal channels, namely the foramen ovale (FO) and the patent ductus arteriosus (PDA), largely bypassing the pulmonary circuit. Although the pulmonary vascular surface area increases during fetal development, pulmonary vascular resistance also increases with gestational age when corrected for body weight, suggesting that pulmonary vascular tone increases during late gestation. After birth, pulmonary blood flow increases dramatically due to a decrease in pulmonary vascular resistance (PVR), which occurs at a variable rate. During birth, critical signals are necessary for the normal rapid fall in PVR to occur, mainly mechanical distension of the lung, a decrease in carbon dioxide tension, and an increase in oxygen tension in the lung. If these signals do not occur the vascular resistance will stay elevated and the result is PPHN.

Typically PPHN is caused by abnormally constricted vasculature as a result of diseased lung parenchyma from pneumonia or meconium aspiration syndrome. However, there are other congenital causes of PPHN that can lead to persistently constricted vasculature without lung disease. Other congenital causes of PPHN can result from a remodeled pulmonary vasculature or hypoplastic vasculature that is often associated with maldeveloped or underdeveloped lungs.

In this review, we will highlight genetic abnormalities that result in abnormalities of pulmonary vasculature that cause PPHN. Importantly, we will first review the normal development of the lung to contextualize the varied presentations of PPHN. PPHN in genetically normal infants has a mortality of 5-10 percent and about 25% of infants with moderate to severe PPHN will exhibit significant neurodevelopmental impairment at 12 to 24 month (Steinhorn, 2010). This group may dramatically differ from infants with congenital causes of PPHN in that there may be a higher mortality and risk for neurodevelopmental impairment in certain anomalies. The ability to identify theses infants early in their clinical course is essential for providing timely counseling to parents and determining whether medical therapy may be beneficial. We will also highlight any of the phenotypic features of congenital syndromes that may assist the clinician in diagnosis.

1.1 Normal lung development

The development of the respiratory system entails both structural development of the lung and lung maturation in order to have normal lung function (Burri, 2006). Lung development occurs during fetal growth in five phases. The embryonic period occurs when the lung first appears as a ventral bud off the esophagus. The lung bud then elongates to form the two mainstem bronchi. Subsequent branching gives rise to the conducting airways. Lobar segments are found by 37 days that then progress to segmental airways by 42 days and further division into subsegmental bronchi by 48 days. The pulmonary vasculature branches off the sixth aortic arch to form a vascular plexus within the mesenchymal of the lung bud. Many of the severe and global tracheal and pulmonary abnormalities occur during this early embryogenesis period.

The second stage involves further branching of about 15 to 20 generations of the airways and occurs during the 7th to 18th week of gestation. This stage is called the pseudoglandular stage. There is some epithelial differentiation that occurs with the appearance of ciliated cells, goblet cells and basal cells. Pulmonary arteries grow in conjunction with the airways with the principal arterial pathways being present by 14 weeks. Pulmonary venous development occurs in parallel but with a different pattern that demarcates lung segments and subsegments. By the end of the pseudoglandular stage, airways arteries and veins are similar at least in pattern to an adult.

The third stage is the cannalicular stage that occurs between 16 and 25 weeks gestation. This represents the transformation of the pre-viable lung to the viable lung that can exchange gas (Zeltner & Burri, 1987). The three major changes that occur during this stage are the appearance of the alveolar air sacs, epithelial differentiation with the appearance of an air-blood barrier, and the presence of surfactant secreting type II cells. The formation of a capillary network to occur in tandem with saccular branching is critical for air exchange. Failure for this to occur can result in alveolar-capillary dysplasia.

The fourth and fifth stages of lung development are the saccular and alveolar stages, respectively. The saccular stage encompasses the period of development from 25 weeks until term. The saccular stage involves the terminal or distal airway that elongates branches and widens until alveolarization is complete. Alveolarization is initiated in the terminal saccules by the appearance of septa in association with capillaries, elastin fibers, and collagen fibers. Alveoli are increasing in number with the most rapid increase from 32 weeks gestation until the first few months after term delivery. New alveoli continue to form until 7-8 years of age.

1.2 Purpose of in utero respiratory movements

Fetal lung fluid is essential for normal lung development. The fetal lung fluid flows up the trachea with fetal breathing movements and a higher pressure in the trachea compared to the amniotic fluid is maintained. This allows a continuously positive outflow of lung fluid and maintenance of lung volume despite high pressures from the surrounding amniotic fluid. The lung is therefore a net secretory organ. The fetal lung fluid maintains a larger lung volume than the normal functional residual capacity of the lung. Animal data have demonstrated that distension of the fetal lung by fluid leads to hyperplasia of the lung while drainage of the fluid leads to pulmonary hypoplasia (Moessinger, Harding, Adamson, Singh, & Kiu, 1990).

In the human fetus, breathing movements are noted as early as 11 weeks of gestation and by 30-40 weeks, it occurs about 30% of the time. Decreased fetal breathing can lower the tracheal pressures allowing lung volume to decrease and result in secondary pulmonary hypoplasia. Abolishing fetal breathing movements in animal experiments by either ablation of the phrenic nerve or spinal cord transection result in pulmonary hypoplasia (Fewell, Lee, & Kitterman, 1981; Wigglesworth, 1981). Increase in carbon dioxide and glucose levels, acidosis and drugs such as caffeine and theophylline are associated with increased fetal breathing movements. Maternal smoking, alcohol and drug use are known to reduce fetal breathing movements.

In the last decade there have been a number of advances in research on fetal tracheal occlusion to maintain fetal lung volume and stretching lung tissue to improve lung growth. A number of animal studies have demonstrated that surgical tracheal occlusion applied during the canalicular and saccular stages of lung development not only improves dry lung weight but also increases airway branching, alveolarization, alveolar surface area, type II pneumocytes and pulmonary vascular growth (Khan, Cloutier, & Piedboeuf, 2007).

2. Major physiological causes of pulmonary hypertension

2.1 Developmental disorders of the lung

Successful lung growth during gestation requires differentiation and branching with development of the pulmonary parenchyma, cartilage and pulmonary vessels all of which are necessary for a successful transition. A number of growth factors, platelet derived growth factors, and vascular endothelial growth factors are required to ensure proper development of pulmonary parenchyma many of which are concurrently assisting the development of the pulmonary vasculature. Therefore when there are abnormalities apparent in the pulmonary parenchyma, one can assume that the pulmonary vessels in the affected lung are also affected resulting in increase pulmonary vascular resistance. In this section we will review the spectrum of lower airway anomalies including pulmonary agenesis/aplasia, congenital cystic adenomatoid malformations, primary pulmonary hypoplasia, secondary pulmonary hypoplasia, and congenital diaphragmatic hernia.

2.1.1 Primary pulmonary hypoplasia

Primary pulmonary hypoplasia (PH) is the underdevelopment of the pulmonary parenchyma of one or both lungs. Pulmonary hypoplasia refers to conditions when the bronchial tree and pulmonary parenchyma are present but with decreased size and number of the airway alveoli and pulmonary vessels present. Pulmonary hypoplasia includes a spectrum of problems which includes hypoplasia, aplasia, or agenesis of selected or all lung segments. The lesions may be lobar, unilateral, or bilateral. Some degree of the pulmonary hypoplasia spectrum is reported in 7 to 26% of all neonatal autopsies (Abudu, Uguru, & Olude, 1988; Aghabiklooei, Goodarzi, & Kariminejad, 2009). Primary pulmonary hypoplasia is rare and is often felt to be sporadic. The etiology and pathogenesis is unknown. It may be caused by an embryologic defect of the lung or vascular tissues or an in utero vascular accident. However, most cases of pulmonary hypoplasia are secondary to conditions that limit fetal lung growth (Correia-Pinto, Gonzaga, Huang, & Rottier, 2010). Secondary causes of pulmonary hypoplasia are much more common than primary forms of pulmonary hypoplasia. These include oligohydramnios, thoracic dysplasia or thoracic space occupying lesions. In a series of 77 cases of pulmonary hypoplasia only 10 were felt to be primary (Page & Stocker, 1982).

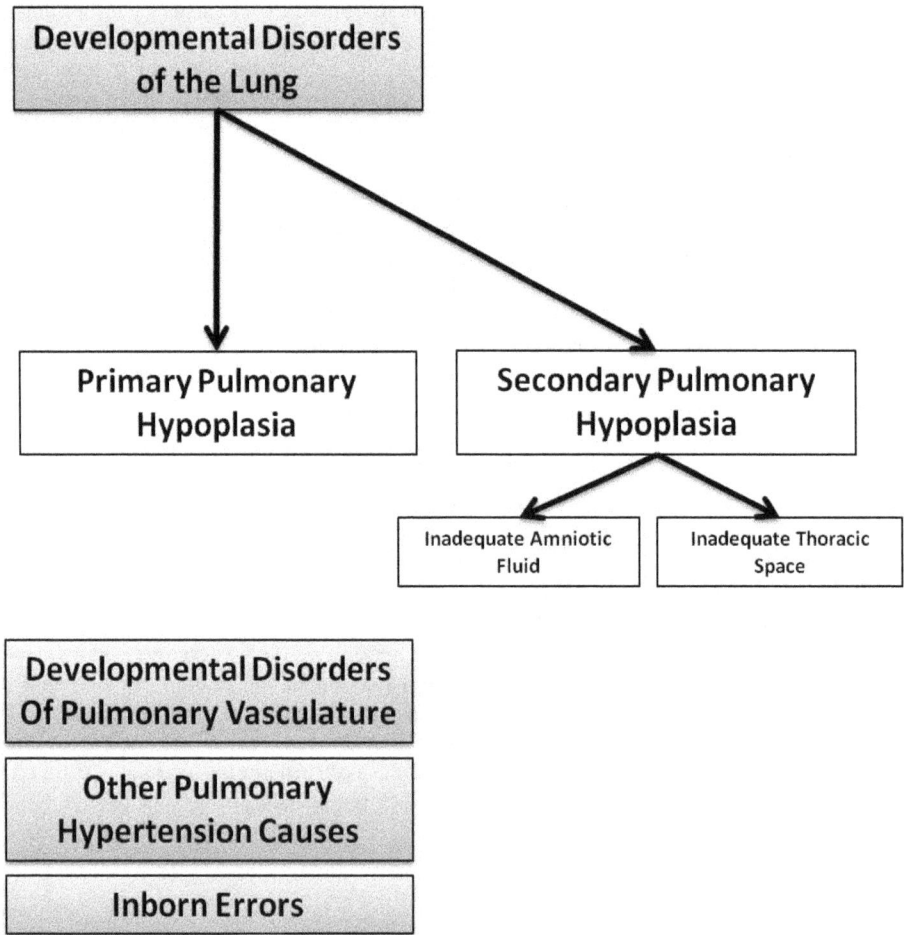

Fig. 1. Categories of causes of PPHN

2.1.1.1 Pulmonary agenesis/aplasia

A rare cause of pulmonary hypoplasia is pulmonary agenesis in which there is unilateral or bilateral absence of the bronchus, pulmonary parenchyma or pulmonary vasculature. Pulmonary aplasia refers to presence of the bronchial tree without development of the parenchyma or pulmonary vasculature. Pulmonary agenesis is typically unilateral in about 70% of cases and bilateral agenesis is lethal at birth. Since unilateral agenesis can be isolated but often presents with other cardiovascular, vertebral, facial urogenital and/or gastrointestinal syndromes. A recent review of 269 cases of pulmonary agenesis from 1937 to 1997 highlighted that 60 had anomalies of the first and second branchial arches and/or radial ray defects (Cunningham & Mann, 1997). As a consequence, pulmonary agenesis has been considered to be a part of the VACTERL association (Cunningham & Mann, 1997; Knowles, Thomas, Lindenbaum, Keeling, & Winter, 1988).

The VACTERL association is an acronym for a condition that includes vertebral defects, anal atresia, cardiac defects, and tracheoesophageal fistula with esophageal atresia, renal dysplasia, and limb defects. VACTERL association is not in itself a diagnosis but a nonrandom association of defects. As such it can be seen as a sporadic occurrence in an otherwise normal family and is more frequently seen in infants born to diabetic mothers (Kallen, Mastroiacovo, Castilla, Robert, & Kallen, 2001). Although many of these patient may have failure to thrive and have some mild delay in early infancy related to their defects, the majority have normal neurodevelopmental outcomes and thus should receive full attempts towards rehabilitation. A phenotypically similar disorder referred to as VACTERL with hydrocephalus due to aqueductal stenosis has been reported and has both autosomal and X-linked recessive inheritance. These infants generally have a poor prognosis in most cases (Evans, Stranc, Kaplan, & Hunter, 1989).

Fryns syndrome displays diaphragmatic abnormalities, coarse facies and distal hypoplasia, and has been reported to have a high incidence (60%) of abnormal lung lobulations including pulmonary agenesis (Fryns, Moerman, Goddeeris, Bossuyt, & Van den Berghe, 1979). Cystic hygroma of the neck is commonly seen on prenatal ultrasounds with the majority delivering stillborn or dying in the early neonatal period. Survival without severe neurodevelopmental impairment has not been reported. All affected individuals have coarse facies and distal digital hypoplasia usually represented by hypoplastic to absent nails and short terminal phalanges.

Hydrolethalus syndrome, also known as the combination of hydrocephalus, micrognathia, and polydactyly commonly has a variety of pulmonary defects including abnormal lung lobulation, malformed or hypoplastic pharynx, with a stenotic or abnormally dilated trachea. The pregnancies of these individuals are complicated by polyhydramnios and intrauterine growth restriction. About 70% are stillborn with live born infants usually surviving a few hours. The disorder has an autosomal recessive inheritance pattern and the defect is found on chromosome 11q23-25.

Pallister-Hall syndrome (PHS) features hypothalamic hamartoblastoma, hypopituitarism, imperforate anus, and postaxial polydactyly (Hall et al., 1980). Infants with PHS can have either pulmonary aplasia or pulmonary agenesis with abnormal lung lobulation. The majority die before age 3, where the most common cause of death in the newborn period is hypoadrenalism (Jones & Smith, 2006). If there are long-term survivors they typically need

L-thyroxine, growth hormone, and corticosteroids from an early age as well as glucose infusions in the neonatal period. The disorder is transmitted in an autosomal dominant inheritance pattern and so a family history is critical. Mutations of GLI3 on 7p13 is responsible for this disorder (Narumi et al., 2010).

Other causes of pulmonary agenesis can occur in conjunction with diaphragmatic agenesis in which either one or both sides of the diaphragm fail to develop. Typically infants with both have associated heart defects, skin tags that are often found on the nares, and in females are found to have a hypoplastic uterus.

Tetraamelia syndrome is characterized by amelia (absence) of all four limbs with agenesis or hypoplasia of the lungs. They often have peripheral pulmonary vessel hypoplasia and death during the neonatal period is common. Other reported findings include low set ears, micrognathia, cleft lib and hydrocephalus. The condition appears to be inherited in an autosomal recessive pattern.

Smith-Lemli-Opitz syndrome (SLOS) has a constellation of features including abnormal pulmonary lobulation such as those with pulmonary agenesis with accompanying severe PPHN. Other key features of SLOS include anteverted nostrils, ptosis of eyelids, syndactyly of the second and third toes, and in males, hypospadias and cryptorchidism (also see 2.1.3.2 Smith-Lemli-Opitz syndrome).

2.1.2 Secondary pulmonary hypoplasia

Secondary PH is much more common than primary PH and can occur from a number of fetal and maternal abnormalities. The two most common cause of secondary PH are conditions in which there is inadequate amniotic fluid or insufficient space in the chest for normal lung development to occur.

2.1.2.1 Inadequate amniotic fluid

Typically the fetus is buoyant in amniotic fluid from 11 weeks gestation to term. Early lung maturation and development depends on the ability of the fetus to have respiratory chest and diaphragmatic effort with excursion of the chest and abdomen. In mid-gestation this involves the exchange of lung fluid and amniotic fluid in and out of the lung to accommodate these activities. The inability to generate such respiratory exercise leads directly to underdevelopment of the lung parenchymal and pulmonary hypoplasia.

2.1.2.1.1 Renal agenesis

One of the most common phenotypes of pulmonary hypoplasia is the Potter sequence in which the fetus' face is distorted and the chest is bell-shaped. Any condition that results in severe oligohydramnios can cause the phenotype if it is prolonged and severe. The most severe would be the lack of production of amniotic fluid from renal agenesis. The physical features of Potter sequence are a direct consequence of the low levels of amniotic fluid. These features include apparent hypertelorism, infraorbital creases, flattened nasal tip, hypoplastic mandible, enlarged and posteriorly rotated ears, redundant dry skin, genu varum, talipes, and metatarsus adductus. The lung volume is correspondingly small with a decrease in the number of airways and alveoli. Also, the size of the alveoli and the pulmonary arterioles are smaller than normal.

Renal agenesis is the complete absence of one or both kidneys. This is separate from any disorder that has remnant or dysfunctional kidneys. Renal agenesis can present as early as 14 weeks with severe oligohydramnios. Up to 40% of infants with bilateral renal agenesis present with stillbirth with the remaining ones being premature and low birth weight. Of the live born infants all have respiratory distress due to pulmonary hypoplasia. Communicating structures in bilateral renal agenesis including complete absence of the ureters and hypoplasia, atresia or absence of the bladder are seen. In females, the vagina and uterus are absent or abnormal in 85% of cases (Gabow, 1993). In males, cryptorchidism and absence or abnormalities of the vas deferens and seminal vesicles are found. In severe cases penile agenesis or penoscrotal transposition have been seen.

Renal agenesis occurs from a defect in embryogenesis early in development (around day 35) or it may occur later as a result of a late occlusion of the renal artery causing involution of the kidney. Because renal agenesis may involve the Wolfian or Mullerian duct, defects of the urogenital sinus are seen together. This would explain the range of defects that involve anal anomalies, caudal and bladder extrophy. An even larger defect involves the entire caudal end of the embryo and result in caudal dysplasia or sirenomelia.

Unilateral renal agenesis may be incidentally discovered on a postnatal examination by palpating the enlarged or displaced remaining kidney or by ultrasound screening. Many individuals are asymptomatic but over 50% of remaining kidneys are found to have anomalies. Associated congenital defects are common. As expected in unilateral renal agenesis many of the defects are seen on the affected side. The ipsilateral uterus and Fallopian tube may be absent and the other uterine and vaginal ducts maybe present including the uterus didelphys (Li, Qayyum, Coakley, & Hricak, 2000). Bladder extrophy, anal atresia, malrotation, Meckel's diverticulum and lumbosacral defects have been reported (Li, et al., 2000). Interestingly the ipsilateral adrenal gland is still found in its usual position unlike in bilateral renal agenesis where adrenal agenesis is common. Prognosis for isolated unilateral renal agenesis is quite good. The remaining kidney often compensates becoming hypertrophic and can have ureteral dilation with vesicoureteral reflux. Most infants that have unilateral renal agenesis are asymptomatic so do not develop pulmonary hypoplasia and therefore do not typically have respiratory problems at birth.

Bilateral renal agenesis is a universally fatal disorder. Of the remaining 60% who are not stillborn, death usually occurs within 24 hours from severe pulmonary hypertension from the pulmonary hypoplasia. There is no effective treatment. Amnio-infusion has been attempted to allow for lung growth but this has not been successful.

Other non-contiguous anomalies that are often seen in both bilateral and unilateral renal agenesis include limb deficiencies, tracheal agenesis, esophageal or duodenal atresia, cleft lip or palate, hydrocephalus and other brain malformations. Amnion nodosum of the placenta is seen as would be expected in oligohydramnios.

There are a number of acrorenal and cerebrorenal defects that are important to recognize. Acrorenal defects include defects that involve the limbs in addition to the kidneys. In particular the hands and feet are often abnormal and may include radial ray defects. Inheritance patterns are variable and some include chromosomal abnormalities as well. Cerebrorenal defects include brain and kidney and include disorders such as PHS, SLOS, and Meckel-Gruber syndrome (MGS). Both PHS and SLOS have been described earlier.

(see 2.1.1.1 Pulmonary Agenesis/Aplasia) MGS is an autosomal recessive disorder and depending on its type is linked to a different chromosomal defect. Type I is linked to 17q22-q23, Type II is linked to 11q and Type III is linked to an 8q deletion (Morgan et al., 2002). The prominent features of MGS include occipital encephalocoele, other structural brain anomalies, ear anomalies, postaxial polydactyly, cleft lip and palate, ambiguous genitalia, biliary and pancreatic dysgenesis (Hsia, Bratu, & Herbordt, 1971). The other renal anomalies can include duplicated ureters, hypoplastic bladder urethral atresia and if the kidneys are present they are often polycystic or dysplastic. This disease is uniformly fatal (Salonen, 1984).

There are also some well-known associations that may involve renal agenesis. CHARGE association stands for coloboma, heart defects, choanal atresia, mental retardation, genital hypoplasia, and ear anomalies. The genital anomalies include renal agenesis, dysplasia or ectopic duplication of the pelvis and ureter, megaureter and reflux. The prognosis depends on the degree of pulmonary hypoplasia as a result of bilateral or unilateral renal agenesis. The inheritance pattern is autosomal dominant with a deletion found on chromosome 8q12.1 (Vissers et al., 2004). MURCS association is an acronym for Mullerian duct aplasia, renal agenesis, and cervicothoracic somatic (vertebral) defects. They can also have a hypoplastic uterus, absent vagina, and short stature. Mutations are sporadic without any inheritance patterns. Prognosis for VACTERL association has been described earlier (see 2.1.1.1 Pulmonary Agenesis/Aplasia).

Renal agenesis also can be seen in over 30 chromosomal disorders including trisomy 13, 18 and 21 (Stevenson, 2006). (See 2.1.2.2.1 Congenital Diaphragmatic Hernia) It can also been found as a result of teratogen exposure in utero including alcohol, cocaine, diabetes, misoprostol, rubella virus, thalidomide, trimethadione, and warfarin (Stevenson, 2006).

Inheritance patterns can be heterogeneous. There have been familial cases of renal agenesis suggesting all types of inheritance as possibilities (Morse, Rawnsley, Crowe, Marin-Padilla, & Graham, 1987). Isolated renal agenesis has been considered to be multifactorial with a low chance of recurrence in first-degree relatives.

2.1.2.2 Inadequate thoracic space

Another cause for development of secondary hypoplasia is the presence of space occupying lesions within the chest. This can be due to herniated bowel from a diaphragmatic hernia, cysts as in congenital cystic adenomatoid malformations, or a hydrothorax. There are a number of syndromes that are associated with each type of lesion and will be reviewed below.

2.1.2.2.1 Congenital diaphragmatic hernia

Congenital diaphragmatic hernia is the absence or underdevelopment of the tendinous or muscular parts of the diaphragm that allow abdominal contents to enter the thoracic cavity. The extrinsic compression of the lung by bowel secondarily results in pulmonary hypoplasia of both lungs with greatest impact on the affected lung (typically the left in 85 % of cases). This pulmonary hypoplasia results in a pulmonary hypertension that is often resistant to medical therapy (Kinsella, Parker, Ivy, & Abman, 2003). Congenital diaphragmatic hernia may be an isolated defect or associated with multiple malformations. Thirty-nine percent have nonpulmonary malformations (Cunniff, Jones, & Jones, 1990). When congenital diaphragmatic hernia is associated with multiple anomalies it is associated with a poor outcome (Dillon, Renwick, & Wright, 2000). Therefore identification of other anomalies when a diaphragmatic hernia is found is critical for prognosis. Fryns syndrome and Pallister-Killian syndrome must be considered in the differential diagnosis (See 2.1.1.1 Pulmonary Agenesis/Aplasia).

2.1.2.2.1.1 Trisomy 13

Trisomy 13 is a constellation of anomalies that include defects of the eye, nose lip, with forebrain abnormalities resulting in holoprosencephaly in association with polydactyly, narrow hyperconvex fingernails, and skin defects of the posterior scalp. Diaphragmatic defects are found in less than 50% of cases. A standard karyotype is sufficient to confirm the diagnosis.

2.1.2.2.1.2 Trisomy 18

Trisomy 18 is the second most common multiple malformation syndrome with an incidence of 0.3 per 100 newborn babies. There are over a 130 different abnormalities that have been reported in the literature (Jones & Smith, 2006). Of the 10 percent of all congenital diaphragmatic hernias that have chromosomal abnormalities the most common is trisomy 18. The most common features of trisomy 18 are the clenched hands where there is overlapping of the index finger over the third, and the fifth finger over the fourth. They have a short sternum with reduced number of ossification centers, a prominent occiput with micrognathia, and a low arch dermal ridge pattern over six or more fingertips, with hypoplasia of the nails, especially on the fifth finger and toes. About 50 percent of babies with trisomy 18 die in the first week and many of the remaining die over the first year. The average survival time is only 14.5 days. A standard karyotype is sufficient to confirm the diagnosis.

2.1.2.2.1.3 Cornelia de Lange syndrome

Brachman-de Lange also known as Cornelia de Lange syndrome can also have diaphragmatic defects with diaphragmatic hernias or hiatal hernias. The syndrome has a characteristic facial feature of busy eyebrows and synophyrs with long curly eyelashes. Infants are initially hypertonic with a long philtrum, a thin downturning upper lip and micromelia of the upper and lower extremities. They have average intelligence quotients of 53 (Jones & Smith, 2006). The natural history usually consists of failure to thrive, with feeding difficulties, hearing loss and speech delay. The syndrome is inherited in an autosomal dominant pattern and the mutation, Nipped-B homolog (NIPBL) is located on 5p13.

2.1.2.2.1.4 Pallister-Killian syndrome

Pallister-Killian syndrome is a dysmorphic condition involving most organ systems, but is also characterized by a tissue-limited mosaicism where most fibroblasts have 47 chromosomes with an extra small metacentric chromosome and the karyotype of lymphocytes is normal. The characteristic combination of clinical manifestations in this syndrome include coarse face, pigmentary skin anomalies, localized alopecia, profound mental retardation and seizures, and the relatively frequent occurrence of diaphragmatic defects and supernumerary nipples (Jones & Smith, 2006).

2.1.2.2.2 Omphalocele

An omphalocele is an abdominal wall defect whereby abdominal viscera are found centrally through a widened umbilical ring and generally covered with a membrane. The size of an omphalocele can vary tremendously but if giant it can result in a higher risk for PPHN. The mechanisms for this are not fully understood but may relate to reduced diaphragmatic function in the absence of most of the abdominal content. The presence of severe pulmonary morbidity is a notable distinguishing feature of omphaloceles in distinction to gastroschisis, another abdominal wall defect that is much less associated with PPHN. Associated conditions with giant omphaloceles include Beckwith-Wiedemann syndrome, Trisomy 13 (see 2.1.2.2.1.1 Trisomy 13), and limb-body wall complex. A case of omphalocele has been described in association with alveolar capillary dysplasia (Argyle, 1989; Hershenson et al., 1985). The limb-body wall complex is characterized by severe scoliosis, pulmonary hypoplasia, and giant omphalocele, the latter of which usually has an intact covering membrane, and sometimes a short umbilical cord, and should be distinguished from an isolated omphalocele because of its poor prognosis (Kamata, Usui, Sawai, Nose, & Fukuzawa, 2008).

2.1.2.2.3 Congenital Pulmonary Lymphangectasia

Congenital pulmonary lymphangectasia (CPL) often presents with severe life threatening respiratory distress at birth. It is the congenital dilation of the superficial lymphatics of the pleura and septa and of the peribronchial and perivascular adventitia. The disease is characterized by inter-communicating, thin-walled, endothelium-lined, fluid-filled cysts of greatly varying diameter, situated in abundant subpleural, peribronchial, and interlobar connective tissue (Romano et al., 2010). The majority of infants are stillborn or die within the first 24 hours of life. Liveborn individuals typically develop acute respiratory distress with tachypnea, cyanosis, subcostal retractions, and prolonged expiration very soon after birth. Most medical therapies are not effective. On chest radiograph show large, punctate areas lesion throughout the lungs with Kerley B lines at the costophrenic angles, and over-aeration of the lung fields with a flattened diaphragm but a normal sized heart. (Arkoff, 1968) These radiographic findings are useful for the clinician to differentiate CPL from meconium aspiration syndrome and pneumonia since these do not have Kerly B lines.

About ⅓ to ½ of all cases are associated with congenital heart defects particularly total anomalous pulmonary venous drainage, hypoplastic left heart syndrome, and premature closure of the foramen ovale. Both CPL and congenital heart defects together are part of asplenia and Noonan syndrome. Single cases have been reported with omphalocoele, malformation of the intestine, cretinism, arachnodactyly, trisomy 13, ureterovesical obstruction, Ehlers-Danlos syndrome, ichthyosis, cystic fibrosis, cystic hyperplasia of the bile ducts, and diaphragmatic hernia. There is a gender discrepancy with a male to female ratio of 2:1 (Fronstin, Hooper, Besse, & Ferreri, 1967). Several sibling pairs have been reported (Scott-Emuakpor, Warren, Kapur, Quiachon, & Higgins, 1981). Old case series of infants with CPL demonstrated a less than 25% survival. Those who survive suffer attacks of chronic respiratory distress cause by respiratory infections, with wheezing and coughing. Lobar pulmonary lymphangiectasia is cured by resection of the affected lobe. In the majority of cases treatment is usually palliative.

2.1.2.2.3.1 Turner syndrome

Turner syndrome is caused by abnormal chromosomal distribution leading to a 45,XO individual. The most consistent features are short stature and gonadal dysgenesis. At birth about 80% have congenital lymphedema over the dorsum of the fingers and toes (Jones & Smith, 2006). They often have a broad chest with widely spaced nipples that may be hypoplastic, inverted or both. Their facial features include prominent auricles, narrow maxillae, and an appearance of a short neck. Chromosomal testing will confirm the 45,XO genotype.

2.1.2.2.3.2 Noonan syndrome

Prominent features of Noonan syndrome include short stature of postnatal onset, congenital heart defect, mental retardation, downward-slanting palpebrae, widely spaced eyes, ptosis, low nasal bridge, pectus deformity, webbed neck, strabismus, nystagmus, protruding upper lip, shield chest, cryptorchidism, other lymphatic abnormalities including hydrops, periperhal lymphedema, and chylous effusions (Allanson, 1987; Noonan, 1999; Witt et al., 1987). This syndrome has an autosomal dominant inheritance, but due to genetic heterogeneity, it occurs sporadically in families. It is frequently associated with pulmonary valve stenosis, hypertrophic cardiomypathy, atrial septal defect, tetralogy of Fallot, aortic coarctation, mitral valve anomalies, and atrioventricular canal (Glauser, Rorke, Weinberg, & Clancy, 1990). Clinical course often includes poor feeding and gastrointestinal dysfunction, which can lead to failure to thrive. More severe feeding problems in infancy are may be associated with increased cognitive problems in childhood, but impairments are rarely severe.

2.1.2.2.4 Congenital Cystic Adenoid Malformation

Congenital Cystic Adenoid malformation (CCAM) is a pulmonary hamartomatous lesion composed of noncartilage-containing terminal respiratory structures resembling terminal bronchioles: There are three subtypes based on morphologies. The first, macrocystic (Type 1), occurs when there are one or more large cysts, between 2 and 10 cm, that are predominately found. The cysts are lined by ciliated pseudostratified columnar epithelium, which occasionally produce mucin. Bronchiolar and alveolar elements are present between the cysts. The second are microcystic (Type 2), which have small uniform cysts, between 0.5 and 2 cm and are lined with cuboidal or columnar epithelium. The final type (Type 3) are solid in which an airless mass is found consisting of almost all bronchiolar and alveolar elements. On gross exam there are no cysts seen but there are microscopic alveolar cysts (Clements & Warner, 1987). Diagnosis of CCAM is often now made on prenatal ultrasound. Respiratory symptoms can be present at birth and pulmonary hypertension can be seen secondary to either compression of the cysts or from rupture and resultant pneumothorax. Type 2 CCAM has the worst prognosis because they are often associated with other defects. In a series of prenatally diagnosed cases of microcystic lesions, bilateral lesion, or fetal hydrops were found, each were associated with a poor prognosis. However, polyhydramnios and mediastinal shift are not associated with a poor prognosis. In fact, there has been some series in which up to 56% of cases of CCAM have partially or complete regressed in utero (Laberge et al., 2001).

2.1.2.2.5 Congenital Lobar Emphysema

CLE is the most common congenital lesion of the lung parenchyma accounting for 50% of the lesions (Correia-Pinto, et al., 2010). Congenital lobar emphysema (CLE) occurs when there is hyperinflation of one or more lobes of the lung due to an intrinsic defect of the bronchopulmonary tree. Most newborns have respiratory distress with or without cyanosis.

Chest asymmetry, decreased breath sounds, and mediastinal shift may be apparent on physical examination. Chest radiograph may initially show an opaque, fluid filled lobe, but follow-up films will eventually demonstrate overdistension and air trapping in the affected lobe with mediastinal shift and compression of the surrounding lung. Prenatally the diagnosis can be made with ultrasound or MRI. CLE only rarely presents with PPHN at birth (Schwartz & Ramachandran, 1997). Concomitant cardiovascular disease however is not uncommon and should be investigated when CLE is detected (Dogan et al., 2004).

2.1.3 Idiopathic pulmonary hypertension

Some conditions that lead to PPHN are not based on obvious developmental abnormalities of the lung or pulmonary vasculature. Biochemical changes in the normal maintenance of pulmonary vascular tone may be responsible for these conditions. Some of these conditions illustrate the complex and delicate balance of ensuring normal pulmonary vascular function at birth and thereafter.

2.1.3.1 Trisomy 21 (Down syndrome)

Down syndrome (DS) is a chromosomal condition characterized by moderate impairment of cognitive ability and physical growth and a particular set of facial characteristics. They have microgenia (a small chin), an unusually round face, macroglossia, and almond shape of they eye caused by an epicanthic fold of the eyelid, upslanting palpebral fissures, short ribs, a single transverse palmar crease, poor muscle tone, and a larger than normal space between the first and second toes. The incidence of pulmonary hypertension in the newborn has been reported in one retrospective series to be as high as 6 percent of all Down syndrome births over a 4-year period (Cua, Blankenship, North, Hayes, & Nelin, 2007). There have been a number of mechanisms to suggest how some neonates develop protracted pulmonary hypertension. One study demonstrated that DS patients might have an abnormal production of nitric oxide (NO) but respond appropriately to exogenous NO administration in the peripheral circulation (Cappelli-Bigazzi et al., 2004). Another study demonstrated less pulmonary vasodilation in response to NO in DS patients versus controls undergoing cardiac catheterization (Cannon et al., 2005). A genetic factor has been postulated to cause abnormal NO production resulting in an increased risk of PPHN. One study looked at the BMPR2 mutation, a gene mutation resulting in increase NO production and showed an increased occurrence in a subset of DS patients (Roberts et al., 2004). The mortality in DS overall is about 3.3% but is much higher (5.8% versus 1.5%) in infants with congenital heart disease compared to those who do not (Weijerman et al., 2010). In a subset of 58 patients with Down syndrome there were 7 who met criteria for PPHN of which 2 died (Cua, et al., 2007). They did not have cardiac defects other than a PDA. There are no other long-term data on DS newborns with PPHN.

2.1.3.2 Smith-Lemli-Opitz syndrome

We have recently described a case of PPHN without obvious pulmonary hypoplasia in an infant with SLOS (Katheria, Masliah, Benirschke, Jones, & Kim, 2010). In SLOS there is defect in cholesterol biosynthesis leading to abnormally low plasma cholesterol levels and elevated concentrations of the cholesterol precursor 7-dehydrocholesterol (7-DHC), the result of a deficiency of 7-DHC reductase. Disruptions in cholesterol metabolism can interrupt key signaling pathways that participate in the normal maintenance of pulmonary vascular tone. Others and we have found that caveolae-dependent signaling may be involved in this process since our patient had altered expression of caveolin-1 suggesting that additional cellular alterations beyond mere changes associated with abnormal sterols in the membrane likely contribute to the pathogenesis of SLOS (Katheria, et al., 2010; Ren et al., 2011).

2.2 Developmental disorders of pulmonary vasculature

2.2.1 Alveolar Capillary Dysplasia with Misalignment of the Pulmonary Veins (ACD/MPV)

This pulmonary disorder is often found in newborns that are born full term with normal Apgar scores at birth and present with respiratory distress and cyanosis within the first 24 hours. The diagnosis is based on the failure of neonates to respond to conventional therapy and is confirmed on pathological evaluation. Histological features include a decreased number of alveolar capillaries, immature alveolar development, increased muscularization of pulmonary arterioles, and malposition of pulmonary vein branches adjacent to pulmonary artery branches. The pathogenesis of ACD/MPV is thought to be due to the failure of fetal lung vascularization to occur in response to some teratogen. This failure of vascularization forces blood to only be able to be drained via the pulmonary veins, which are malaligned. The obstruction that is created leads to the occlusive changes seen in the pulmonary arterial circulation. While the majority of cases have been sporadic events, there are about 10% of those that are found in siblings suggesting a heritable form of the disease (Langston, 1991). Extra-pulmonary findings are present in about 50 to 80% of cases (Sen, Thakur, Stockton, Langston, & Bejjani, 2004). These include genitourinary, gastrointestinal, and cardiovascular systems. Also disruption of right-left symmetry has been reported in about 25% of cases (Sen, et al., 2004). It has also been seen in infants with Down syndrome (Sen, et al., 2004). There is no genetic test available, diagnosis is based on lung biopsy alone.

2.2.2 Anomalous pulmonary veins

Impairment of venous return to the left heart can result in inadequate blood flow through the pulmonary vasculature, which can predispose to pulmonary hypertension. Therefore any review of genetic causes of pulmonary hypertension must include cardiac conditions with anomalies of the pulmonary veins. Anomalies of the pulmonary veins can depend on the location, number and patency of the pulmonary veins. The main abnormalities are an abnormal pulmonary vein connection where one of more of the pulmonary veins connects to a systemic vein or to the right atrium. Absence of connections between the pulmonary veins and the left atrium is total anomalous pulmonary venous return (TAPVR). In partial anomalous pulmonary venous return (PAPVR), one to three of the pulmonary veins connects to the systemic veins. The most common abnormal connection is where the right pulmonary vein or veins connects into the superior or inferior vena cava. One candidate genetic locus with autosomal dominant inheritance of TAPVR involves the short arm of chromosome 4 and may be a vascular epithelial growth factor receptor, thought to have a role in vasculogenesis. No syndromic phenotype has been described for this defect however.

An anatomic variant of PAPVR is scimitar syndrome in which all or some of the right pulmonary veins enter the inferior vena cava at or below the level of the diaphragm. Other associated features of scimitar syndrome include right lung hypoplasia or horseshoe lung, secondary dextrocardia, hypoplasia of the right pulmonary artery, and pulmonary sequestration (Stevenson, 2006). Noncardiac malformations include vertebral anomalies, horseshoe kidneys and rectovaginal fistula. Scimitar syndrome can be diagnosed by the presence of a characteristic curvilinear pattern created on a chest radiograph by the pulmonary veins that drain to the inferior vena cava. Infants who present with Scimitar syndrome can develop pulmonary hypertension refractory to medical therapy requiring prompt cardiac surgery. However, infants often have postoperative pulmonary venous obstruction. There have been variations in survival reports in the literature with mortality rates ranging from 16 to 64% (Dupuis, Charaf, Breviere, & Abou, 1993; Huddleston, Exil, Canter, & Mendeloff, 1999; Huddleston & Mendeloff, 1999).

Two other syndromes associated with partial anomalous venous return are Turner syndrome (See Turner Syndrome 2.1.2.2.3.1) and Holt-Oram syndrome. Holt-Oram syndrome or cardiac limb syndrome has an autosomal dominant inheritance pattern. The infants typically have malformation of the upper extremities. The thumbs may be absent, hypoplastic, thriphalangeal or bifid. Syndactyly often occurs between the thumb and the index finger. There may be dysplasia or aplasia of the radius or upper arm. There is a mutation on the TBX5 gene, which is linked to chromosome 12q24.1 in about 25% of familial cases and 50% of sporadic cases. There are no neurodevelopmental sequelae that have been reported. Outcome is dependent on the severity of the cardiac lesion.

In TAPVR, the pulmonary venous return to the systemic circulation may occur above the diaphragm, below the diaphragm or intracardiac. Two syndromes frequently associated with TAPVR are Cat eye syndrome and Smith Lemli Opitz syndrome. (see Smith Lemli Opitz syndrome, 2.1.3.2) Cat eye syndrome or coloboma of iris-anal atresia syndrome is hallmarked by the anal atresia and colobomata of the iris. The facies are characterized by hypertelorism, downslant of the palpebral fissures, with a low root of the nose. There may be pre-auricular tags and/or fistulas. Generally the colobomas are bilateral and they may have microphthalmos. However, only 9 of 100 reported cases had both features (Rosias et al., 2001). Cardiac defects are found in about 1/3 of cases and can include in addition to TAPVR, persistence of the left superior vena cava, ventral septal defects (VSD), and atrial septal defects (ASD) (Schinzel et al., 1981). There is usually mild mental retardation although there have been some with reported normal intelligence but emotional disturbance problems. The etiology is a result of an extra chromosome derived from two identical segments of chromosome 22 or a tiny piece of the long arm of 22 (22pter; q11) (Jones & Smith, 2006). Fluorescent in situ hybridization studies have been used successfully to document typical as well as atypical cases as well.

2.2.3 Adams-Oliver syndrome (AOS)

Adams-Oliver syndrome presents with aplasia cutis congenital, terminal transverse defects of limbs and in some cases severe pulmonary hypertension. Postmortem examination of an AOS patient with pulmonary hypertension showed defective vascular smooth muscle cell/pericyte coverage of the vasculature associated with 2 blood vessel abnormalities (Patel et al., 2004). Pericyte absence correlated with vessel dilatation whereas hyperproliferation of pericytes correlated with vessel stenosis. These findings suggested a unifying pathogenic mechanism for the abnormalities seen in AOS.

Condition	Defects
Down Syndrome	Congenital diaphragmatic hernia Alveolar capillary hypoplasia Renal agenesis
Turner Syndrome	Cystic hygroma Anomalous pulmonary venous drainage
Trisomy 18	Congenital diaphragmatic hernia Renal agenesis
Trisomy 13	Congenital diaphragmatic hernia Renal agenesis Omphalocele
Smith-Lemli-Opitz Syndrome	Pulmonary agenesis, abnormal lobulation Primary pulmonary hypertension
Fryns syndrome	Congenital diaphragmatic hernia Pulmonary agenesis, abnormal lobulation Cystic hygroma

Table 1. Common conditions with multiple causes of PPHN

2.3 Inborn errors

2.3.1 Introduction

Single gene defects can lead to pulmonary under- or maldevelopment. Some causes are not associated with any obvious dysmorphisms and may be difficult to diagnose clinically aside for the severity of disease. The congenital surfactant deficiencies belong to one major class that lead to severe respiratory failure with severe PPHN.

2.3.2 Congenital surfactant deficiencies

Pulmonary surfactant is critical for postnatal adaptation of the newborn as it reduces the surface tension of the lung and prevents atelectasis that leads to lung injury. In fact, surfactant replacement therapy is one of the first therapies given to infants with PPHN to improve oxygenation. Surfactant is a complex of proteins and phospholipids in which each component is critical for a variety of functions. The protein components A, B, C, D make up about 10% by weight of pulmonary surfactant. We will review a number of mutations that are associated with disorders of pulmonary surfactant metabolism.

Neonates with defects in surfactant metabolism present can present acutely or in a more chronic and variable presentation. In the first presentation neonates develop respiratory failure shortly after birth that requires significant ventilator support and is minimally or transiently responsive to surfactant and often require extracorporeal membrane oxygenation (ECMO). Secondary pulmonary hypertension develops early and may only be partially responsive to inhaled NO. Chest X-rays show a diffuse haziness mimicking respiratory distress syndrome (RDS). This presentation is typical of infants with mutations in SFTPB or ABCA3, but has also been occasionally seen in infants with mutation in SFTPC and NKX2.1 as well (Garmany et al., 2006; Nogee, Wert, Proffit, Hull, & Whitsett, 2000; Shulenin et al., 2004).

In the second less severe but variable presentation has been seen in infants with mutations in SFTPC, ABCA3 and NKX2.1. These children may present in the newborn period with milder respiratory symptoms that is often misdiagnosed as transient tachypnea of the newborn or congenital pneumonia and later develop a gradual onset of respiratory insufficiency, hypoxemia, failure to thrive and interstitial lung disease on chest radiographs. While some cases have a concurrent history of viral illnesses or aspiration, these features are not always consistent, suggesting that the variability in severity of the course of the disease is not dependent on the type of mutation making early accurate prognosis difficult.

2.3.2.1 Surfactant protein-B deficiency

Surfactant protein-B (SP-B) is a rare autosomal recessive disorder with an incidence of about 1 per million live births. Over 30 mutations in the SFTPB region have been identified resulting in partial to complete absence of the SP-B protein. The most common mutation, 121ins2, is associated with about 70% of the cases of SP-B deficiency, and is most often found in those of European descent (Nogee, Wert, Proffit, Hull, & Whitsett, 2000). The condition is lethal in the newborn period with the inability to oxygenate and ventilate and often infants are unable to come off ECMO successfully. SP-B deficiency has not been identified in infants less than 30 weeks gestation.

2.3.2.2 ABCA3 deficiency

ABCA3 is highly expressed in lung tissue, but also in the heart, brain, pancreas, kidneys and platelets. Similar to SP-B deficiency it is also autosomal recessive and when it presents in the acute form it is universally fatal. However it has also been seen in a chronic form often in premature infants whose respiratory dysfunction is more severe than would be anticipated for gestational age (Shulenin et al., 2004). This suggests that ABCA3 may be a marker for the risk as severity of RDS in newborns. Some studies suggest that ABCA3 deficiency may be the most common of the surfactant metabolism disorders. While the exact role of ABCA3 in surfactant metabolism is unknown, data from humans and mice suggest that ABCA3 mediates transport of phospholipids into lamellar bodies to produce surfactant. Disruption of this transport leads to reduce surfactant function.

2.3.2.3 Surfactant protein-C disorders

Surfactant protein-C (SP-C) is a lung is a lung specific protein that lowers the surface tension of the alveolae. The natural history is variable but less often presents as acute respiratory failure. The protein is encoded by the gene SFTPC in which about 35 different mutations have been described in both familial and sporadic cases (Brown, Dohm, Bernardino de la Serna, & Barron, 2011). It can be inherited in an autosomal dominant pattern.

2.3.2.4 Thyroid transcription factor

Thyroid transcription factor is expressed in the brain, thyroid gland, and the lung and is critical for normal development. It has autosomal dominant inheritance and is expressed in the NKX2.1 gene and mutations present a constellation of hypothyroidism, choreoathetosis, and respiratory disease (Hamvas, 2010). The respiratory disease can manifest as RDS in the newborn period or as recurrent pulmonary infection or interstitial lung disease in later childhood. Similar to SFTPC about half the mutations are spontaneous. The natural history is variable.

All of the surfactant disorders can be tested with genetic analysis for the various mutations, thereby avoiding more invasive testing such as lung biopsies. Diagnosis for these disorders is critical for prognosis and genetic counseling for future pregnancies. The only therapy for any of the surfactant disorders is lung transplant with a 5-year survival of only 50%. Most of the short-term mortality is due to infection which in the long term accompanies other risks such as malignancies and the development of bronchiolitis obliterans. Even those who have survived the neonatal period have gross motor delays and need for nasogastric or gastrostomy feedings. The difficulties with the quality of life and excessive care these infants require prompt about half of the families eligible for transplantation to choose compassionate care for their infants.

3. Conclusions

The proper clinical diagnosis of pulmonary hypertension requires the integration of clinical, physiologic and echocardiographic information. Readily identifying accompanying clinical syndromes that are associated with severe PPHN is essential to making critical decisions on the extent and intensity of care. A sound knowledge of the pathophysiology of PPHN can help the clinician make sense of the varied presentations of PPHN particularly when syndromic features are recognized.

4. References

Abudu, O. O., Uguru, V., & Olude, O. (1988). Contribution Of Congenital Malformation To Perinatal Mortality In Lagos, Nigeria. *International Journal Of Gynaecology And Obstetrics*, Vol.27, No.1, pp. 63-67, 0020-7292 (Print) 0020-7292 (Linking).

Aghabiklooei, A., Goodarzi, P., & Kariminejad, M. H. (2009). Lung Hypoplasia And Its Associated Major Congenital Abnormalities In Perinatal Death: An Autopsy Study Of 850 Cases. *Indian Journal Of Pediatrics*, Vol.76, No.11, pp. 1137-1140, 0973-7693 (Electronic) 0019-5456 (Linking).

Allanson, J. E. (1987). Noonan Syndrome. *Journal Of Medical Genetics*, Vol.24, No.1, pp. 9-13, 0022-2593 (Print) 0022-2593 (Linking).

Argyle, J. C. (1989). Pulmonary Hypoplasia In Infants With Giant Abdominal Wall Defects. *Pediatric Pathology*, Vol.9, No.1, pp. 43-55, 0277-0938 (Print) 0277-0938 (Linking).

Arkoff, R. S. (1968). Congenital Pulmonary Lymphangiectasis. *California Medicine*, Vol.109, No.6, pp. 464-466, 0008-1264 (Print) 0008-1264 (Linking).

Brown, N. J., Dohm, M. T., Bernardino De La Serna, J., & Barron, A. E. (2011). Biomimetic N-Terminal Alkylation Of Peptoid Analogues Of Surfactant Protein C. *Biophysical Journal*, Vol.101, No.5, pp. 1076-1085, 1542-0086 (Electronic) 0006-3495 (Linking).

Burri, P. H. (2006). Structural Aspects Of Postnatal Lung Development - Alveolar Formation And Growth. *Biology Of The Neonate*, Vol.89, No.4, pp. 313-322, 0006-3126 (Print) 0006-3126 (Linking).

Cannon, B. C., Feltes, T. F., Fraley, J. K., Grifka, R. G., Riddle, E. M., & Kovalchin, J. P. (2005). Nitric Oxide In The Evaluation Of Congenital Heart Disease With Pulmonary Hypertension: Factors Related To Nitric Oxide Response. *Pediatric Cardiology*, Vol.26, No.5, pp. 565-569, 0172-0643 (Print) 0172-0643 (Linking).

Cappelli-Bigazzi, M., Santoro, G., Battaglia, C., Palladino, M. T., Carrozza, M., Russo, M. G., Calabro, R. (2004). Endothelial Cell Function In Patients With Down's Syndrome.

The American Journal Of Cardiology, Vol.94, No.3, pp. 392-395, 0002-9149 (Print) 0002-9149 (Linking).

Clements, B. S., & Warner, J. O. (1987). Pulmonary Sequestration And Related Congenital Bronchopulmonary-Vascular Malformations: Nomenclature And Classification Based On Anatomical And Embryological Considerations. *Thorax,* Vol.42, No.6, pp. 401-408, 0040-6376 (Print) 0040-6376 (Linking).

Correia-Pinto, J., Gonzaga, S., Huang, Y., & Rottier, R. (2010). Congenital Lung Lesions-- Underlying Molecular Mechanisms. *Seminars In Pediatric Surgery,* Vol.19, No.3, pp. 171-179, 1532-9453 (Electronic) 1055-8586 (Linking).

Cua, C. L., Blankenship, A., North, A. L., Hayes, J., & Nelin, L. D. (2007). Increased Incidence Of Idiopathic Persistent Pulmonary Hypertension In Down Syndrome Neonates. *Pediatric Cardiology,* Vol.28, No.4, pp. 250-254, 0172-0643 (Print) 0172-0643 (Linking).

Cunniff, C., Jones, K. L., & Jones, M. C. (1990). Patterns Of Malformation In Children With Congenital Diaphragmatic Defects. *The Journal Of Pediatrics,* Vol.116, No.2, pp. 258-261, 0022-3476 (Print) 0022-3476 (Linking).

Cunningham, M. L., & Mann, N. (1997). Pulmonary Agenesis: A Predictor Of Ipsilateral Malformations. *American Journal Of Medical Genetics,* Vol.70, No.4, pp. 391-398, 0148-7299 (Print) 0148-7299 (Linking).

Dillon, E., Renwick, M., & Wright, C. (2000). Congenital Diaphragmatic Herniation: Antenatal Detection And Outcome. *The British Journal Of Radiology,* Vol.73, No.868, pp. 360-365, 0007-1285 (Print) 0007-1285 (Linking).

Dogan, R., Dogan, O. F., Yilmaz, M., Demircin, M., Pasaoglu, I., Kiper, N., . . . Boke, E. (2004). Surgical Management Of Infants With Congenital Lobar Emphysema And Concomitant Congenital Heart Disease. *The Heart Surgery Forum,* Vol.7, No.6, pp. E644-649, 1522-6662 (Electronic) 1098-3511 (Linking).

Dupuis, C., Charaf, L. A., Breviere, G. M., & Abou, P. (1993). "Infantile" Form Of The Scimitar Syndrome With Pulmonary Hypertension. *American Journal Of Cardiology,* Vol.71, No.15, pp. 1326-1330, 0002-9149 (Print) 0002-9149 (Linking).

Evans, J. A., Stranc, L. C., Kaplan, P., & Hunter, A. G. (1989). Vacterl With Hydrocephalus: Further Delineation Of The Syndrome(S). *American Journal Of Medical Genetics,* Vol.34, No.2, pp. 177-182, 0148-7299 (Print) 0148-7299 (Linking).

Fewell, J. E., Lee, C. C., & Kitterman, J. A. (1981). Effects Of Phrenic Nerve Section On The Respiratory System Of Fetal Lambs. *Journal Of Applied Physiology: Respiratory, Environmental And Exercise Physiology,* Vol.51, No.2, pp. 293-297, 0161-7567 (Print) 0161-7567 (Linking).

Fronstin, M. H., Hooper, G. S., Besse, B. E., & Ferreri, S. (1967). Congenital Pulmonary Cystic Lymphangiectasis. Case Report And A Review Of 32 Cases. *American Journal Of Diseases Of Children,* Vol.114, No.3, pp. 330-335, 0002-922x (Print) 0002-922x (Linking).

Fryns, J. P., Moerman, F., Goddeeris, P., Bossuyt, C., & Van Den Berghe, H. (1979). A New Lethal Syndrome With Cloudy Corneae, Diaphragmatic Defects And Distal Limb Deformities. *Human Genetics,* Vol.50, No.1, pp. 65-70, 0340-6717 (Print) 0340-6717 (Linking).

Gabow, P. A. (1993). Autosomal Dominant Polycystic Kidney Disease. *American Journal Of Kidney Diseases : The Official Journal Of The National Kidney Foundation,* Vol.22, No.4, pp. 511-512, 0272-6386 (Print) 0272-6386 (Linking).

Garmany, T. H., Moxley, M. A., White, F. V., Dean, M., Hull, W. M., Whitsett, J. A., Hamvas, A. (2006). Surfactant Composition And Function In Patients With Abca3 Mutations. *Pediatric Research,* Vol.59, No.6, pp. 801-805, 0031-3998 (Print) 0031-3998 (Linking).

Glauser, T. A., Rorke, L. B., Weinberg, P. M., & Clancy, R. R. (1990). Congenital Brain Anomalies Associated With The Hypoplastic Left Heart Syndrome. *Pediatrics,* Vol.85, No.6, pp. 984-990, 0031-4005 (Print) 0031-4005 (Linking).

Hall, J. G., Pallister, P. D., Clarren, S. K., Beckwith, J. B., Wiglesworth, F. W., Fraser, F. C., Reed, S. D. (1980). Congenital Hypothalamic Hamartoblastoma, Hypopituitarism, Imperforate Anus And Postaxial Polydactyly--A New Syndrome? Part I: Clinical, Causal, And Pathogenetic Considerations. *American Journal Of Medical Genetics,* Vol.7, No.1, pp. 47-74, 0148-7299 (Print) 0148-7299 (Linking).

Hamvas, A. (2010). Evaluation And Management Of Inherited Disorders Of Surfactant Metabolism. *Chinese Medical Journal,* Vol.123, No.20, pp. 2943-2947, 0366-6999 (Print) 0366-6999 (Linking).

Hershenson, M. B., Brouillette, R. T., Klemka, L., Raffensperger, J. D., Poznanski, A. K., & Hunt, C. E. (1985). Respiratory Insufficiency In Newborns With Abdominal Wall Defects. *Journal Of Pediatric Surgery,* Vol.20, No.4, pp. 348-353, 0022-3468 (Print) 0022-3468 (Linking).

Hsia, Y. E., Bratu, M., & Herbordt, A. (1971). Genetics Of The Meckel Syndrome (Dysencephalia Splanchnocystica). *Pediatrics,* Vol.48, No.2, pp. 237-247, 0031-4005 (Print) 0031-4005 (Linking).

Huddleston, C. B., Exil, V., Canter, C. E., & Mendeloff, E. N. (1999). Scimitar Syndrome Presenting In Infancy. *The Annals Of Thoracic Surgery,* Vol.67, No.1, pp. 154-159; Discussion 160, 0003-4975 (Print) 0003-4975 (Linking).

Huddleston, C. B., & Mendeloff, E. N. (1999). Scimitar Syndrome. *Advances In Cardiac Surgery,* Vol.11, pp. 161-178, 0889-5074 (Print) 0889-5074 (Linking).

Jones, K. L., & Smith, D. W. (2006). *Smith's Recognizable Patterns Of Human Malformation* (6th Ed.). Philadelphia: Elsevier Saunders.

Kallen, K., Mastroiacovo, P., Castilla, E. E., Robert, E., & Kallen, B. (2001). Vater Non-Random Association Of Congenital Malformations: Study Based On Data From Four Malformation Registers. *American Journal Of Medical Genetics,* Vol.101, No.1, pp. 26-32, 0148-7299 (Print) 0148-7299 (Linking).

Kamata, S., Usui, N., Sawai, T., Nose, K., & Fukuzawa, M. (2008). Prenatal Detection Of Pulmonary Hypoplasia In Giant Omphalocele. *Pediatric Surgery International,* Vol.24, No.1, pp. 107-111, 0179-0358 (Print) 0179-0358 (Linking).

Katheria, A. C., Masliah, E., Benirschke, K., Jones, K. L., & Kim, J. H. (2010). Idiopathic Persistent Pulmonary Hypertension In An Infant With Smith-Lemli-Opitz Syndrome. *Fetal And Pediatric Pathology,* Vol.29, No.6, pp. 373-379, 1551-3823 (Electronic) 1551-3815 (Linking).

Khan, P. A., Cloutier, M., & Piedboeuf, B. (2007). Tracheal Occlusion: A Review Of Obstructing Fetal Lungs To Make Them Grow And Mature. *Journal Of Medical Genetics. Part C, Seminars In Medical Genetics,* Vol.145c, No.2, pp. 125-138, 1552-4868 (Print) 1552-4868 (Linking).

Kinsella, J. P., Parker, T. A., Ivy, D. D., & Abman, S. H. (2003). Noninvasive Delivery Of Inhaled Nitric Oxide Therapy For Late Pulmonary Hypertension In Newborn

Infants With Congenital Diaphragmatic Hernia. *The Journal Of Pediatrics*, Vol.142, No.4, pp. 397-401, 0022-3476 (Print) 0022-3476 (Linking).

Knowles, S., Thomas, R. M., Lindenbaum, R. H., Keeling, J. W., & Winter, R. M. (1988). Pulmonary Agenesis As Part Of The Vacterl Sequence. *Archives Of Disease In Childhood*, Vol.63, No.7 Spec No, pp. 723-726, 1468-2044 (Electronic) 0003-9888 (Linking).

Laberge, J. M., Flageole, H., Pugash, D., Khalife, S., Blair, G., Filiatrault, D., Wilson, R. D. (2001). Outcome Of The Prenatally Diagnosed Congenital Cystic Adenomatoid Lung Malformation: A Canadian Experience. *Fetal Diagnosis And Therapy*, Vol.16, No.3, pp. 178-186, 1015-3837 (Print) 1015-3837 (Linking).

Langston, C. (1991). Misalignment Of Pulmonary Veins And Alveolar Capillary Dysplasia. *Pediatric Pathology*, Vol.11, No.1, pp. 163-170, 0277-0938 (Print) 0277-0938 (Linking).

Li, S., Qayyum, A., Coakley, F. V., & Hricak, H. (2000). Association Of Renal Agenesis And Mullerian Duct Anomalies. *Journal Of Computer Assisted Tomography*, Vol.24, No.6, pp. 829-834, 0363-8715 (Print) 0363-8715 (Linking).

Moessinger, A. C., Harding, R., Adamson, T. M., Singh, M., & Kiu, G. T. (1990). Role Of Lung Fluid Volume In Growth And Maturation Of The Fetal Sheep Lung. *The Journal Of Clinical Investigation*, Vol.86, No.4, pp. 1270-1277, 0021-9738 (Print) 0021-9738 (Linking).

Morgan, N. V., Gissen, P., Sharif, S. M., Baumber, L., Sutherland, J., Kelly, D. A., Johnson, C. A. (2002). A Novel Locus For Meckel-Gruber Syndrome, Mks3, Maps To Chromosome 8q24. *Human Genetics*, Vol.111, No.4-5, pp. 456-461, 0340-6717 (Print) 0340-6717 (Linking).

Morse, R. P., Rawnsley, E., Crowe, H. C., Marin-Padilla, M., & Graham, J. M., Jr. (1987). Bilateral Renal Agenesis In Three Consecutive Siblings. *Prenatal Diagnosis*, Vol.7, No.8, pp. 573-579, 0197-3851 (Print) 0197-3851 (Linking).

Narumi, Y., Kosho, T., Tsuruta, G., Shiohara, M., Shimazaki, E., Mori, T., Fukushima, Y. (2010). Genital Abnormalities In Pallister-Hall Syndrome: Report Of Two Patients And Review Of The Literature. *American Journal Of Medical Genetics. Part A*, Vol.152a, No.12, pp. 3143-3147, 1552-4833 (Electronic) 1552-4825 (Linking).

Nogee, L. M., Wert, S. E., Proffit, S. A., Hull, W. M., & Whitsett, J. A. (2000). Allelic Heterogeneity In Hereditary Surfactant Protein B (Sp-B) Deficiency. *American Journal Of Respiratory And Critical Care Medicine*, Vol.161, No.3 Pt 1, pp. 973-981, 1073-449x (Print) 1073-449x (Linking).

Noonan, J. (1999). Noonan Syndrome--Then And Now. *Cardiology In The Young*, Vol.9, No.6, pp. 545-546, 1047-9511 (Print) 1047-9511 (Linking).

Page, D. V., & Stocker, J. T. (1982). Anomalies Associated With Pulmonary Hypoplasia. *The American Review Of Respiratory Disease*, Vol.125, No.2, pp. 216-221, 0003-0805 (Print) 0003-0805 (Linking).

Patel, M. S., Taylor, G. P., Bharya, S., Al-Sanna'a, N., Adatia, I., Chitayat, D., Human, D. G. (2004). Abnormal Pericyte Recruitment As A Cause For Pulmonary Hypertension In Adams-Oliver Syndrome. *American Journal Of Medical Genetics. Part A*, Vol.129a, No.3, pp. 294-299, 1552-4825 (Print) 1552-4825 (Linking).

Ren, G., Jacob, R. F., Kaulin, Y., Dimuzio, P., Xie, Y., Mason, R. P., Tulenko, T. N. (2011). Alterations In Membrane Caveolae And Bk(Ca) Channel Activity In Skin

Fibroblasts In Smith-Lemli-Opitz Syndrome. *Mol Genet Metab*, pp. 1096-7206 (Electronic) 1096-7192 (Linking).

Roberts, K. E., Mcelroy, J. J., Wong, W. P., Yen, E., Widlitz, A., Barst, R. J., Morse, J. H. (2004). Bmpr2 Mutations In Pulmonary Arterial Hypertension With Congenital Heart Disease. *The European Respiratory Journal : Official Journal Of The European Society For Clinical Respiratory Physiology*, Vol.24, No.3, pp. 371-374, 0903-1936 (Print) 0903-1936 (Linking).

Romano, A. A., Allanson, J. E., Dahlgren, J., Gelb, B. D., Hall, B., Pierpont, M. E., Noonan, J. A. (2010). Noonan Syndrome: Clinical Features, Diagnosis, And Management Guidelines. *Pediatrics*, Vol.126, No.4, pp. 746-759, 1098-4275 (Electronic) 0031-4005 (Linking).

Rosias, P. R., Sijstermans, J. M., Theunissen, P. M., Pulles-Heintzberger, C. F., De Die-Smulders, C. E., Engelen, J. J., & Van Der Meer, S. B. (2001). Phenotypic Variability Of The Cat Eye Syndrome. Case Report And Review Of The Literature. *Genetic Counseling*, Vol.12, No.3, pp. 273-282, 1015-8146 (Print) 1015-8146 (Linking).

Salonen, R. (1984). The Meckel Syndrome: Clinicopathological Findings In 67 Patients. *American Journal Of Medical Genetics*, Vol.18, No.4, pp. 671-689, 0148-7299 (Print) 0148-7299 (Linking).

Schinzel, A., Schmid, W., Fraccaro, M., Tiepolo, L., Zuffardi, O., Opitz, J. M., Pagon, R. A. (1981). The "Cat Eye Syndrome": Dicentric Small Marker Chromosome Probably Derived From A No.22 (Tetrasomy 22pter To Q11) Associated With A Characteristic Phenotype. Report Of 11 Patients And Delineation Of The Clinical Picture. *Human Genetics*, Vol.57, No.2, pp. 148-158, 0340-6717 (Print) 0340-6717 (Linking).

Schwartz, M. Z., & Ramachandran, P. (1997). Congenital Malformations Of The Lung And Mediastinum--A Quarter Century Of Experience From A Single Institution. *Journal Of Pediatric Surgery*, Vol.32, No.1, pp. 44-47, 0022-3468 (Print) 0022-3468 (Linking).

Scott-Emuakpor, A. B., Warren, S. T., Kapur, S., Quiachon, E. B., & Higgins, J. V. (1981). Familial Occurrence Of Congenital Pulmonary Lymphangiectasis. Genetic Implications. *American Journal Of Diseases Of Children*, Vol.135, No.6, pp. 532-534, 0002-922x (Print) 0002-922x (Linking).

Sen, P., Thakur, N., Stockton, D. W., Langston, C., & Bejjani, B. A. (2004). Expanding The Phenotype Of Alveolar Capillary Dysplasia (Acd). *Journal Of Pediatrics*, Vol.145, No.5, pp. 646-651, 0022-3476 (Print) 0022-3476 (Linking).

Shulenin, S., Nogee, L. M., Annilo, T., Wert, S. E., Whitsett, J. A., & Dean, M. (2004). Abca3 Gene Mutations In Newborns With Fatal Surfactant Deficiency. *The New England Journal Of Medicine*, Vol.350, No.13, pp. 1296-1303, 1533-4406 (Electronic) 0028-4793 (Linking).

Steinhorn, R. H. (2010). Neonatal Pulmonary Hypertension. *Pediatric Critical Care*, Vol.11, No.2 Suppl, pp. S79-84, 1529-7535 (Print) 1529-7535 (Linking).

Stevenson, R. E. (2006). *Human Malformations And Related Anomalies* (2nd Ed.). Oxford ; New York: Oxford University Press.

Vissers, L. E., Van Ravenswaaij, C. M., Admiraal, R., Hurst, J. A., De Vries, B. B., Janssen, I. M., Van Kessel, A. G. (2004). Mutations In A New Member Of The Chromodomain Gene Family Cause Charge Syndrome. *Nature Genetics*, Vol.36, No.9, pp. 955-957, 1061-4036 (Print) 1061-4036 (Linking).

Weijerman, M. E., Van Furth, A. M., Van Der Mooren, M. D., Van Weissenbruch, M. M., Rammeloo, L., Broers, C. J., & Gemke, R. J. (2010). Prevalence Of Congenital Heart Defects And Persistent Pulmonary Hypertension Of The Neonate With Down Syndrome. *European Journal Of Pediatrics,* Vol.169, No.10, pp. 1195-1199, 1432-1076 (Electronic) 0340-6199 (Linking).

Wigglesworth, J. S. (1981). Pulmonary Hypoplasia With Phrenic Nerve Agenesis. *The Journal Of Pediatrics,* Vol.98, No.4, pp. 667-668, 0022-3476 (Print) 0022-3476 (Linking).

Witt, D. R., Hoyme, H. E., Zonana, J., Manchester, D. K., Fryns, J. P., Stevenson, J. G., Hall, J. G. (1987). Lymphedema In Noonan Syndrome: Clues To Pathogenesis And Prenatal Diagnosis And Review Of The Literature. *American Journal Of Medical Genetics,* Vol.27, No.4, pp. 841-856, 0148-7299 (Print) 0148-7299 (Linking).

Zeltner, T. B., & Burri, P. H. (1987). The Postnatal Development And Growth Of The Human Lung. Ii. Morphology. *Respiration Physiology,* Vol.67, No.3, pp. 269-282, 0034-5687 (Print) 0034-5687 (Linking).

14

Pulmonary Hypertension in Patients with Chronic Kidney Disease

Alessandro Domenici, Remo Luciani, Francesco Principe,
Francesco Paneni, Giuseppino Massimo Ciavarella and Luciano De Biase
Department of Cardiovascular, Renal and Pulmonary Diseases,
Sant'Andrea Hospital, Sapienza University of Rome,
Italy

1. Introduction

An unexpectedly high prevalence of pulmonary hypertension (PH) has been detected by Doppler echocardiography in chronic kidney disease (CKD) patients and found to be associated with overall poor outcome. A number of pathogenetic mechanisms appears to act synergistically in producing such a condition, the relative importance of which is a matter of ongoing investigation. This chapter will review the literature on the topic and summarizes what can be drawn from published studies. Our work and experience at Sant'Andrea University Hospital is also extensively reported and area for future research addressed.

2. The facts

2.1 Pulmonary hypertension in CKD patients on maintenance hemodialysis

Quite surprisingly, PH remained an overlooked issue in CKD patients until very recent years. Moving from an analysis of the backround diseases in their series of patients with PH, Yigla and co-workers were the first to report, in a seminal paper (Yigla et al., 2003), a PH prevalence as high as 39.7% in patients receiving haemodialysis (HD) through a surgically created arterio-venous fistula (AVF). These authors found PH to be associated with cardiac output (CO) and anemia. They were also the first to report that temporary occlusion of the AVF by compression results in a reduction of both CO and systolic pulmonary artery pressure (PAP_s), that PH may actually increase in pre-dialysis patients after renal replacement therapy (RRT) initiation, and that it might reduce after successful renal transplantation (Tx). This findings prompted other studies from the same group, focusing on the possible role of pulmonary calcifications (Yigla et al., 2004) and endothelin-1 (ET-1) and nitric oxide (NO) (Nakhoul et al., 2005) in the pathogenesis of PH in HD patients. In the first study, in a group of HD patients, 57% of whom with PH, no correlation was found with pulmonary calcification detected by technetium-99m diphosphonate scanning. In the second study they found ET-1 level to be higher in HD patients, both with and without PH, than in controls; no correlation with PAP_s could be demonstrated, however. Indeed, lower NO metabolites were detected in HD patients with PH than in those without and in controls, as well as a blunted increase during the HD session. Two years later, another group reported on PH in chronic renal failure (CRF) patients

(Havlucu et al., 2007). Despite severe exclusion criteria, they found a echocardiographically estimated $PAP_s \geq 35$ mmHg in 14 out of 25 (56%) patients already on HD and in 9 out of 23 (39%) patients not yet on dialysis. Patients with PH showed significantly higher CO, higher serum levels of parathyroid hormone (PTH), higher calcium-phosphate product and a longer CRF duration. They also found that the presence of an AVF was associated with a higher risk of PH, and that Doppler estimated AVF flow correlated with PAP_s. Patients were revaluated at least 6 months later: quite interestingly, while patients still in pre-dialysis had deteriorated, in those who had started HD in the meanwhile PAP_s, blood pressure (BP) and serum PTH had overall decreased and ejection fraction increased. In a very similar study (Abdelwhab & Elshinnawy, 2008), PH was detected in 20 out of 45 (44%) patients on HD and in 10 out of 31 (32%) pre-dialysis patients on conservative treatment. Dialysis patients with PH had higher AVF blood flow, higher prevalence of left ventricular diastolic dysfunction and higher NT-proBNP and TXB_2 levels. A role for inflammation in the pathogenesis of PH in HD was addressed by researchers from Taiwan (Yu et al., 2009). In this study high sensitivity-C reactive protein (hs-CRP) and a number of cytokines were measured in 39 patients on long standing maintenance HD and correlated with the presence of PH. The prevalence of PH was remarkably high (61%), and patients with PH exhibited higher CO, higher AVF blood flow rate and, intriguingly, poorer residual renal function (RRF) and dialytic solute clearances. Serum levels of hs-CRP, IL-1β, TNF-α, IL-6 were significantly higher in patients with PH than in those without.

In all these studies, echocardiography was performed within one hour from the completion of the HD procedure, in order to possibly avoid the effect of volume overload, almost always present immediately before the haemodialysis treatment in the most commonly used thrice weekly in-centre schedule. PAP_s was measured according to the modified Bernoulli equation: PAP = 4 x (peak tricuspid regurgitant jet velocity)^2 + 10 mmHg (estimated right atrial pressure, RAP). Patients with cardiac, pulmonary or systemic diseases known to associate with PH were *a priori* excluded in these earlier studies. A somewhat different approach was used in a prospective study from Texas, USA (Ramasubbu et al, 2010), including 90 HD patients (64% afro-american, 18% Hispanic and 18% Caucasian), dialyzed trough arterio-venous graft (44%), AVF (40%) or catheters (16%). Patients underwent comprehensive echocardiographic examination before the haemodialysis session, because it was felt that the pre-dialysis status of the patients more closely reflects the chronic volume status than the immediate post dialysis "dry weight" state. Furthermore, PH was defined as a peak tricuspid regurgitant (TR) jet velocity ≥ 2,5 m/sec, and as "more severe PH" when TR jet velocity was ≥ 3 m/sec. Forty-two patients (42%) met the definition of PH, 18 of whom (20%) of more severe grade. Quite surprisingly, patients with PH did have a significantly lower BMI. As expected, on the other hand, patients with PH were found to have larger right atrial (RA) and right ventricular (RV) sizes, higher RAP, and a trend towards decreased RV function and more left ventricular (LV) hypertrophy. Mean LVEF tended to be lower with increasing PAP_s, but was still overall preserved. There was a trend to larger left atrial (LA) size with increasing PAP_s, consistent with significantly higher estimates of left sided filling pressures. After 12 months, 14 patients (15,6%) had died. Mortality was significantly higher in patients who had PH (26%), particularly in those with a TR jet velocity ≥ 3 m/sec. Patients who died had been longer on HD, and they had larger RA and RV sizes, worse RV function, more severe TR, significantly higher RAP, PAP_s and pulmonary capillary wedge pressure (PCWP). This study provides evidence that development of PH in HD patients may well reflect the consequence of chronic volume overload and chronically elevated left heart filling pressures, suggesting that elevated PCWP may play a major role in PAP increase. Of note, in this study population 77% of the patients exhibited abnormal LV diastolic function, possibly the result of LVH and myocardial stiffness.

Three studies attempt to explore specifically the role of the AVF in determining PH in CKD patients. The first published study (Acarturk et al, 2008) used mean PAP calculated from the right ventricular outflow tract acceleration time according to the Mahan's equation (mPAP in mmHg =79 – 0.45 x acceleration time in ms); AVF blood flow rate was estimated by Doppler sonography. Thirty-two patients were included, 24 with a radial and 8 with a brachial AVF created 32±34 months before evaluation. PH (defined as mPAP > 25 mmHg,) was detected in 14 patients (43%). Results confirmed the already reported relationship between PAP and cardiac index (CO normalized to body surface area) and disclosed a higher cardiac index in patients with PH. No direct relationship between AVF blood flow rate and mPAP could be demonstrated, however. The second study (Beigi et al, 2009), did find a statistically significant positive correlation between AVF flow and PAP in 34 patients studied before AVF creation and at least 6 months apart. The mean AVF flow was 1322 ml/min in patients without PH and 2750 ml/min in patients with PH, the latter being clearly higher than currently regarded as necessary and safe, even more when considering that the authors reported a negative correlation between PAP and ejection fraction (EF) before as well as after the creation of AVF. The third study (Ünal et al, 2010) included 20 patients evaluated before AVF creation and 23±2 months later, failed to find an effect of AVF creation on PAP, which indeed tend to decrease after AVF creation and initiation of RRT, and a correlation between PAP and AVF blood flow rate (truly not given). A further study with an original design has been recently published (Kiykim et al, 2010). Seventy-four HD patients dialyzed through permanent tunnelled jugular central venous catheter (CVC) were studied echocardiographically immediately before and at the end of a HD session with two different dialysis membrane – cellulose acetate and high-flux polysulfone – in a cross-over design. Pre-HD PH prevalence was remarkably high (68,8%, moderate in 40,5%). A significant PAP reduction and a significant correlation with UF volume was observed only when patients where dialyzed with the more biocompatible polysulfone membrane, suggesting a role for biocompatibility on short-term PAPs.

2.2 Pulmonary hypertension in patients on Peritoneal Dialysis

Apart from the data on 5 patients on peritoneal dialysis (PD) included in the control group of the first study from Yigla and co-workers (Yigla et al, 2003), none of whom found to have PH, the first study of PH in PD patients was published in 2007 (Kumbar et al, 2007). In this retrospective study including 36 patients undergoing echocardiographic evaluation on clinical indication, a PH prevalence of 42% was found. Due to the selection bias, however, patients with congestive heart failure and/or coronary artery disease were probably overrepresented in the study; indeed, patients with PH exhibited more dilated left ventricular chamber and their mean EF (46±19 %) would have represented a reason for exclusion in most of the previously published studies. An unexplained higher PH prevalence in patients on continuous cycling PD (CCPD) as compared to continuous ambulatory PD (CAPD) was noted. Duration of PD was not reported, but overall residual renal function was marginal. Two years later, to date the largest study on PH in PD patients was published (Ünal et al, 2009). One hundred and thirty five, quite young (47±13 years old) patients on CAPD (64 females) were studied and, notably, this is the first study which included a bioelectrical impedance analysis to estimate the ratio of extracellular water (ECW) to total body water (TBW) and thus stratified patients according to volume status. PH was found in 17 patients (12,6%), who showed also significantly higher ECW/TBW ratio and lower serum albumin, triglyceride and ejection fraction. No differences were found between patients with PH and patients without in terms of age, gender, smoking, diabetes or hypertension, use of erythropoietin (EPO), duration of dialysis, systolic and diastolic blood pressure, body mass index (BMI), white blood cell count, haemoglobin (Hb), serum creatinine, solute clearances, residual glomerular filtration rate (GFR), alkaline phosphatise, intact parathyroid hormone (iPTH), hs-CRP, LDL and total cholesterol, calcium-phosphate product, amount of ultrafiltration (UF), left ventricular mass (LVM), and hypertrophy (LVH) and plasma level of asymmetric dimethylarginine (ADMA). Echocardiographically estimated PAP_s correlated with ECW/TBW ratio, LVM and LVMI, and, inversely, with serum albumin, trygliceride, Hb and EF. In multivariate analysis, serum albumin, ECW/TBW and LVMI were found to be independent risk factors for PH. According to bioelectrical impedance analysis no patient was hypovolemic, 51 (37,8%) of the 135 patients were hypervolemic and 84 (62,2%) were normovolemic. Hypervolemic patients had lower Hb levels, higher mean systolic PAP and a significantly higher prevalence of PH (27,5% vs 3,6%, p=0.001). These findings are highly suggestive of a major role for fluid overload in determining PH in PD patients and the same should hold true for all CKD disease patients, regardless of dialysis modality, and even for those on conservative pre-dialysis treatment. An Italian study (Fabbian et al, 2011) including 29 patients on HD and 27 patients on PD found PH in 22 patients (39%), and confirmed a higher prevalence in patient on HD (58,6% versus 18,5%, p=0.002). Patients with PH had been longer on RRT, had higher inter-dialytic weight gain, lower diastolic pressure and ejection fraction than those without. PH positively correlated with diastolic left ventricular volume (r = 0.32, p=0.013) and negatively with EF (r = -0.54, p< 0.0001).

2.3 Pulmonary hypertension and mortality

The impact of PH on mortality of patients undergoing chronic HD was investigated by Yigla and co-workers (Yigla et al, 2009) in a retrospective study including 127 HD patients representative of the national cohort of patients on HD in Israel. Including also patients with already known cardiac disease, but using a higher threshold cut-off value (≥ 45 mmHg) for PH definition, the prevalence of PH in the whole cohort was found to be 29,1%, and it was present before dialysis initiation in 13,4%, while developed after HD initiation in 15,7%. In latter group, the time interval to the first echocardiographic study showing PH was less than 1 year in 75% of the cases. No differences in baseline cardiac status could be demonstrated between patients without PH at any time and patients developing PH after the initiation of HD, that instead was significantly worse in patients with pre-existing PH. The overall 1-, 3-, and 5-year survival was 90.6, 66.9 and 52.8 %, respectively. Survival of patients with PH was significantly shorter than that of those without (78.6, 42.9 and 25.2 %, log-rank test p=0.0001), regardless PH was present before dialysis initiation or developed thereafter. The age of non survivors at HD initiation was meaningfully higher, however, yet a survival advantage was found in 20 patients without PH matched to the group with PH developed after dialysis initiation for age, gender, aetiology of kidney disease, location of vascular access and comorbidity.

Very interestingly, when PAP$_s$ was analyzed as a continuous variable, as it is, the authors were able to demonstrate an adjusted hazard ratio (HR) for mortality of 1.5 for each 10 mmHg increase in PAP$_s$ (95% CI 1.2-1.9, p=0.0007). One pitfalls of this study is that patients who have had only one echocardiographic evaluation while on HD, showing no PH, were assumed and analyzed as having normal pre-HD PAP$_s$, which is not necessarily true, as suggested by several papers reporting the possibility of actual modification of PAP in a substantial proportion of patients on RRT, which holds true in our experience.

2.4 Pulmonary hypertension and renal transplantation

The association between PH before transplantation and subsequent outcome was first addressed by a study from the Mayo Clinic College of Medicine, Rochester, MN, USA (Issa et al., 2008). In this retrospective analysis of 215 dialysis patients who have had an echocardiographic evaluation before renal transplantation, mean PAP$_s$ was found to be 34±10 mmHg (range 21-71) in the whole cohort; 146 patients (68%) have PAP$_s$ < 35 mmHg (regarded as normal), 47 (22%) have moderately high PAP$_s$ (36-50 mm Hg) and 22 (10%) markedly elevated PAP$_s$ (> 50 mm Hg), suggestive of severe PH. Longer time on dialysis was the strongest correlate of higher PAP$_s$ pre-transplant (r= 0.252, p< 0.001), PH being detected in 25% of patients who had never been on RRT (pre-emptive Tx) or had received dialysis for less than 1 year, in 38% of those who had been on dialysis longer than 1 but less 2 years, and in 58% of those who have been on dialysis for more than 2 years before transplantation. Patients with severe PH had a significantly higher risk of death (HR 3.75, 1.17-11.97, p=0.025) early after Tx than patients with lower PAP$_s$. Age was associated with both PAP$_s$ and mortality in this study. A significantly lower prevalence of PH (17%) was found in a cohort of 500 younger patients studied as a part of pre-transplant evaluation (Bozbas et al, 2009), and again PH was associated with longer duration of dialysis and HD as the RRT modality versus PD. Amongst echocardiographic data, LVEF was significantly lower and right and left atria diameters greater in patients with PH than in those without. The prevalence of LVH was higher in patients with PH, while the percentage of patient with diastolic dysfunction was not significantly different. Another recently published study (Zlotnick et al, 2010) investigated the possible relationship between pre-transplant echocardiograpically detected PH and early graft function. In 55 patients, 21 of whom (38%) with pH, the incidence of the composite outcome of delayed or slow graft function was found to be significantly higher in patients with pre-transplant PH (43 vs 6%, p=0.002), supporting the hypothesis that pre-transplant pulmonary hypertension could represent an independent predictor of early graft dysfunction.

3. What we have done

Sant'Andrea Hospital is a tertiary 450-bed University Hospital which began its activity in 2003. At that time the burden of cardio-renal syndromes was increasingly recognized as an emerging epidemic and prompted a strict and motivated cooperation between Cardiologists and Nephrologists. In that context all patients with kidney disease underwent first a comprehensive cardiovascular evaluation by one experienced Cardiologist (L.D.B.), who acts as the referring physician responsible for individually tailored work up, treatment and follow up of patients with renal diseases. The first patients with CKD at our Institution were those referred to the nephrology outpatient clinic, the nephrology ward and the outpatients dialysis facility. At the same time many patients with cardiac diseases were referred for a nephrological consultation due to evidence of renal dysfunction. This interplay helped to disclose a number of interesting and quite novel findings. Among these, the unexpected, and at that time largely underrecognized, high prevalence of elevated pulmonary artery pressure as detected by Doppler echocardiography was one of the main framework. At the beginning most CKD patients on maintenance RRT at our hospital had started dialysis elsewhere, with quite large differences of previous duration of RRT and co-morbidities burden. Pivotal to the evaluation of their cardiac status was conventional and tissue Doppler imaging (TDI) trans-thoracic echocardiography, performed by two sonographer-experienced Cardiologists (F.P. & G.M.C.). In more detail, patients with stage 5 CKD on RRT underwent two-dimensional and M-mode study using an Acuson Sequoia® C 256 ultrasound machine. Left ventricular diameters and wall thickness were measured according to the American Society of Echocardiography, left ventricular volumes were estimated using the z-derived method. LVEF was calculated using the Teicholz formula and further confirmed with Simpson's technique in the 4-chamber view. Pulsed-wave Doppler of mitral inflow velocity was performed. The maximal tricuspid regurgitation velocity was measured by continuous wave Doppler echocardiography from the apical 4-chamber view. The highest peak velocity was recorded and the average peak velocity from 3 beats were calculated and used to calculate systolic pulmonary pressure according to the modified Bernoulli equation. Pulmonary hypertension was defined as a value of systolic pulmonary pressure > 35 mmHg at rest. Right ventricular diameters were measured in the long axis view. EF of the right ventricle was calculated by using the Simpson's formula from the apical 4-chamber view. Early (E) and late (A) right ventricular inflow velocity were measured with pulse-wave Doppler by placing the sample volume in between the tips of the tricuspid valve in the apical 4-chamber window. TDI spectral signal was acquired from the apical 4-chamber view, with the sample volume placed along the lateral and septal tricuspid annulus. The systolic myocardial velocity (Sm), protodiastolic myocardial velocity (Em), and late peak diastolic myocardial velocity (Am) were measured. The E/Em ratio, an index of ventricular filling pressure, was calculated. Ejection time, isovolumic relaxation and contraction time were also measured. Regional TDI myocardial performance index (MPI) was calculated. Average regional TDI MPI of the right ventricle was calculated as follow: (MPI $_{lateral}$ + MPI $_{septal}$) /2. Right ventricular dysfunction (RVD) was defined by an average regional MPI value > 2 SD from the mean of the values derived from 100 healthy subjects (MPI>0.53). An early analysis included 68 patients on RRT, 54 (79%) on thrice weekly HD and 14 (21%) on PD, who did not differ in age, gender, height, weight, BMI, BSA, blood pressure, heart rate, serum calcium, phosphate, Ca x P product, uric acid, Hb, total cholesterol, triglyceride and total protein. Patients on PD had however significantly higher HDL cholesterol, lower serum albumin, shorter duration of RRT and more preserved residual renal function (RRF) than their HD counterpart. Patients on HD showed a significantly higher left and right ventricular wall thickness, higher PAP$_s$ (35±8 versus 28±9 mmHg) and higher left ventricular mass index (p<0.01). A significant correlation was found between PAP$_s$ and some measures of diastolic and systolic function of the right ventricle, such as isovolumic relaxation time (IVRT) (r=0.414, p=0.003) and Sm (r= -0.454, p=0.001). Both these measures were significantly more compromised in the HD cohort. As long as CKD patients new to dialysis entered our RRT program, we were able to extend our observation in a larger study (Paneni et al, 2010), including 94 patients on HD, 62 dialyzed trough a radial AVF and 32 trough a brachial AVF, and 26 on PD, most of whom on nightly automated PD (APD), compared with 100 healthy controls matched for age, gender and BMI. Patients on RRT did not differ with regards to the prevalence of hypertension and diabetes and type of medications used. Duration of dialysis tended to be longer in HD patients (45 ± 3 months versus 37 ± 3 in patients on PD) but this difference was no longer statistically significant. LV diameters and volumes were higher in dialysis patients than in controls. LVEF was significantly lower in HD patients than in PD patients and controls. No significant differences in the indices of systolic and diastolic function were found between HD patients with radial or brachial AVF. PAP_s was significantly higher in HD patients than in PD patients and controls (38.9 ± 6.8, 29.7 ± 6.7 and 21.7 ± 6.8 mmHg, respectively, p< 0.001). Patients on HD presented larger right ventricular diameters than PD patients and controls; RVEF was significantly reduced in dialysis patients as compared to controls, but to a different extent in the HD and PD group. TDI indices of diastolic and systolic function were significantly lower in patients undergoing HD, and the impairment was more pronounced in those with a brachial AVF. Compared to PD patients, patients on HD showed a prolonged IVRT and higher E/EM ratio. Lateral and septal Sm velocities were reduced among HD patients, the greatest reduction being observed in patients with a brachial AVF. When right ventricular dysfunction was defined by a TDI MPI > 2 SD from the mean value derived from healthy controls, RVD was identified in 79 (65,8%) dialysis patients, the prevalence being significantly higher in HD as compared to PD patients (71.3 versus 34.6%, p<0.001). RVD was significantly more prevalent in HD patients with a brachial versus radial AVF (90.6 versus 61.3%, p<0.001). TDI MPI of the right ventricle showed significant correlation with systolic PAP (r = 0.45, p<0.01), Sm velocity measured at both lateral and septal tricuspid annulus , Em velocity, Am velocity, right and left ventricular EF. Linear regression analysis adjusted for age, gender, heart rate, duration of dialysis, dialysis adequacy and PAP_s, showed that HD treatment was independently associated with average TDI MPI of the right ventricle (β = 0.34, p<0.001). Logistic regression analysis adjusted for the same confounding showed that patients on HD have an increased risk of RVD as compared to patient on PD (OR 6.3 95% CI 2-19.5, p<0.001). Our preliminary data deriving from longitudinal follow up examinations show that "aggressive" correction of over hydration, as addressed by bio-impedance spectroscopy, may result in significant reduction of PAP_s and improvement of most indices of diastolic and systolic function of both ventricle, thus supporting a major role for chronic volume overload in determining overall cardiac compromise in our CKD patients.

4. Summary

4.1 Diagnosis

The gold standard for the diagnosis of PH is right heart catheterization (RHC), usually performed as a pre-operative tool in cardiac surgery, for hemodynamic evaluation of the critically ill patient, or in the suspicion of severe PH. To the best of our knowledge, no study has been published to date systematically performing RHC in patients with kidney diseases. The whole literature on PH in CKD patients employed rather uniform echocardiographic criteria to detect PAP_s. Reliance on echocardiography to diagnose PH has recently been mitigated, especially when pre-load is not controlled. The most recent consensus conference on PH, held in Dana Point in 2008, do not mention anymore echocardiographic parameters for the diagnosis of PH, while citing for the first time dialysis-dependent CKD as a self-standing entity among group 5, PH with unclear multifactorial mechanisms. It appears however unlikely that RHC will be largely used in this subset of patients, as long as the less invasive ultrasound study will refine to provide clinically adequate informations. To date, unfortunately, only the study from Ünal and co-workers on PD patients (Ünal et al, 2009) included an imperfect yet objective measure of the hydration status, which should be included in future studies on PH in CKD patients.

4.2 The role of the AV haemodialysis access

When PH was first detected in a high percentage of patients on maintenance HD, the possibility that AV access could play a major role in the development of PH was greatly emphasized. Subsequent studies, yet including relatively small numbers of patients, fail to demonstrate a major impact of AVF creation on PH in the short-medium term, with the possible exception of very high flow fistulas, in most cases brachial. It is our opinion that caution should be paid not to get excessively high, yet unnecessary, flow when creating arterio-venous access for RRT.

4.3 PH and dialysis modality

That the AV access cannot tell the whole story is clearly indicated by the absence of PH in about 50% of HD patients carrying an AVF and, on the other side, by the occurrence of PH in CKD patients without. PH prevalence and severity has been consistently reported to be lower in PD patients than in their HD counterpart (Domenici et al, 2010). One possible and little investigated explanation could well be the usually higher RRF of patients on PD, at least in the first years of RRT. A role for the differences in biocompatibility and intermittency schedules of different dialysis modalities seems likely, but has not been adequately explored.

4.4 PH, inflammation and endothelial dysfunction

A correlation between inflammation markers and PAP_s has been suggested, but this link has not been investigated in a longitudinal perspective. The pathogenetic relevance of endothelial dysfunction in CKD appears likely, as suggested by the increasing evidence of a common pathway in sleep disordered breathing, PH, early renal Tx outcome and markers of endothelial dysfunction.

4.5 PH and renal Tx

Current limited evidence suggests that echocardiographically-estimated PAP_s and RV function should be part of the pre-transplant evaluation, because of their prognostic relevance. Successful renal Tx is associated with normalization of PAP_s and improvement of cardiac function in most, but not all, transplanted patients.

5. Area for future research

The prevalence and the clinical correlates of PH in CKD needs to be better defined in larger prospective studies, which should take into account volume status and RRF. Patients with lower degree of renal impairment should be included, as well as patients with renal diseases but preserved glomerular filtration rate (GFR), such as nephrotics. PH has been recently detected in conjunction with sleep disordered breathing, a common co-morbidity in CKD patients that independently portends an unfavourable outcome. The prevalence and clinical relevance of PH in critically ill patients, its role as a risk factor for acute kidney injury (AKI) and its relevance to outcome warrants to be investigated. Studies focusing on the impact of different dialytic strategies and/or pharmacologic tools to efficaciously treat this condition in patients with CKD are urgently needed.

6. References

Abdelwhab, S. & Elshinnawy, S. (2008). Pulmonary hypertension in chronic renal failure patients. *Am J Nephrol*, Vol. 28, pp. 990-997

Acarturk, G.; Albayrak, R.; Melek, M.; Yuksel, S.; Uslan, I.; Atli, H.; Colbay, M.; Unlu, M.; Fidan, F.; Asci, Z.; Cander, S.; Karaman, O. & Acar, M. (2008). The relationship between arteriovenous fistula blood flow rate and pulmonary artery pressure in hemodialysis patients. *Int Urol Nephrol*, Vol. 40, N°2,pp. 509-513

Beigi, A.A.; Sadeghi, A.M.; Khosravi, A.R.; Karami, M. & Masoudpour, H. (2009). Effects of the arteriovenous fistula on pulmonary artery pressure and cardiac output in patients with chronic renal failure. *J Vasc Access*, Vol. 10, N°3, pp. 160- 166

Bozbas, S.S.; Akcay, S.; Altin, H.; Bozbas, E.; Karacaglar, E.; Kanyilmaz, S.; Sayin, H.; Muderrisoglu, H. & Haberal, M. (2009). Pulmonary hypertension in patients with end-stage renal disease undergoing renal transplantation. *Transplant Proc*, Vol. 41, pp. 2753-2756

Domenici, A.; Luciani, R. & Principe, F. (2010). Pulmonary hypertension in dialysis patients. *Peritoneal Dialysis International*, Vol. 30, N°2, pp. 251-252

Fabbian, F.; Cantelli, S.; Molino, C.; Pala, M.; Longhini, C. & Portaluppi, F. (2011). Pulmonary hypertension in dialysis patients: a cross-sectional Italian study. *International Journal of Nephrology*, Vol. 2011, Article ID 28475, doi:10.4061/2011/283475

Havlucu, Y.; Kursat, S:; Ekmekci, C.; Celik, P.; Serter, S.; Bayturan, O. & Dinc, G. (2007). Pulmonary hypertension in patients with chronic renal failure. *Respiration*, Vol. 74, pp. 503-510

Issa, N.; Krowka, M.J.; Griffin, M.D.; Hickson, L.T.J.; Stegall, M.D. & Cosio, F.G. (2008). Pulmonary hypertension is associated with reduced patient survival after kidney transplantation. *Transplantation*, Vol. 86, N° 10, pp. 1384-1388

Kiykim, A.A.; Horoz, M.; Ozcan, T.; Yildiz, I.; Sari, S. & Genctoy G. (2010). Pulmonary hypertension in hemodialysis patients without arteriovenous fistula: the effect of dialyzer composition. *Renal Failure*, Vol. 32, N° 10, pp. 1148-1152

Kumbar, L.; Fein, P; Rafiq, M.A.; Borawski, C.; Chattopadhyay, J. & Avram, M.M. (2007). Pulmonary hypertension in Peritoneal Dialysis patients. *Advances in Peritoneal Dialysis*, Vol. 23, pp. 127-131

Nakhoul, F.; Yigla, M.; Gilman, R.; Reisner, S.A. & Abassi, Z. (2005). The pathogenesis of pulmonary hypertension in hemodialysis patients via aterio-venous access. *Nephrol Dial Transplant*, Vol. 20, (2005), pp. 1686-1692

Paneni, F.; Gregori, M.; Ciavarella, G.M.; Sciarretta, S.; De Biase, L.; Marino, L.; Tocci, G.; Principe, F.; Domenici, A.; Luciani, R.; Punzo, G.; Menè, P. & Volpe, M. (2010).

Right ventricular dysfunction in patients with end-stage renal disease. *Am J Nephrol*, Vol. 32, pp. 432-438

Ramasubbu, K.; Deswal, A.; Herderjugen, C.; Aguilar, D. & Frost, A.E. (2010). A prospective echocardiographic evaluation of pulmonary hypertension in chronic hemodialysis patients in the United States: prevalence and significance. *International Journal of General Medicine*, Vol. 3, pp. 279-286

Ünal, A.; Sipahioglu, M.; Oguz, F.; Kaya, M.; Tokgoz, B.; Buyukoglan, H.; Oymak, O. & Utaz, C. (2009). Pulmonary hypertension in peritoneal dialysis patients: prevalence and risk factors. *Perit Dial Int*, Vol. 29, pp. 191-198

Ünal, A.; Tasdemir, K.; Oymak, S.; Duran, M.; Kocyigit, I.; Oguz, F.; Tokgoz, B.; Sipahioglu, M.H.; Utas, C. & Oymak, O. (2010). The long-term effects of arteriovenous fistula creation on the development of pulmonary hypertension in hemodialysis patients. *Hemodialysis International*, Vol. 14, pp. 398-402

Yigla, M.; Nakhoul, F.; Sabag, A.; Tov, N.; Gorevich, B., Abassi, Z. & Reisner, S.A. (2003). Pulmonary hypertension in patients with end-stage renal disease. *Chest*, Vol. 123, N°5, pp. 1577-1582

Yigla, M.; Keidar, Z.; Safadi, I.; Tov, N:, Reisner, S.A. & Nakhoul, F. (2004). Pulmonary calcification in hemodialysis patients: correlation with pulmonary artery pressure. *Kidney International*, Vol. 66, (2004), pp. 806-810

Yigla, M.; Fruchter, O.; Aharonson, D.; Yanay, N.; Reisner, S.A.; Lewin, M. & Nakhoul F. (2009). Pulmonary hypertension is an independent predictor of mortality in hemodialysis patients. *Kidney Int*, Vol. 75, pp. 969-975

Yu, T.M.; Chen Y.H.; Hsu, J.Y.; Sun, C.S.; Chuang, Y.W.; Chen, C.H.; Wu, M.J.; Cheng, C.H. & Shu, K.S. (2009). Systemic inflammation is associated with pulmonary hypertension in patients undergoing haemodialysis. *Nephrol Dial Transplant*, Vol. 24, pp. 1946-1951

Zlotnick, D.M.; Axelrod, D.A.; Chobanian, M.C.; Friedman, S.; Brown, J.; Catherwood, E. & Costa, S.P. (2010). Non-invasive detection of pulmonary hypertension prior to renal transplantation is a predictor of increased risk for early graft dysfunction. *Nephrol Dial Transplant*, Vol 25, pp. 3090-3096

Part 5

Special Considerations in Evaluation and Management of Pulmonary Hypertension

15

Pregnancy and Pulmonary Arterial Hypertension

Jean M. Elwing and Ralph J. Panos
Pulmonary, Critical Care, and Sleep Division, Department of Internal Medicine
University of Cincinnati, School of Medicine
Cincinnati Veterans Administration Hospital
Cincinnati, OH,
USA

1. Introduction

Pregnancy in women with pulmonary arterial hypertension (PAH) due to defined or unknown causes is associated with greatly increased maternal morbidity. Significant respiratory, cardiac, and hematologic adaptations occur during pregnancy that may exacerbate the hemodynamic consequences of PAH and may precipitate malignant dysrhythmias and acute right ventricular overload and failure. Because of these potentially fatal consequences, the European Society of Cardiology and the American College of Cardiology/American Heart Association dissuade conception in women with PAH and recommend termination should pregnancy occur (Oakley 2003). Recent reviews suggest that significant progress has been achieved in the treatment and management of PAH during pregnancy (Bedard 2009). From 1978 to 1996 the overall maternal mortality rate was 38% and declined to 25% from 1997 to 2007 (Bedard 2009). Despite this improvement, mortality rates remain significantly elevated and the consideration of pregnancy in women with PAH should be thoroughly reviewed and discussed prior to conception (Roberts 1990) and, for those women with PAH who become pregnant or are diagnosed with PAH during pregnancy, a multidisciplinary management team with expertise in high risk pregnancy, maternal-fetal medicine, and pulmonary hypertension is warranted (Kiely 2010).

In this chapter, we will review the maternal physiological changes that occur during pregnancy and their effects on pulmonary vascular and cardiac function, physical examination findings and diagnostic studies of PAH during pregnancy, the epidemiology and outcomes of pregnancy in women with PAH, and current pharmacologic and management strategies for the treatment of these patients.

2. Physiologic changes during pregnancy (Table 1)

2.1 Respiratory

Profound changes in respiratory physiology occur during pregnancy. Basal oxygen consumption increases by 50 ml/min by term (Thornberg 2000). This increased oxygen demand is met by augmentation of minute ventilation. Alveolar ventilation increases due to progesterone, effects of reduced osmolality, increased angiotensin II and vasopressin (Thornberg 2000). The elevation in alveolar ventilation is caused primarily by a 25-40% increase in tidal volume (Fujitani 2005) and produces a fall in alveolar P_{CO2} from 38 torr to 30 torr at term (Thornberg 2000). The total lung capacity may decline slightly but does not change significantly during pregnancy. In contrast, functional residual capacity declines by 20-30% due to elevation of the diaphragm by the gravid uterus, reduced downward pull by the abdomen, and alterations in the chest wall that diminish outward recoil (Hegewald 2011).

Pulmonary	
Total Lung Capacity	Same to slightly decreased <5%
Functional Residual Capacity	Decreases 20-30% (200-300 ml)
Residual Volume	Decreases 20-25% (200-400 ml)
Inspiratory Capacity	Increases 5-10% (200-350 ml)
Cardiovascular	
Blood volume	Increases 50%
Systemic vascular resistance	Decreases 20%
Pulmonary vascular resistance	Decreases 25%
Systolic blood pressure	Decreases 5-10 mm Hg
Diastolic blood pressure	Decreases 10-15 mm Hg
Heart rate	Increases 10-15 bpm
Stroke volume	Increases
Cardiac output	Increases 30-50%
Left ventricular ejection fraction	Increases
Central venous pressure	Same
Pulmonary pressures	Same
Hematologic	
Levels of factors II, V, VII, VIII, IX, X, XII, fibrinogen and von Willebrand factor	Increase
Protein S activity	Declines
Resistance to activated protein C	Increases
Circulating prothrombin fragments (PF1+2), thrombin-antithrombin complexes, microparticles	Increase

(adapted from Hegewald 2011, Hameed 2007)

Table 1. Physiologic Changes during Pregnancy

2.2 Pulmonary vasculature

Blood volume expands up to 40% by term (Thornberg 2000) and most of the increase is due to plasma volume increases (Madden 2009). In addition, the red cell mass enlarges by 30% (Thornberg 2000). Cardiac output (CO) increases by more than 50% by mid-third trimester due to augmentation of stroke volume, quickened heart rate, reduced afterload, and increased left ventricular (LV) outflow area (Thornberg 2000, Capeless 1989, Duvekot 1994, Mashini 1987, Vered 1991). Heart rate accelerates gradually throughout gestation whereas engorgement of stroke volume (SV) stabilizes by 20 weeks (Atkins 1981). SV increases due to cardiac remodeling with enlargement of all four chambers, elevation in end diastolic volume, and maintenance of ejection fraction (Thornberg 2000, Fujitani 2005). Cross sectional echocardiographic studies of left ventricular mass and function demonstrate a greater than 50% increase in LV mass during pregnancy; LV diastolic function also increases during the first two trimesters but then declines during the last trimester (Kametas 2001). Despite the elevated CO, systolic and diastolic arterial blood pressure decline and pulse pressure widens slightly during pregnancy. With the increase in CO and decrease in blood pressure, peripheral vascular resistance declines over the first trimester and remains low for the remainder of pregnancy without further reduction. Aortic diameter and compliance, venous capacitance, and blood volume all increase (Thornberg 2000).

Although pulmonary blood flow increases dramatically during pregnancy, a reduction in pulmonary vascular resistance (PVR) maintains pulmonary arterial pressure (PAP) constant throughout pregnancy. Serial pulsed Doppler echocardiographic studies of 13 women during pregnancy demonstrated the mean PAP before pregnancy was 13.8 mm Hg and did not change throughout pregnancy; however, pulmonary blood flow increased from 4.88 to 7.19 L/min during pregnancy with a decline in pulmonary vascular resistance from 2.85 to 2.17 resistance units. PVR returned to normal by 6 months post partum. (Robson 1991)

CO may increase by 25-30% during the second stage of labor due to uterine contractions and by up to 80% immediately post partum due to autotransfusion of blood from the uterus to the systemic circulation (Madden 2009). Postpartum, heart rate, systemic vascular resistance, and cardiac output decrease and cardiac enlargement begins to regress. Blood volume normalizes quickly and hemodynamic parameters including cardiac output, stroke volume, ventricular volume, myocardial contractility, and pulmonary and systemic vascular resistance return to pre-pregnancy levels over several weeks whereas cardiac remodeling occurs over several months (Weiss 2000, Capeless 1991, Duvekot 1994).

2.3 Hematologic

There is a significant increase in procoagulant activity during pregnancy due to increases in clotting factor concentrations and decreases in quantity and activity of physiological anticoagulants (Brenner 2004). The levels of factors II, V, VII, VIII, IX, X, XII, fibrinogen and von Willebrand factor increase whereas protein S activity declines and resistance to activated protein C develops (Brenner 2004, Montavon 2008). There are also increases in circulating prothrombin fragments (PF1+2) and thrombin-antithrombin complexes. Microparticles shed from the cell membranes of maternal endothelial cells and platelets are also associated with enhanced thrombosis. Throughout pregnancy, the risk of venous thrombosis is increased 4-10 fold and is 3-4 fold higher post partum compared with pregnancy (Brenner 2004, Montavon 2008). The platelet count generally decreases during pregnancy because of hemodilution and increased destruction (Thornton 2010). In women with pre-existing PAH, these hematologic changes may predispose to *in situ* thrombosis within the already deranged pulmonary vasculature exacerbating elevations in pulmonary vascular resistance and precipitating right ventricular strain and potentially failure.

3. History and physical examination

3.1 History

Cardiopulmonary symptoms are common throughout pregnancy. Progressive fatigue, weariness, and breathlessness frequently occur during pregnancy. Palpitations related to tachycardia are often experienced. Other common symptoms of pregnancy include pedal edema, fatigue, and reduced exercise tolerance (Hameed 2007). Supine hypotension may occur in up to 10% of pregnant women and may cause lightheadedness, dizziness, and occasionally syncope (Hameed 2007). The symptoms of PAH are very similar and may include exertional breathlessness or syncope, fatigue, dizziness, lower extremity edema, palpitations, chest discomfort, and tachycardia. The strong similarity between the clinical manifestations of normal pregnancy and the symptoms of PAH confound the recognition and diagnosis of PAH during pregnancy.

A careful clinical history helps to identify or exclude recognized causes of PAH. A thorough medication history including prior use of anorexigens or chemotherapeutic agents should be elicited (Rubin 2005). Serologies can establish prior exposures to HIV and hepatitis B and C. A history of prior or familial thrombosis should prompt consideration of chronic thrombo-embolic disease. Other pulmonary processes such as concurrent interstitial lung disease should be pursued with imaging studies such as high resolution chest computed tomography and pulmonary function testing. A thorough history of skin, joint, and muscle symptoms as well as serologic testing can determine the presence of a concurrent connective tissue disorder. A careful history and evaluation for congenital and acquired cardiac disorders should be considered because many women with PAH during pregnancy have known or undiagnosed cardiac disease.

3.2 Physical examination

Cardiac auscultatory changes are present in over 90% of pregnant women and are usually physiologic flow murmurs caused by cardiac dilation, increased blood volume, and elevated cardiac output. Tricuspid or pulmonic regurgitation occurs in over 90% of pregnant women and 28% have echocardiographic evidence of mitral regurgitation (Hameed 2007). Pregnancy-associated flow murmurs frequently occur during mid-systole and are present at the left lower sternal border and pulmonic areas (Hurst 1958, O'Rourke 1970). In women with PAH, signs of right ventricle enlargement or overload may include the presence of a right ventricular lift, prominent P_2, right sided S_4 gallop, and the murmur of tricuspid regurgitation. Tricuspid valve insufficiency may be manifest by elevated jugular venous pressure, hepatojugular reflux, and a pulsatile liver. Thus, the cardiac findings of normal pregnancy and PAH are very similar and the lack of distinguishing clinical features may delay further studies to diagnose the presence of elevated pulmonary pressures.

3.3 Electrocardiogram

PAH may cause right ventricular hypertrophy or strain which can be detected by electrocardiographic changes. The electrocardiographic manifestations of cor pulmonale are relatively specific, 86%, but not sensitive, 51%, for PAH and do not correlate with the severity of PAH (Oswald-Mammosser 1987; Himelman 1988). Electrocardiographic features that suggest PAH include: A) P pulmonale, P-wave amplitude > 2.5 mm in leads II, III, and/or aVF; B) S_1, S_2, S_3 pattern; C) an $S_1 Q_3$ pattern; D) incomplete or complete right bundle branch block; E) evidence of RVH: R axis deviation $\geq 100°$, dominant R wave in lead $V_1 \geq 7$ mm in amplitude, ST segment depression and T wave inversion in leads V_1 to V_4, and deep S waves in leads V_5, V_6, I and aVL with a QRS duration < 0.12 s; and F) low voltage QRS (Barbera et al 2003; Harrigan and Jones 2002). Pregnancy is associated with electrocardiographic changes that may obfuscate the electrocardiographic recognition of PAH: A) left axis deviation; B) reduced QRS voltage; C) T-wave inversion in lead III; D) Q-waves and inverted P-waves in lead III that may normalize with inspiration; E) sinus tachycardia; F) presence of premature atrial and ventricular beats; and G) other dysrhythmias (Hameed 2007). Thus, pregnancy-associated changes in the electrocardiogram may obscure the electrocardiographic manifestations of PAH, delaying or thwarting its recognition and diagnosis.

4. Effects of normal pregnancy related vascular changes on pre-existing PAH

PAH is associated with increased PAP due to elevated PVR caused by vascular remodeling and local thrombus formation that can produce cor pulmonale and RV failure. Individuals with pre-existing PAH have difficulty tolerating the physiologic changes of pregnancy especially the elevation of heart rate and circulating blood volume. CO may have been reduced by increased PVR and the right ventricle may not be able to increase output due to the elevated afterload. The subsequent decrease in left ventricular preload may further accentuate the decline in systemic blood pressure due to an inability to compensate for the reduction in SVR that occurs during pregnancy. The fixed pulmonary vasculature of PAH may preclude or attenuate the physiologic decline in PVR that occurs during pregnancy to accommodate the increase in pulmonary blood volume and flow. Any augmentation of PVR (due to *in situ* or metastatic pulmonary vascular thrombosis, hypoxemia, acidosis, or hypercarbia) increases RV work and may trigger pulmonary hypertensive crisis, RV failure, acute reduction in LV preload, and precipitous reduction in systemic blood pressure (Warnes 2004, Madden 2009).

Pregnancy-related physiologic changes in coagulation may accentuate *in situ* thrombosis within the pulmonary vasculature or pulmonary emboli that may further impede pulmonary blood flow and precipitate a critical reduction in RV function and systemic hypotension (Madden 2009).

Diagnosis of unrecognized PAH during pregnancy may be difficult as many of the cardiac changes of pregnancy may mask or mimic the findings of PAH. The presence of PAH may be manifest by signs and symptoms of right heart failure, PAH crisis with acute RV failure, dysrhythmias, and pulmonary thromboembolic disease. Exertional breathlessness out of proportion to that expected during pregnancy may be the sole symptom of PAH. The differential diagnosis includes pre-existing cardiac abnormalities, patent foramen ovale, asthma, peripartum cardiomyopathy, and thromboembolic disease.

5. Screening for PAH before or during pregnancy

A retrospective review of 27 patients undergoing echocardiography and right heart catheterization (RHC) during pregnancy from 1990 to 2000 showed that echocardiography significantly over-estimated the presence and severity of PAH (Penning 2001). Over three quarters of these patients had structural heart defects and most were due to congenital cardiac disease. Nearly one third of patients with PAH estimated by echocardiography had normal pressures at the time of RHC. This overestimation of the presence of PAH by echocardiography may be due to the methodology used to calculate PAP: the gradient between the right atrium and right ventricle was determined using the modified Bernoulli equation, $4v^2$, and the right atrial pressure was estimated from the degree of collapse of the inferior vena cava (IVC) during inspiration (Hemnes 2009). However, the increase in blood volume during pregnancy may reduce respiratory variation in IVC diameter and lead to overestimation of right atrial (RA) pressure causing the calculated PAP to be falsely elevated. The average sPAP (systolic PAP) determined echocardiographically was 59.6 mm Hg but was only 54.8 when measured hemodynamically ($p<0.005$). In another study of 18 patients undergoing RHC and echocardiography, one third of patients diagnosed with PAH by echocardiography had normal pressures on RHC. Although the echocardiographically estimated sPAP was 66.3 mm Hg and the average sPAP measured at RHC was 62.7 mm Hg, the two measurements correlated significantly. These studies show that Doppler echocardiography is not specific for the determination of PAH and up to one third of individuals with elevated PAP's by echocardiography may have normal pulmonary pressures measured by RHC. Thus, invasive hemodynamic measurement is essential for the diagnosis and subsequent management of PAH during pregnancy.

6. Preconception counseling

6.1 Clinical outcomes: Morbidity and mortality-maternal and fetus

In a systemic review of 73 pregnant women with PAH from 1997 to 2007, 29 (40%) had idiopathic PAH, 29 (40%) had PAH associated with congenital heart disease, and 15 (21%) had other causes of PAH (Bedard 2009). The diagnosis of idiopathic PAH was known prior to pregnancy in only 45% of the women, whereas over 75% of women with other causes of PAH were known to have PAH prior to conception. Of those with idiopathic PAH, the mortality rate was 17%, 2 died during pregnancy and 3 died post partum. The causes of death included refractory right heart failure, circulatory collapse, and PAH crisis. Of those with PAH associated with congenital heart disease, 8 (28%) died during the post partum period due to right heart failure, pulmonary thromboembolism (PTE), cardiac arrest, PAH crisis, and bacterial endocarditis. Five patients (33%) with other causes of PAH died, 1 during pregnancy and 4 post partum. Right heart failure and PTE were the major causes of death. Neonatal or fetal death occurred in 9.6% and premature delivery occurred in nearly all pregnancies.

7. Management of pulmonary hypertension during pregnancy

7.1 General medical management

Currently, there are no clear consensus guidelines for the management of PAH in pregnancy; however, several case series have been published in the last two decades that provide guidance for the evaluation, treatment, and monitoring of this high risk patient group. If PAH is suspected, a thorough evaluation should ensue. RHC is required for definitive confirmation of the diagnosis of PAH as well as the assessment of disease severity (McLaughlin 2009). A multidisciplinary team approach to the care of PAH in pregnancy has been utilized successfully (Garabedian 2010). This approach is associated with improved survival compared with historical data (Kiely 2010, Smedstad 1994). The multidisciplinary team includes physicians and staff with expertise in pulmonary vascular disease, hematology, maternal-fetal medicine, high risk obstetrics, and obstetric anesthesia.

The pharmacotherapeutic management of PAH requires a multifaceted approach with the goal of lowering RV afterload by reducing pulmonary vascular resistance, prevention of thromboembolism, optimization of RV preload, and maintainence of RV inotropy. Initial pharmacologic management utilizes pulmonary vasodilators to reduce RV afterload. Several pulmonary vasodilators are currently approved for the medical management of PAH; however, all therapeutic options for PAH are not advisable for use in patients during pregnancy because of the teratogenicity of selected agents. (Figure 1)

7.2 PAH specific therapy with pulmonary vasodilators

PAH occurs due to an imbalance of pulmonary vasodilatory and constrictor mediators in the pulmonary vasculature causing vasoconstriction, remodeling of the pulmonary vessel wall, and thrombosis *in situ* (Voelkel 1997). Aberrations of many physiologic pathways likely contribute to these pulmonary vascular changes and the subsequent development of pulmonary hypertension. Three of these pathways are targets for currently approved PAH therapies and include the endothelin, prostacyclin, and nitric oxide pathways (Humbert 2004).

Endothelin is a potent pulmonary vasoconstrictor (Yanisagawa 1988). Endothelin receptor antagonists (ERAs) improve outcomes in non-pregnant pulmonary arterial hypertension patients (Rubin 2002, Galiè 2008); however, the use of ERAs is not recommended for treatment of PAH in pregnancy because of their known teratogenicity (pregnancy risk category X).

Prostacyclin is a potent pulmonary vasodilator with anti-proliferative (Clapp 2002) and anti-thrombotic effects (Moncada 1976). The prostacyclin analog, epoprostenol, was the first available PAH specific therapy and has been shown to improve functionality, pulmonary hemodynamics, and survival in non-pregnant PAH patients (Barst 1996). Epoprostenol is the most frequently reported treatment for PAH in pregnancy (Bédard 2009). Epoprostenol is classified as a pregnancy risk category B drug and has not been associated with fetal abnormalities in recent literature reviews (Stewart 2001, Bédard 2009, Kiely 2010). More recently approved prostacyclin analogues include treprostinil and iloprost. Treprostinil carries a pregnancy category B risk classification with limited data regarding safety data in pregnancy. Iloprost has been shown to be associated with adverse fetal effects in animals (pregnancy risk category C) but has been used successfully without adverse human fetal effects in a series of 9 patients (Kiely 2010).

Nitric oxide is a known pulmonary vasodilator (Pepke-Zaba 1991). The nitric oxide pathway can be targeted for the treatment of pulmonary hypertension by exogenous delivery of nitric oxide or augmentation of nitric oxide dependent cyclic GMP mediated pulmonary vasodilatation by inhibiting the breakdown of cyclic GMP by phosphodiesterase type 5 (PDEI-5) (Humbert 2004). Phosphodiesterase inhibition with sildenafil has been used to treat

PAH in pregnancy with no reported complications (Goland 2010, Kiely 2010). The currently approved PDEI-5s for the treatment of PAH are pregnancy risk category B.

Over the last two decades, multiple clinical series and case reports have described outcomes and management of PAH in pregnancy. A systematic review of the published literature from 1997 to 2007 found 47 case reports with a total of 73 parturients affected by PAH (Bédard 2009). Advanced PAH therapies were utilized in 72% of the reported patients. Prostacyclin analogues were the most commonly used form of PAH therapy. In patients with idiopathic PAH treated with epoprostenol, the mortality rate was 20% (Bédard 2009). Overall mortality in PAH patients managed from 1978-96 compared with patients managed from 1997-2007 has improved. Mortality has decreased in patients with idiopathic PAH (30% to 17%), congenital heart disease associated PAH (36% to 28%) and other forms of precapillary PAH (56% to 33%) in the modern era (P = 0.047) (Bédard 2009).

Prior to the initiation of pharmacologic treatment, detailed discussion of the risks and benefits of the various therapeutic options should be undertaken. Based upon the current available literature, initiation of a prostacyclin with careful upward titration of the dose as tolerated is advisable (Bédard 2009, Kiely 2010, Garabedian 2010). The addition of oral sildenafil has been used successfully in the past and could be considered adjunctive therapy (Goland 2010, Kiely 2010).

7.3 Maternal and fetal monitoring

The optimal monitoring strategy for PAH in pregnancy is unclear at the present time. Initial evaluation and commencement of PAH therapy, i.e. prostacyclin, likely will require observation in the inpatient setting or prolonged intense monitoring as an outpatient. Subsequently, close outpatient monitoring may be considered in the appropriate patient. Successful outpatient monitoring has been reported in a series of 9 women with PAH during 10 pregnancies managed at a quaternary care hospital in the United Kingdom (Kiely 2010). These patients were evaluated in the outpatient setting every 4 weeks until week 28 gestation followed by every 2 weeks until week 30 gestation and then weekly until 24 hours prior to scheduled delivery unless clinical worsening occurred that required hospitalization. Each outpatient assessment included a history, examination, routine laboratory assessment, electrocardiogram, and an exercise tolerance assessment. Maternal cardiac echocardiogram was repeated if clinically indicated (Kiely 2010). Once hospitalized, continuous monitoring of maternal heart rate and oxygen saturation was performed in all patients. Repeat right heart catheterization remains debatable and is not universally utilized during pregnancy for evaluation of clinical worsening and/or at the time of delivery (Kiely 2010, Bonnin 2005).

In a systematic review of outcomes in PAH in pregnancy from 1978-1996 the overall neonatal survival ranged from 87% to 89% (Weiss 1998). Fetal monitoring and ultrasound biometry (Garabedian 2010, Kiely 2010) often is utilized to monitor fetal growth and development. If a fetal abnormality or growth restriction is suspected, further assessment is employed to guide management (Kiely 2010).

7.4 Thromboprophylaxis

Pregnancy is a hypercoagulable state (Brenner 2004) associated with an increased risk of thromboembolic disease. Currently, there is no standard thromboprophylaxis regimen recommended in PAH patients during pregnancy prior to delivery. Anticoagulation risks and benefits should be assessed on an individual basis and may not be well tolerated in select patient groups such as those with Eisenmenger's Syndrome (Pitts 1977) or other bleeding diatheses. Warfarin use is contraindicated in pregnancy due to its known teratogenicity (pregnancy risk category X.) Both unfractionated heparin (Bédard 2009) and low molecular weight heparin (LMWH) (Kiely 2010, Goland 2010, Garabedian 2010) have been successfully used for thromboprophylaxis and treatment in pregnant PAH patients. If full dose anticoagulation is chosen, transition to prophylactic dosing should occur prior to delivery and may be resumed after delivery if there is no contraindication (Kiely 2010).

7.5 Maintenance of optimal preload and management of anemia

Volume status should be monitored closely and maintenance of euvolemia should be attempted (Piazza 2005). Diuretic therapy may be necessary (Bédard 2009) but should be used with caution during the peripartum period when patients are at risk for rapid volume shifts and acute hemorrhagic anemia. If acute hemorrhage occurs, addressing the underlying cause and resuscitation is paramount to maintain hemodynamic stability (Krasuski 2004). If induction of labor is required, oxytocin, prostaglandin $F_{2\alpha}$ should be infused slowly and intravenous boluses avoided because they may induce pulmonary vasoconstriction (Dagher 1993, Pinder 2002) which would be poorly tolerated.

7.6 Inotropic support

The third trimester of pregnancy, labor, and delivery are associated with a marked increase in cardiac work (Madden 2009). In women with PAH, the already taxed RV may not be able to meet these demands. Management of RV failure in this setting may require urgent delivery, dose escalation of pulmonary vasodilators to reduce RV afterload, and possibly direct inotropic support (Piazza 2005).

8. Timing of labor and mode of delivery

Timing of delivery is usually based upon the maternal and fetal tolerance of pregnancy. The risk for maternal deterioration increases as pregnancy progresses and is greatest after the majority of pregnancy-induced hemodynamic changes have occurred (approximately the 20th to 24th week of gestation) (Cheek 2001). Frequently, delivery is preterm either due to maternal worsening or planned delivery at 32-34 weeks gestation (Bédard 2009, Kiely 2010).

The optimal mode of labor and delivery remains unclear in patients with PAH and should be tailored to fit the individual patient's needs. A review of 15 consecutive pregnancies in women with PAH managed at a referral center in France from 1992 - 2002 revealed an overall mortality of 36% and there was not a clear survival advantage associated with any particular mode of delivery. Scheduled cesarean section delivery with regional anesthesia via epidural or spinal-epidural is reported as the preferred delivery mode in two series. The advantages of this approach are daytime scheduling and avoidance of marked hemodynamic changes that may occur with vaginal delivery and general anesthesia (Bonnin

2005, Kiely 2010). Regional anesthesia with cesarean section has been used successfully in several other reported cases (Bédard 2009, Khan 1996, Stewart 2001, Goland 2010). If epidural or spinal-epidural anesthesia is chosen, incrementally increasing epidural anesthesia is advocated to avoid rapid hemodynamic changes (Smedstad 1994). Additionally, the use of bolus spinal anesthesia is not recommended due to the potential for hemodynamic compromise.

Vaginal delivery without epidural anesthesia may not be well tolerated as it is associated with dramatic increases in cardiac work due to 12% increases in cardiac output in the first stages of labor and 34% in advanced labor at full cervical dilatation (Hunter 1992). If vaginal delivery is the chosen mode, epidural anesthesia with low-dose analgesia is recommended to reduce the adverse hemodynamic demands of labor (Slomka 1988, Smedstad 1994). Furthermore, if oxytocin, prostaglandin $F_{2\alpha}$, is used to induce labor it should be infused slowly to prevent the negative hemodynamic consequences caused by its pulmonary vasoconstrictive properties (Slomka 1988).

General anesthesia has been used successfully in the delivery of patients with PAH (Garabedian 2010, Bonnin 2005); however, general anesthesia may be associated with pulmonary vasoconstriction and other adverse hemodynamic changes associated with mechanical ventilation that may be deleterious in this patient population (Blaise 2003).

9. Post partum management

The postpartum period is the most critical time for pregnant PAH patients because the risk of morbidity and mortality is greatest due to a marked increase in pulmonary vascular resistance and cardiac output (Madden 2009). The majority of these hemodynamic alterations resolve in the first 2 weeks after delivery with complete normalization over the next 6 months (Cheek 2001). Monitoring post partum patients with PAH in a critical care setting is advocated for at least several days (Bonnin 2005) to a week (Kiely 2010) after delivery to ensure continued stability. Close monitoring with further escalation of pulmonary vasodilators, addition of inotropic support, and packed red blood cell transfusions may be required during this vulnerable time. The use of full dose anticoagulation is widely utilized in the post partum period and initiated 12-24 hours post partum based on the mode of delivery if there is no contraindication (James 2006).

Once the patient with PAH has been monitored and durable hemodynamic stability achieved postpartum, she can be maintained on appropriate PAH therapies (McLaughlin 2009) and discharged from the hospital with continued management in the outpatient setting (Kiely 2010).

10. Summary

Despite moderate advances in the management of PAH, pregnancy with concurrent PAH remains extremely high risk with significant morbidity and mortality (Bonnin 2005). Counseling regarding risks of pregnancy and early termination remain the recommended interventions. If a woman with PAH chooses to proceed with pregnancy, a detailed discussion of risks should be undertaken. Thorough evaluation and management utilizing a multi-professional team (Kiely 2010, Smedstad 1994) and full diagnostic assessment of PAH is recommended.

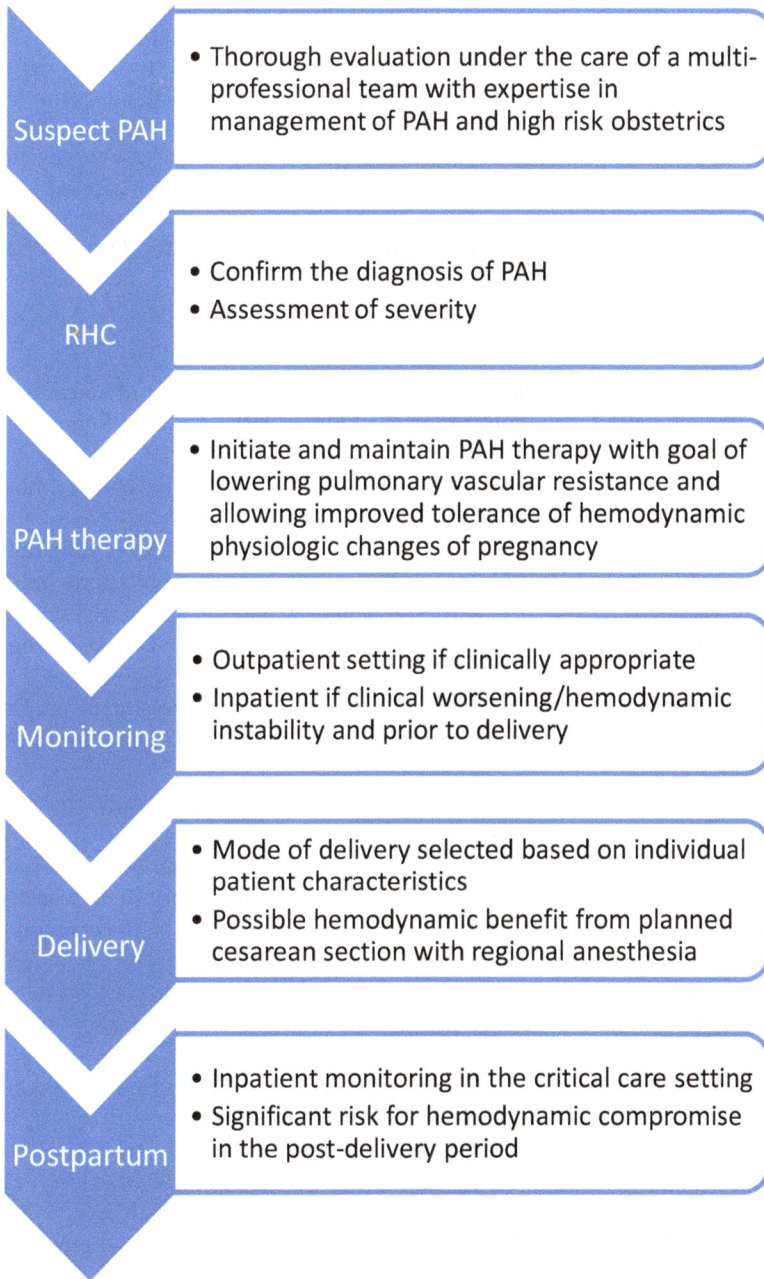

Fig. 1. Right heart catheterization (RHC), Pulmonary arterial hypertension (PAH)

PAH therapy should be initiated and gradually increased to maintain hemodynamic stability. Inpatient monitoring is recommended in cases of worsening and prior to scheduled delivery (Kiely 2010). The optimal mode of delivery is not clear at this time but scheduled cesarean section with regional anesthesia has been used successfully in multiple case reports (Bédard 2009, Khan 1996, Stewart 2001, Goland 2010). The post partum period is the most critical time for worsening and death because of the rapid reversal of the physiologic hemodynamic changes of pregnancy. As these alterations resolve, post partum patients with PAH should be monitored in a critical care setting for several days to a week after delivery and supported medically. After discharge, continued close monitoring is recommended as women with PAH are at risk for decompensation for several months after delivery.

11. References

Atkins AF, Watt JM, Milan P, Davies P, Crawford JS. A longitudinal study ofcardiovascular dynamic changes throughout pregnancy. Eur J Obstet Gynecol Reprod Biol. 1981 Oct;12(4):215-24.

Barbera JA, Peinado VI, Santos S. Pulmonary hypertension in chronic obstructive pulmonary disease. Eur Respir J. 2003 May; 21:892-905.

Barst RJ, Rubin LJ, Long WA, McGoon MD, Rich S, Badesch DB, Groves BM, Tapson VF, Bourge RC, Brundage BH, et al. A comparison of continuous intravenous epoprostenol (prostacyclin) with conventional therapy for primary pulmonary hypertension. The Primary Pulmonary Hypertension Study Group. N Engl J Med. 1996 Feb 1;334(5):296-302.

Bédard E, Dimopoulos K, Gatzoulis MA. Has there been any progress made on pregnancy outcomes among women with pulmonary arterial hypertension? Eur Heart J.2009 Feb;30(3):256-65.

Blaise G, Langleben D, Hubert B: Pulmonary arterial hypertension: Pathophysiology and anesthetic approach. Anesthesiology 2003; 99:1415-32.

Bonnin M, Mercier FJ, Sitbon O, Roger-Christoph S, Jaïs X, Humbert M, Audibert F, Frydman R, Simonneau G, Benhamou D. Severe pulmonary hypertension during pregnancy: mode of delivery and anesthetic management of 15 consecutive cases. Anesthesiology. 2005 Jun;102(6):1133-7; discussion 5A-6A.

Brenner B. Haemostatic changes in pregnancy. Thromb Res. 2004; 114(5-6):409-14.

Capeless EL, Clapp JF. Cardiovascular changes in early phase of pregnancy. Am J Obstet Gynecol. 1989 Dec;161(6 Pt 1):1449-53.

Capeless EL, Clapp JF. When do cardiovascular parameters return to their preconception values? Am J Obstet Gynecol. 1991 Oct;165(4 Pt 1):883-6.

Cheek TG, Gutsche BB. Maternal physiologic alteration during pregnancy, Shnider and Levinson's Anesthesia for Obstetrics. Edited by Hugues SC, Levinson G, Rosen MA. Philadelphia, Lippincott Williams & Wilkins, 2001, pp 3–18.

Clapp LH, Finney P, Turcato S, Tran S, Rubin LJ, Tinker A. Differential effects of stable prostacyclin analogues on smooth muscle proliferation and cyclic AMP generation in human pulmonary artery. Am J Respir Cell Mol Biol 2002;26:194-201.

Dagher E, Dumont L, Chartrand C, Blaise G: Effects of PGE1 in experimental vasoconstrictive pulmonary hypertension. Eur Surg Res 1993; 25:65–73.

Duvekot JJ, Peeters LL. Maternal cardiovascular hemodynamic adaptation to pregnancy. Obstet Gynecol Surv. 1994 Dec;49(12 Suppl):S1-14.

Fujitani S, Baldisseri MR. Hemodynamic assessment in a pregnant and peripartum patient. Crit Care Med. 2005 Oct;33(10 Suppl):S354-61.

Galiè N, Olschewski H, Oudiz RJ, Torres F, Frost A, Ghofrani HA, Badesch DB, McGoon MD, McLaughlin VV, Roecker EB, Gerber MJ, Dufton C, Wiens BL, Rubin LJ; Ambrisentan in Pulmonary Arterial Hypertension, Randomized, Double-Blind, Placebo-Controlled, Multicenter, Efficacy Studies (ARIES) Group. Ambrisentan for the treatment of pulmonary arterial hypertension: results of the ambrisentan in pulmonary arterial hypertension, randomized, double-blind, placebo-controlled, multicenter, efficacy (ARIES) study 1 and 2. Circulation. 2008 Jun 10;117(23):3010-9. Epub 2008 May 27.

Garabedian MJ, Hansen WF, Gianferrari EA, Lain KY, Fragneto RY, Campbell CL, Booth DC. Epoprostenol treatment for idiopathic pulmonary arterial hypertension in pregnancy. J Perinatol. 2010 Sep;30(9):628-31.

Goland S, Tsai F, Habib M, Janmohamed M, Goodwin TM, Elkayam U. Favorable outcome of pregnancy with an elective use of epoprostenol and sildenafil in women with severe pulmonary hypertension. Cardiology. 2010;115(3):205-8.

Hameed AB, Sklansky MS. Pregnancy: maternal and fetal heart disease. Curr Probl Cardiol. 2007 Aug;32(8):419-494.

Harrigan HA, Jones K. ABC of clinical electrocardiography: Conditions affecting the right side of the heart. BMJ 2002; 324:1201-1204.

Hegewald MJ, Crapo RO. Respiratory Physiology in Pregnancy. Clin Chest Med. 2011 32:1-13.

Hemnes AR, Forfia PR, Champion HC. Assessment of pulmonary vasculature and right heart by invasive haemodynamics and echocardiography. Int J Clin PractSuppl. 2009 Sep;(162):4-19.

Himelman RB, Struve SN, Brown JK, et al. Improved recognition of cor pulmonale in patients with severe chronic obstructive pulmonary disease. Amer J Med 1988; 84:891-898.

Humbert M, Sitbon O, Simonneau G. Treatment of pulmonary arterial hypertension. N Engl J Med. 2004 Sep 30;351(14):1425-36.

Hunter S, Robson SC. Adaptation of the maternal heart in pregnancy. Br Heart J. 1992 Dec;68(6):540-3. Review.

Hurst J, Staton J, Hubbard D. Precordial murmurs during pregnancy and lactation. N Engl J Med 1958; 259(11):515-517.

James AH, Abel DE, Brancazio LR. Anticoagulants in pregnancy. Obstet Gynecol Surv. 2006 Jan;61(1):59-69; quiz 70-72. Review.

Kametas NA, McAuliffe F, Hancock J, Chambers J, Nicolaides KH. Maternal left ventricular mass and diastolic function during pregnancy. Ultrasound Obstet Gynecol. 2001 Nov;18(5):460-6.

Khan MJ, Bhatt SB, Kryc JJ. Anesthetic considerations for parturients with primary pulmonary hypertension: review of the literature and clinical presentation. Int J Obstet Anesth. 1996 Jan;5(1):36-42.

Kiely DG, Condliffe R, Webster V, Mills GH, Wrench I, Gandhi SV, Selby K,Armstrong IJ, Martin L, Howarth ES, Bu'lock FA, Stewart P, Elliot CA. Improved survival in pregnancy and pulmonary hypertension using a multiprofessional approach. BJOG. 2010 Apr;117(5):565-74.

Krasuski R, Smith B, Wang A, et al. Anemia is a powerful independent predictor of mortality in patients with pulmonary hypertension. Circulation. 2004;110(17):III-559.

Madden BP. Pulmonary hypertension and pregnancy. Int J Obstet Anesth. 2009 Apr;18(2):156-64.

Mashini IS, Albazzaz SJ, Fadel HE, Abdulla AM, Hadi HA, Harp R, Devoe LD.Serial noninvasive evaluation of cardiovascular hemodynamics during pregnancy. AmJ Obstet Gynecol. 1987 May;156(5):1208-13.

McLaughlin VV, Archer SL, Badesch DB, Barst RJ, Farber HW, Lindner JR, Mathier MA, McGoon MD, Park MH, Rosenson RS, Rubin LJ, Tapson VF, Varga J. American College of Cardiology Foundation Task Force on Expert Consensus Documents; American Heart Association; American College of Chest Physicians; American Thoracic Society, Inc; Pulmonary Hypertension Association. J Am Coll Cardiol. 2009 Apr 28;53(17):1573-619.

Moncada S, Gryglewsli R, Bunting S,Vane JR. An enzyme isolated from arteries transforms prostaglandin endoperoxides to an unstable substance that inhibits platelet aggregation. Nature 1976;263:663-5.

Montavon C, Hoesli I, Holzgreve W, Tsakiris DA Thrombophilia and anticoagulation in pregnancy: indications, risks and management. J Matern Fetal Neonatal Med. 2008 Oct;21(10):685-96.

O'Rourke RA, Ewy GA, Marcus FI, et al. Cardiac auscultation in pregnancy. Med Ann Dist Columbia 1970; 39(2): 92-94.

Oakley C, Child A, Jung B, Presbitero P, Tornos P, Klein W, Alonso Garcia MA, Blomstrom-Lundqvist C, de Backer G, Dargie H, Deckers J, Flather M, Hradec J, Mazzotta G, Oto A, Parkhomenko A, Silber S, Torbicki A, Trappe HJ, Dean V, Poumeyrol-Jumeau D. Expert consensus document on management of cardio-vascular diseases during pregnancy. Eur Heart J 2003; 24:761-781.

Oswald-Mammosser M, Oswald T, Nyankiye E, et al. Non-invasive diagnosis of pulmonary hypertension in chronic obstructive pulmonary disease. Comparison of ECG, radiological measurements, echocardiography and myocardial scintigraphy. Eur J Respir Dis 1987; 71:419-429.

Penning S, Robinson KD, Major CA, Garite TJ. A comparison of echocardiography and pulmonary artery catheterization for evaluation of pulmonary artery pressures in pregnant patients with suspected pulmonary hypertension. Am J Obstet Gynecol. 2001 Jun;184(7):1568-70.

Pepke-Zaba J, Higenbottam TW, Dinh-Xuan AT, et al. Inhaled nitric oxide as a cause of selective pulmonary vasodilatation in pulmonary hypertension. Lancet 1991;338: 1173-4.

Piazza G, Goldhaber SZ. The Acutely Decompensated Right Ventricle: Pathways for Diagnosis and Management Chest 2005;128;1836-1852.

Pinder AJ, Dresner M, Calow C, Shorten GD, O'Riordan J, Johnson R: Haemodynamic changes caused by oxytocin during caesarean section under spinal anaesthesia. Int J Obstet Anesth 2002; 11:156–9.

Pitts JA, Crosby WM, Basta LL. Eisenmenger's syndrome in pregnancy: does heparin prophylaxis improve the maternal mortality rate? Am Heart J. 1977 Mar;93(3):321-6.

Roberts NV, Keast PJ. Pulmonary hypertension and pregnancy--a lethal combination. Anaesth Intensive Care. 1990 Aug;18(3):366-74. Review.

Robson SC, Hunter S, Boys RJ, Dunlop W. Serial changes in pulmonary haemodynamics during human pregnancy: a non-invasive study using Dopplerechocardiography. Clin Sci (Lond). 1991 Feb;80(2):113-7.

Rubin LJ, Badesch DB, Barst RJ, et al. Bosentan therapy for pulmonary arterial hypertension. N Engl J Med 2002;346:896-903.

Rubin LJ, Badesch DB. Evaluation and management of the patient with pulmonary arterial hypertension. Ann Intern Med. 2005 Aug 16;143(4):282-92.

Slomka F, Salmeron S, Zetlaoui P, Cohen H, Simonneau G, Samii K: Primary pulmonary hypertension and pregnancy: anesthetic management for delivery. Anesthesiology 1988; 69:959–61.

Smedstad KG, Cramb R, Morison DH. Pulmonary hypertension and pregnancy: A series of eight cases. Can J Anaesth 1994; 41:502–12.

Stewart R, Tuazon D, Olson G, Duarte AG. Pregnancy and primary pulmonary hypertension: successful outcome with epoprostenol therapy. Chest. 2001 Mar;119(3):973-5.

Thornburg KL, Jacobson SL, Giraud GD, Morton MJ. Hemodynamic changes in pregnancy. Semin Perinatol. 2000 Feb;24(1):11-4.

Thornton P, Douglas J. Coagulation in pregnancy. Best Pract Res Clin Obstet Gynaecol. 2010 Jun;24(3):339-52.

Vered Z, Poler SM, Gibson P, Wlody D, Pérez JE. Noninvasive detection of the morphologic and hemodynamic changes during normal pregnancy. Clin Cardiol. 1991Apr;14(4):327-34.

Voelkel NF, Tuder RM, Weir EK. Pathophysiology of primary pulmonary hypertension. In: Rubin L, Rich S, eds. Primary pulmonary hypertension. New York: Marcel Dekker, 1997:83-129.

Warnes CA. Pregnancy and pulmonary hypertension. Int J Cardiol. 2004 Dec;97 Suppl 1:11-3.

Weeks SK, Smith JB. Obstetric anaesthesia in patients with primary pulmonary hypertension. Can J Anaesth 1991; 38:814–6.

Weiss BM, Hess OM. Pulmonary vascular disease and pregnancy: current controversies, management strategies, and perspectives. Eur Heart J. 2000; 21(2):104-15.

Weiss BM, Zemp L, Seifert B, Hess OM: Outcome of pulmonary vascular disease in pregnancy: A systematic overview from 1978 through 1996. J Am Cardiol 1998; 31:1650-7.

Yanisagawa M, Kurihara H, Kimura S,et al. A novel potent vasoconstrictor peptide produced by vascular endothelial cells. Nature 1988;332:411-5.

16

Perioperative Management of Pulmonary Hypertension

Philip L. Kalarickal, Sabrina T. Bent,
Michael J. Yarborough, Kavitha A. Mathew and Charles Fox
Department of Anesthesiology, Tulane University School of Medicine, New Orleans, LA
United States of America

1. Introduction

Pulmonary hypertension is the manifestation of a disorder of the pulmonary vascular bed, which results in obstruction of pulmonary blood flow. Although many different causes exist, hypertension in the pulmonary circulation is the result of increased vascular resistance, increased vascular bed flow, or both. The signs and symptoms of pulmonary hypertension are nonspecific and subtle. Left untreated, patients will experience progressive symptoms of dyspnea and right heart failure culminating in a markedly curtailed survival [Gaine, 2000]. Idiopathic pulmonary arterial hypertension is a relatively rare disease of unknown cause [Lloyd et al, 1995]; however, in the perioperative arena the majority of patients encountered with pulmonary hypertension have acquired it secondary to a cardiac or a pulmonary disease process. Left sided ventricular or atrial disease and left sided valvular heart disease are common causes of pulmonary hypertension. Both of these conditions elevate left atrial pressure and passively increase pulmonary venous pressure, pulmonary artery pressure (PAP), and pulmonary vascular resistance (PVR). Multiple respiratory diseases lead to the development of pulmonary hypertension via a hypoxia-induced vasoconstriction [Phillips et al, 1999]. Regardless of causation, all pathways lead to an altered vascular endothelium and smooth muscle function through cellular remodeling [MacLean, 1999; Tuder et al, 2001]. This results in increased vascular contractility or lack of vascular relaxation in response to various endogenous vasodilator substances. Detailed discussion of the pathology, pathophysiology, evaluation and treatment are provided elsewhere in this text and via consensus statements from the American College of Cardiology/American Heart Association. [McLaughlin et al, 2009]

From a clinical anesthesia standpoint, although mild pulmonary hypertension rarely impacts anesthetic management, severe or moderate pulmonary hypertension can lead to acute right heart failure (RHF) and cardiogenic shock. The perioperative management of patients with pulmonary hypertension varies depending upon the pathological features present, functional clinical classification (Table 1), hemodynamics, and success of current medical therapy. This chapter will provided an overview of the pre-operative evaluation, intraoperative considerations, management strategies and postoperative considerations.

Class I	Class II	Class III	Class IV
Patients with pulmonary hypertension but without resulting limitation of physical activity Ordinary physical activity does not cause undue dyspnea or fatigue, chest pain or near syncope	Patients with pulmonary hypertension resulting in minimal limitation of physical activity These patients are comfortable at rest, but ordinary physical activity causes undue dyspnea or fatigue, chest pain or near syncope	Patients with pulmonary hypertension resulting in marked limitation of physical activity These patients have no discomfort at rest, but less than ordinary physical activity causes undue dyspnea or fatigue, chest pain or near syncope	Patients with pulmonary hypertension resulting in inability to perform any physical activity without symptoms These patients manifest signs of right heart failure Dyspnea and fatigue may be present at rest, and discomfort is increased by any physical activity

* Modified from the New York Heart Association classification of patients with cardiac disease.

Table 1. Functional Assessment of the patient with pulmonary hypertension.

2. Preoperative evaluation and preparation

Surgery for patients with pulmonary hypertension is associated with significant morbidity and mortality regardless of the anesthetic technique utilized [Krowka et al, 2004; Martin et al, 2002; Ramakrishna et al, 2005; Roberts & Keast 1990; Tan et al 2001; Weiss & Atanassoff, 1993]. For example, patients with Eisenmenger's syndrome undergoing cesarean section have had mortality reported as high as 70% [Kahn, 1993]. Although there is not an overabundance of literature regarding the development of postoperative pulmonary complications following noncardiac surgery, the few studies that do exist demonstrate the risk associated with procedures. Therefore, medical optimization is critical. During perioperative risk assessment, one should take into account the type of surgery, the patient's functional status, the severity of the pulmonary hypertension, the function of the right ventricle and any co-morbidities. Superficial procedures and non-orthopedic procedures will be associated with less hemodynamic and sympathetic nervous system perturbations than more invasive procedures. Orthopedic procedures with bony involvement can be quite stimulating for the patient and will increase the risk of increases in PVR and RV failure. Thoracic surgery is associated with changes in intrathoracic pressures, lung volumes and oxygenation, which may cause acute increases in PVR and decreased RV function [Ross AF et al., 2010]. Laparoscopic surgery requires pneumoperitoneum which may be poorly tolerated because it can decrease preload and increase afterload. Procedures associated with rapid blood loss may be poorly tolerated.

2.1 History and physical exam

Preoperative evaluation should include a thorough history and physical examination with special attention paid to signs and symptoms of right ventricular dysfunction. Symptoms are typically nonspecific with the most frequent being progressive dyspnea. The signs present depend on disease severity with dyspnea at rest, low cardiac output with metabolic acidosis, hypoxemia, evidence of right heart failure (large V wave on jugular vein, peripheral edema, hepatomegaly), and syncope being useful indicators [Blaise et al, 2003]. Laboratory studies should be directed according to the procedure that the patient is undergoing and the medication profile of the patient. Tests that should be strongly considered include electrocardiography, chest radiographs, echocardiography, and possibly right heart catheterization. In addition, depending on severity of the pulmonary hypertension, the following studies may also be useful, especially in the initial workup or depending on causes:

pulmonary function testing, arterial blood gas analysis, ventilation/perfusion scanning, pulmonary angiography, spiral computed tomography, serologic testing, and liver function testing. The ECG may demonstrate signs of right ventricular hypertrophy, such as tall right precordial R waves, right axis deviation and right ventricular strain [Nauser & Stites, 2001], but ECG changes alone cannot determine disease severity or prognosis [Ahearn et al, 2002; Bossone et al, 2002]. The chest radiograph may show evidence of right ventricular hypertrophy (decreased retrosternal space) or prominent pulmonary vasculature.

Among the myriad of available tests, echocardiography is the screening method of choice. Echocardiography may be useful to show right ventricular hypertrophy and to estimate pulmonary arterial pressure [Blaise et al, 2003]. Right heart catheterization is the gold standard for measuring pulmonary arterial pressures, however. Evidence of significant right ventricular dysfunction should prompt reevaluation of the need for surgery [Pearl, 2005]. All attempts to lower pulmonary arterial pressure should be done prior to surgery. Treatment options include oxygen, bronchodilators, vasodilators and inotropes. In addition to the careful evaluation of the patient's current therapeutic regimen for pulmonary hypertension, all other medications should be reviewed for possible interactions with others that may need to be instituted while under anesthesia. Likewise, it is important to maintain the patient's current therapeutic regimen as withdrawal of medications can lead to rebound pulmonary hypertension and RV dysfunction. Although medications such as inhaled prostacyclin (epoprostenol or Flolan®) are associated with impaired platelet aggregation, they have not been implicated in clinically significant bleeding. Due to the short half-life of this medication, epoprostenol should not be stopped at any time in the perioperative period. The anesthesiologist must ensure preoperative maximization of the patient's therapeutic options has been accomplished and coordinate, if needed, a strategy for continuance of chronic pulmonary hypertension therapy perioperatively.

2.2 Perioperative care team coordination

The major physiologic consideration for patients with pulmonary hypertension is the effect of increased PVR on right ventricular function. The induction and maintenance of general anesthesia coupled with positive pressure ventilation can cause dramatic hemodynamic effects in the patient with pulmonary arterial hypertension. These patients have an increased risk of developing significant cardiac dysfunction and have an increased risk of perioperative cardiovascular complications [Carmosino et al, 2007; Subramaniam & Yared, 2007]. Because of this, after preoperative data have been collected and reviewed, it is imperative that the anesthesiologist understands the causes and pathophysiology of the patient's disease so that a therapeutic perioperative regimen and anesthetic plan can be established. Although major advancements in treatment have prolonged survival and improved these patients' quality of life, no current therapy cures this disease. Depending on the severity and chronicity of the disease, the patient may or may not respond to vasodilator therapy. Owing to the complexity of most pulmonary hypertension treatment protocols, preoperative evaluation and optimization by the patient's primary pulmonary physician is desirable whenever possible. The perioperative medical treatment of this disease frequently involves a multidisciplinary (respiratory therapists, pharmacists, nurses, pulmonologist, anesthesiologist, surgeon, etc…) approach and, depending upon the level of specialization of your institution, coordination of these efforts could take considerable 'lead' time. Most patients with PHTN will be categorized as American Society of Anesthesiologists (ASA) Physical Status 4 (Table 2).

ASA Physical Status 1	A patient with mild systemic disease
ASA Physical Status 2	A patient with mild systemic disease
ASA Physical Status 3	A patient with severe systemic disease
ASA Physical Status 4	A patient with severe systemic disease that is a constant threat to life
ASA Physical Status 5	A moribund patient who is not expected to survive without the operation
ASA Physical Status 6	A declared brain-dead patient whose organs are being removed for donor purposes
ASA E	Emergency operation of any variety (used to modify one of the above classifications, i.e., ASA-4E)

Table 2. ASA Physical Status classifications from the American Society of Anesthesiologists

3. Perioperative risk

The patient with pulmonary hypertension (PHTN) is at elevated risk for morbidity and mortality in the perioperative period [Cuenco et al, 1999; Kuralay et al, 2002; Tay et al, 1999; Rodriguez et al 1998]. There is a relative paucity of literature studying outcomes in this population presenting for noncardiac surgery, however, the evidence that does exist points to significantly increased potential for complications in the perioperative period. Ramakrishna et al. presented the results from an overview of 145 patients with PHTN presenting for noncardiac surgery. A 42% rate of early (<30 days) morbidity and a 9.7% rate of early mortality in this population have been reported. [Ramakrishna et al, 2005] Clinical characteristics associated with early morbidity and mortality are shown in Table 3.

Clinical characteristics of early mortality	Clinical characteristics of early morbidity
1. Right axis deviation	1. NYHA class at least 2
2. Right ventricular hypertrophy	2. History of pulmonary embolism
3. RVSP/SBP ratio above 0.6	3. Obstructive sleep apnea
4. Intraoperative use of epinephrine or dopamine	4. High-risk surgery
	5. Anesthesia duration at least 3 h
	6. Intraoperative use of epinephrine or dopamine

Table 3. Clinical characteristics associtated with increased morbility and mortality in PHTN patients. (Ramakrishna et al, 2005) NYHA = New York Heart Association, RVSP = right ventricular systolic pressure, SBP = systolic blood pressure.

Lai et al. performed a case-control study examining using 67 cases of patients with pulmonary systolic pressures greater than 70 mm Hg compared to controls with normal pulmonary pressures. [Lai et al, 2007] As shown in table 4, the pulmonary hypertension group demonstrated greater postoperative heart failure (9.7 vs. 0%, $p = .028$), delayed tracheal extubation (21 vs. 0%, $p = .004$) and greater in hospital mortality (9.7 vs. 0%, $p = .004$).

A review of a large U.S. database by Memtsoudis et al. was undertaken to identify mortality in patients undergoing total hip arthroplasty (THA) and total knee arthroplasty (TKA).[Memtsoudis et al., 2010] The authors identified 1359 THA and 2184 TKA patients that also carried the diagnosis of pulmonary hypertension. In comparison to a matched sample without pulmonary hypertension, the THA patients demonstrated a 4-fold increased adjusted risk of in-hospital mortality and the TKA patients demonstrated a 4.5-fold increase (p< .001).

	Control (n=62)	PH (n=62)	P-value
Morbidity (%)	2 [3.2]	15 [24.2]*	0.002
Heart failure (%)	0 [0]	6 [9.7]	0.028
Delayed tracheal extubation >24 h (%)	2 [3.2]	13 [21]	0.004
Stroke (%)	0 [0]	1 [1.6]	NS
Myocardial ischaemia/infarction (%)	0 [0]	1 [1.6]	NS
Major arrhythmia (%)	0 [0]	2 [3.2]**	NS
Mortality (in-hospital death, %)	0 [0]	6 [9.7]***	0.028

Table 4. Postoperative morbidity in patients with Pulmonary Hypertension compared to controls. (Lai et al., 2007) PH= Pulmonary Hypertension (Pulm Syst. BP >70mm Hg)

In summary, patients with PHTN are at considerably increased risk in the perioperative period morbidity and mortality.

4. Intraoperative considerations

The right ventricle (RV) is a crescent shaped, thin walled, compliant muscle intended for volume work, not pressure work. Chronic PHTN leads to right ventricular hypertrophy as a compensatory mechanism. However, the ability of the RV to adapt is finite and may eventually lead to RV failure. Unlike the muscular left ventricle, a hypertrophied RV may not tolerate the acute rises in PVR that are associated with pain, surgical stimulation and positive pressure ventilation. RV failure and dilatation can lead to left ventricular compression and diminished cardiac output. This in turn leads to decreased coronary blood flow and perfusion pressure and can become a viscous cycle that can be difficult to overcome. The goals of management are to optimize PAP's, RV preload and to avoid RV ischemia and failure. During anesthesia and surgery, there are significant alterations in all the above parameters and appropriate vigilance and monitoring is essential. Proper operating room monitoring for patients with pulmonary hypertension usually involves placement of arterial and/or pulmonary artery catheters and/or a transesophageal echocardiography probe. Intra-arterial blood pressure monitoring is necessary for beat-to-beat blood pressure monitoring to ensure adequate myocardial perfusion pressures and for frequent blood gas analysis. A pulmonary artery catheter can be used in addition to PCWP to give an indication of left ventricular preload in the patient with PHTN whose cardiac output is limited by right ventricular function. Central venous pressure may be a more accurate guide for volume administration. Additionally, PVR, SVR, and cardiac outputs can be measured and used as guides for volume, vasodilator, or inotropic therapy. Care should be taken in placing these catheters as these patients are reliant on atrial contraction for adequate preload and cardiac output. Arrhythmias associated with catheter insertion may not be tolerated well by the patient. Finally, transesophageal echocardiography can be useful to assess the preload and contractility of both right and left ventricles.

4.1 Echocardiography and pulmonary hypertension

Echocardiography can be useful for both diagnosis and monitoring of disease progression in pulmonary hypertension (PH). Although transthoracic echocardiography is most widely used for this purpose, transesophageal echocardiography (TEE) can be useful for patients with poor acoustic windows and for intraoperative monitoring. Compared to other monitoring modalities, TEE can be particularly useful in narrowing the differential for intraoperative hemodynamic instability (hypovolemia, hypervolemia, right or left ventricular ischemia/failure) and in formulating a therapeutic plan.

Multiple echocardiographic methods, M-mode, 2D and real-time 3D have been utilized to assess PH. The echocardiographic findings associated with PH include: (i) a diminished or absent atrial wave of the pulmonary valve, (ii) mid-systolic closure or notching of the pulmonary valve, (iii) enlarged right atrial or right ventricular (RV) chambers, (iv) intraventricular septal flattening, (v) paradoxical systolic motion of the intraventricular septum (IVS) toward the left ventricle, (vi) a dilated inferior vena cava with reduced respiratory variability, (vii) increased IVS/posterior left ventricular (LV) wall ratio (>1), (viii) increased RV end-diastolic volume index, (ix) increased RV end-systolic volume index, and (x)decreased RV ejection fraction.[Bossone et al, 2005; Mookadam et al., 2010; Morikawa et al., 2011]   Methods to determine pulmonary arterial pressure include: measurement of the tricuspid annular plane systolic excursion (TAPSE), two-dimensional strain, tissue Doppler echocardiography, the speckle tracking method, acceleration time across the pulmonic valve, the pulmonary artery regurgitant jet method and the tricuspid regurgitant jet method. (Janda et al, 2011) The tricuspid regurgitant jet method is the most commonly used for determination of the pulmonary artery systolic pressure (PASP). The simplified Bernoulli equation, $P_1 - P_2 = 4V^2$, where $P_1 - P_2$ is the pressure gradient and V is the peak velocity, is used to approximate the PASP by continuous wave Doppler across the tricuspid valve regurgitant jet. In this case, RVSP $\approx$ PASP = $4V^2$ + RAP, where RVSP is the right ventricular systolic pressure and RAP is the right atrial pressure. The RVSP approximates PASP when no pulmonary valve stenosis or right ventricular outflow obstruction exists. [Janda et al., 2011; Sciomer et al., 2011]   Figure 1 demonstrates the enlarged right ventricle, deviated intraventricular septum and compressed left ventricle.

Although right heart catheterization (RHC) remains the gold standard for assessment of hemodynamics in PH, advantages of echocardiography include wide availability, noninvasive modality, and costs. Intraoperatively, TEE allows dynamic interpretation and assessment of the therapeutic management of PH. Disadvantages include the need for specialized training for interpretation, modest diagnostic accuracy and correlation to PH as compared to RHC.[Fisher et al., 2009; Janda et al., 2011] Janda et al found the summary correlation coefficient of systolic pulmonary artery pressure (PASP) by echocardiography as compared with PASP by RHC to be 0.70 (95% CI 0.67 to 0.73) as well as a summary sensitivity and specificity of 83% (95% CI 73 to 90) and 72% (95% CI 53 to 85), respectively for diagnostic accuracy of echocardiography for pulmonary hypertension. (Janda et al, 2011) The variability of echocardiography to correlate to RHC is in part due to the underlying disease, lung conditions, time of the examination, and the skills of the echocardiographer.

[Mookadam et al, 2010; Pedoto & Amar, 2009; Sciomer et al., 2007] Underestimation of PASP by echocardiography resulting in improper classification of PH (mild, moderate, severe) is more likely than overestimation, however inaccuracy in both under and overestimation occur with similar frequency. [Fisher et al., 2009] Improvement in obtaining the tricuspid regurgitant jet peak velocity has been found with the use of an intravenous bolus of agitated saline. [Bossone et al., 2005; McLaughlin et al., 2009; Mookadam et al, 2010] Despite the technical challenges and inaccuracies associated with echocardiography, it remains as useful tool for the diagnosis, monitoring, and management of PH.

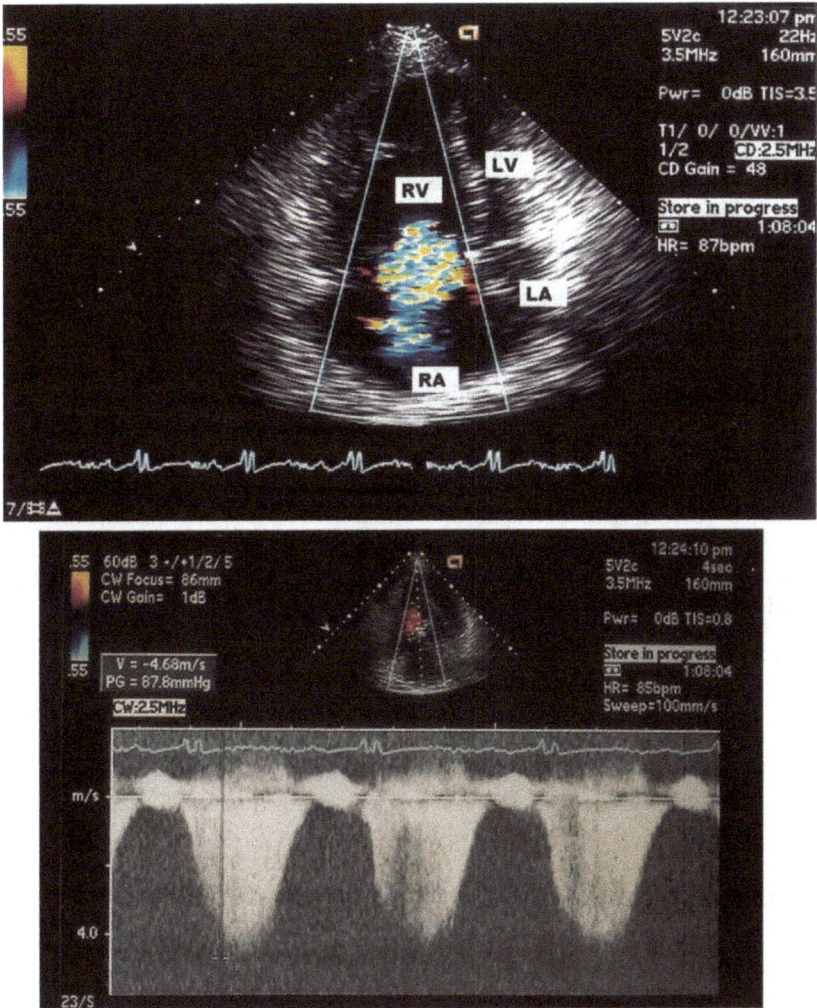

Fig. 1. Top: Apical four-chamber view (systole) showing enlarged right-side chambers with compressed and geometric distortion of an intrinsically normal LV secondary to marked RV pressure overload; severe TR. RA-right atrium; LA- left atrium. Bottom: Peak TR velocity of 4.68 m/s, with a peak gradient of 87.8 mm Hg indicating severe PH. (Bossone et al., 2005)

4.2 Anesthetic technique and pharmacological considerations

Outside of case reports, very little literature exists evaluating management strategies for intraoperative and postoperative management of the patient with pulmonary hypertension. Various management techniques have been described with success including regional, general, and peripheral nerve blockade. [Armstrong, 1992; Martin et al., 2002] The choice of technique is not as important as the ability to adhere to the goals of avoidance of elevations in PVR and right ventricular failure.

4.2.1 Regional anesthesia

Regional techniques, including peripheral nerve blockade and neuraxial blockade (epidural, spinal anesthesia) have been successfully utilized in patients with severe pulmonary hypertension. Among the benefits are avoidance of the stimulation of direct laryngoscopy and endotracheal intubation. Even with adequate IV hypnotics, opioids and neuromuscular blockade, it is difficult to avoid increases in sympathetic nervous system activity with direct laryngoscopy. These increases could lead to increases in PVR and potential acute right heart failure. Additionally, during a general anesthetic, with the variable stimulation during the operative procedure, the anesthesiologist is continually managing the balance between excessive sympathetic outflow, increased PVR and potential acute right heart failure on one hand and excessive depth of anesthesia, low cardiac output, low coronary perfusion and cardiovascular collapse on the other hand. (Hohn L et al., 1999) The healthy patient tolerates these variations well, but the patient with severe PH has limited reserve to tolerate acute increases in PVR or decreased coronary perfusion. A peripheral nerve block technique can limit anesthesia to the specific location of the surgery and avoid the need for the stimulation of intubation and reduced likelihood of sympathectomy and low blood pressure as one would achieve with general anesthesia. An important distinction is that a sympathectomy is still possible when utilizing a regional anesthesia technique such as epidural or spinal anesthesia. This may lead to arterial and venous dilation and reduced preload and cardiac output compromising coronary perfusion.

When utilizing regional or peripheral techniques, it is important to ensure adequate ventilation and oxygenation to prevent increases in PVR. For example, sedation provided to allow the patient to tolerate placement of a peripheral nerve block or to tolerate laying on the narrow, stiff operating table may lead to hypoxemia and hypercarbia secondary to hypoventilation. On the other hand, lack of sedation can promote anxiety, pain and sympathetic stimulation. Finding the appropriate balance can be a challenge for the anesthesiologist.

4.2.2 General anesthesia

For major surgery, general anesthesia is still the method of choice and allows for control of ventilation. Commonly used intravenous anesthetics such as propofol and thiopental are associated with hypotension and some myocardial depression. Their use should be judicious. Etomidate has much less an effect on SVR, PVR and myocardial contractility and may be a more useful hypnotic for patient with severe pulmonary hypertension. Use of volatile anesthetics is associated with decreased SVR, myocardial contractility and potential arrhythmias all of which can impair right ventricular myocardial perfusion and also right ventricular cardiac output. A balanced technique utilizing high dose narcotics to blunt the cardiovascular response to surgical stimulation and minimal volatile anesthetics can limit these adverse effects. Additionally, the anesthesiologist should strive to use basic physiology to his advantage. These principles include utilization of 100% oxygen for its pulmonary vasodilator effects, and aggressive treatment of hypercarbia, acidosis, and hypothermia as these all cause pulmonary vasoconstriction. Certain anesthetic agents such as nitrous oxide and ketamine have been associated with increases in PVR and should be used with caution [Rich et al., 1994; Schulte-Sasse et al., 1982].

Intraoperative management of the right ventricle can be made on the presence of RV failure and the presence of systemic *hyper-* or *hypo*tension. Initially, one should ensure that oxygenation, ventilation, and acid/base status are optimized. Treatment options for PHTN include both intravenous (IV) and inhaled agents. Intravenous vasodilators, such as nitroglycerin, sodium nitroprusside, beta blockers, calcium channel blockers, and certain prostaglandin preparations will cause dilation of *both* the pulmonary and systemic vascular beds and can be useful in the setting of PHTN with systemic hypertension. The advantages to IV preparations are the relative decreased cost, easier availability of medications, longer duration of action and ease of administration in comparison to inhaled agents.

Milrinone is a phosphodiesterase-3 inhibitor and prevents the breakdown of cyclic adenosine monophosphate (cAMP). It has shown to reduce both PVR and SVR in addition to causing increases in myocardial contractility [Tanake et al, 1991]. If the clinical picture is of pulmonary hypertension with systemic hypotension, IV vasodilators may cause worsening of systemic blood pressure, subsequent RV hypoperfusion, ischemia and failure. In this situation, the patient may benefit from therapy selective for the pulmonary vasculature such as inhaled nitric oxide (INO) or prostacyclin.

INO diffuses from the alveoli to the pulmonary capillaries and acts via stimulation of guanylate cyclase and increasing cyclic guanosine monophosphate (cGMP) leading to vasodilation. INO does not produce systemic vasodilatation because nitric oxide is inactivated when bound to hemoglobin. It also has the benefit of improving ventilation–perfusion matching by increasing perfusion to areas of the lung that are well ventilated. INO has been shown to improve PHTN in cardiopulmonary bypass settings [Ichinose et al., 2004; Kavanaugh & Pearl, 1995]. Prostacyclin, available in inhaled and i.v. forms, stimulates adenylate cyclase and increases cAMP and release of endothelial NO leading to decreases in PAP, right atrial pressures, and increased cardiac output. An example of a prostacyclin nebulized delivery system that can be integrated into the anesthesia circuit is shown in Figure 2. [Jerath, 2010] Combination therapy, with both INO and prostacyclin, has been shown to augment the effects compared to monotherapy [Atz et al., 2002; Petros et al., 1995]. Due to the extremely short half-life of these medications, one should ensure that the medication is delivered continuously without interruption to minimize the risk of rebound pulmonary hypertension. Weaning from these medications should be performed gradually with frequent assessment of pulmonary artery pressures and the right ventricle. A disadvantage of INO compared to inhaled prostacyclin is its cost. A recent analysis revealed that INO is approximately 20 times more expensive than prostacyclin ($3000/day vs. $150/day). [De Wet, 2006]. Table 5 lists the medical management options, including common doses, for intraoperative pulmonary hypertension. Lastly, in patients refractory to the above therapies, right ventricular assist device implantation should be considered.

1. Ensure good oxygenation, avoid hypercarbia, acidosis and hypothermia
2. Inhaled nitric oxide 20–40 ppm.
3. Milrinone (phosphodiesterase III inhibitor) is 50mcg/kg bolus, then 0.5–0.75mcg•kg^{-1}•min^{-1}
4. Dipiridamole is 0.2–0.6 mg/kg i.v. over 15 min. Repeat after 12 h.
5. Inhaled prostacyclin: Continuous administration of 50 ng•kg^{-1}•min^{-1}. Reconstitute prostacyclin in sterile glycine diluent to 30,000 ng/ml (1.5mg of prostacyclin in 50 ml of diluent). For an 80 kg patient, 50 ng/kg per min is 8 ml of this solution per hour. It is nebulized into inspiratory limb (see Figure 2).
6. Intravenous prostacyclin (if inhaled is not available) is 4–10 ng•kg^{-1}•min^{-1}.
7. Wean the above medications slowly to prevent rebound pulmonary hypertension.
8.   Regional anesthesia can be provided using peripheral nerve blockade, brachial plexus block, and lumbar plexus block.
9.   Epidural anesthesia should be induced slowly. Mixtures of local anesthetics and opioids should be given to reduce the dose of local anesthetics and hypotension.
10. Hypotension should be treated according to causes. Phenylephrine and norepinephrine have been used to treat persistent systemic hypotension. Norepinephrine has the advantage of being both a vasoconstrictor and positive inotropic agent. In hypotension, dobutamine and vasopressin have also been advocated for treatment of hypotension [Pearl, 2005; Subramaniam & Yared 2007].

Table 5. Management options for intraoperative PHTN (modified from Blaise et al., 2003).

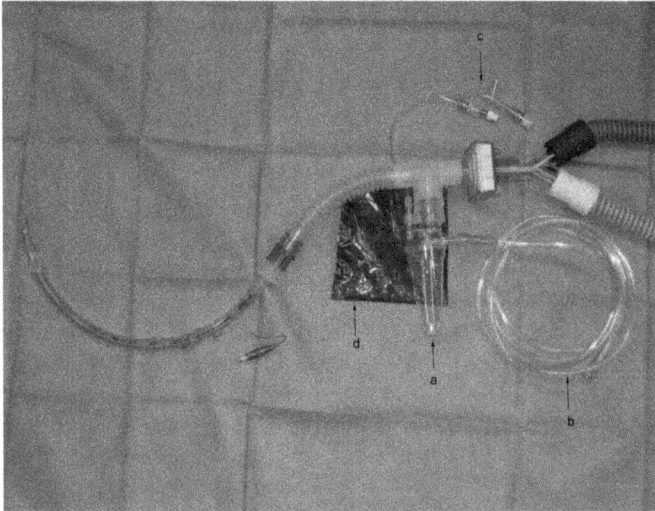

Fig. 2. Inhaled prostacyclin delivery system. Reconstituted prostacyclin is delivered by a Lo-Flo MiniHeart nebulizer (a), which is driven by a separate oxygen source at 2 L/min (b). The nebulizer output is 8 mL/h, which allows for 1–3 h of continuous nebulization.
The nebulizer should be supported by an IV pole or ventilator side arm to prevent spillage.
An IV port (c) allows the chamber to be refilled without disconnecting from the anesthetic circuit. Prostacyclin is photosensitive and requires the nebulizing chamber to be covered from ambient light (d). [Jerath, 2010]

5. Postoperative management

These patients warrant intensive care monitoring in the postoperative period with experienced critical care personnel. As the analgesic and sympathetic nervous system effects of opioids, volatile anesthetics, and regional anesthetics, the patient can develop sudden worsening of PHTN and RV ischemia. Weaning from the ventilator and extubation should be done gradually with close attention to adequate oxygenation, ventilation and analgesia. Even routine events such as bucking on the ventilator due to tracheal stimulation, while tolerated in the average patient, can lead to acute rises in PVR and RV failure in the patient with severe PHTN [Rodriguez & Pearl, 1998].

6. Conclusion

Due to advances in the management of PHTN, it appears likely that these patients will be encountered more frequently in the perioperative period for procedures incidental to their primary disease process. These patients present challenging clinically scenarios secondary to the complexity of their PHTN and are at increased risk for significant perioperative complications. The ideal perioperative care of these patients requires a multidisciplinary approach with appropriate planning for pre-procedure optimization, appropriate resources and monitoring intra-operatively as well as intensive care unit monitoring in the post-operative period. This aggressive approach can test the expertise and resources of medical institutions. Although no curative agent has been identified, the practitioners' knowledge of the existing treatment options, pathophysiology, and the implications of various anesthetic agents and techniques are required to ensure the highest level of patient safety and care.

7. References

Ahearn GS, Tapson VF, Rebeiz A, Greenfield JC Jr. Electrocardiography to define clinical status in primary pulmonary hypertension and pulmonary hypertension secondary to collagen vascular disease. (2002). *Chest*. Vol. 122, No. 2, (August, 2002), pp. 524–527, ISSN: 0012-3692

Armstrong P. Thoracic epidural anaesthesia and primary pulmonary hypertension. (1992). *Anaesthesia*. Vol. 47, No. 6, (June, 1992), pp. 496–499, ISSN: 0003-2409

Atz AM, Lefler AK, Fairbrother DL, et al. Sildenafil augments the effect of inhaled nitric oxide for postoperative pulmonary hypertensive crises. (2002). *Journal of Thoracic and Cardiovascular Surgery*. Vol. 124, No. 3, (September, 2002), pp. 628–629, ISSN: 0022-5223

Blaise G, Langleben D, Hubert B. Pulmonary arterial hypertension: pathophysiology and anesthetic approach. (2003). *Anesthesiology*. Vol. 99, No. 6, (December, 2003), pp. 1415–1432, ISSN: 0003-3022

Bossone E, Bodini BD, Mazza A, Allegra L. Pulmonary Arterial Hypertension, The Key Role of Echocardiography. (2005). *CHEST*. Vol. 127, No. 5, (May, 2005), pp. 1836-1843, ISSN: 0012-3692Bossone E, Paciacco G, Iarussi D, et al. The prognostic role of the ECG in primary pulmonary hypertension. (2002). *Chest*. Vol. 121, No. 2, (February, 2002), pp. 513–518, ISSN: 0012-3692

Carmosino MJ, Friesen RH, Doran A, Ivy DD. Perioperative complications in children with pulmonary hypertension undergoing noncardiac surgery or cardiac catheterization.

(2007). *Anesthesia and Analgesia.* Vol. 104, No. 3, (March, 2007), pp. 521–527, ISSN: 0003-2999

Cuenco J, Tzeng G, Wittels B. Anesthetic management of the parturient with systemic lupus erythematosus, pulmonary hypertension, and pulmonary edema. (1999). *Anesthesiology.* Vol. 91, No. 1, (August, 1999), pp. 568–570, ISSN: 0003-3022

Davies MJ, Beavis RE. Epidural anaesthesia for vascular surgery in a patient with primary pulmonary hypertension. (1984). *Anaesthesia and Intensive Care.* Vol. 12, No. 2, (May, 1984), pp. 115–117, ISSN: 0310-057X

De Wet CJ, Affleck DJ, Jacobsohn E, Avidan MS, Tymkew H, Hill ll, Zanaboni PB, Moazami N, Smith JR. Inhaled prostacyclin is safe, effective, and affordable in patients with pulmonary hypertension, right heart dysfunction,and refractory hypoxemia after cardiothoracic surgery. (2004). *The Journal of Thoracic and Cardiovascular Surgery.* Vol 127, No. 4, (Aril 2004), pp. 1058-67, ISSN: 0022-5223

Fisher MR, Forfia PR, Chamera E, et al. Accuracy of Doppler Echocardiography in the Hemodynamic Assessment of Pulmonary Hypertension. (2009). *American Journal of Respiratory and Critical Care Medicine.* Vol. 179, No. 7, (April, 2009), pp. 615-21, ISSN: 1073-449X

Gaine S. Pulmonary hypertension. (2000). *JAMA.* Vol. 284, No. 24, (December, 2000), pp. 3160–3168, ISSN: 0098-7484

Ichinose F, Roberts JD, Zapol WM. Inhaled nitric oxide: a selective pulmonary vasodilator – current uses and therapeutic potential. (2004). *Circulation.* Vol. 109, No. 25, (June, 2004), pp. 3106–3111, ISSN: 0009-7322

Janda S, Shahidi N, Gin K, Swiston J. Diagnostic accuracy of echocardiography for pulmonary hypertension: a systematic review and meta-analysis. (2011). *Heart.* Vol. 97, No. 8, (April, 2011), pp. 612-622, ISSN: 1355-6037

Kahn ML. Eisenmenger's syndrome in pregnancy. (1993). *New England Journal of Medicine.* Vol. 329, No. 12, (September, 1993), p. 887, ISSN: 0028-4793

Kavanaugh BP, Pearl RG. Inhaled nitric oxide in anesthesia and critical care medicine. (1995). *International Anesthesiology Clinics.* Vol. 33, No.1, (Winter, 1995), pp. 181–210, ISSN: 0020-5907

Krowka MJ, Mandell MS, Ramsay MA, et al. Hepatopulmonary syndrome and portopulmonary hypertension: a report of the multicenter liver transplant database. (2004). *Liver Transplantation.* Vol. 10, No. 2, (February, 2004), pp. 174–182, ISSN: 1527-6465

Kuralay E, Demirkilic U, Oz BS, et al. Primary pulmonary hypertension and coronary artery bypass surgery. (2002). *Journal of Cardiac Surgergy.* Vol. 17, No. 1, (January, 2002), pp. 79–80, ISSN: 0886-0440

Lai HC, Lai HC, Wang KY et al. Severe pulmonary hypertension complicates postoperative outcome of non-cardiac surgery. (2007). *British Journal of Anesthesia.* Vol. 99, No. 2, (August, 2007), pp. 184-90, ISSN: 1471-6771

Loyd JE, Butler MG, Foroud TM, et al. Genetic anticipation and abnormal gender ratio at birth in familial primary pulmonary hypertension. (1995). *American Journal of Respiratory and Critical Care Medicine.* Vol. 152, No. 1, (July, 1995), pp. 93–97, ISSN: 1073-449X

MacLean MR. Endothelin-1 and serotonin: mediators of primary and secondary pulmonary hypertension? (1999). *Journal of Laboratory and Clinical Medicine*. Vol. 134, No. 2. (August 1999), pp. 105–144, ISSN: 0022-2143

Martin JT, Tautz TJ, Antognini JF. Safety of regional anesthesia in Eisenmenger's syndrome. (2002). *Regional Anesthesia and Pain Medicine*. Vol. 27, No. 5, (September, 2002), pp. 509–513, ISSN: 1098-7339McLaughlin VV, Archer SL, Badesch DB, et al. ACCF/AHA 2009 expert consensus document on pulmonary hypertension: a report of the American College of Cardiology Foundation Task Force on Expert Consensus Documents and the American Heart Association: developed in collaboration with the American College of Chest Physicians, American Thoracic Society, Inc., and the Pulmonary Hypertension Association. *Circulation*. Vol. 119, No. 16, (April, 2009), pp. 2250-94, ISSN: 0009-7322

Memtsoudis, SG, Ma Y, Chiu, YL et al. Perioperative Mortality in Patients with PulmonaryHypertension Undergoing Major Joint Replacement. (2010). *Anesthesia and Analgesia*. Vol. 111, No. 5, (November, 2010), pp. 1110-6, ISSN: 0003-2999

Mookadam F, Jiamsripong P, Goel R, Warsame TA, Emani UR, Khandheria BK. Critical Appraisal on the Utility of Echocardiography in the Management of Acute Pulmonary Embolism. (2010). *Cardiology in Review*. Vol. 18, No. 1, (January 2010), pp. 29-37, ISSN: 1061-5377

Morikawa T, Murata M, Okuda S, et al. Quantitative Analysis of Right Ventricular Function in Patients with Pulmonary Hypertension Using Three-Dimensional Echocardiography and a Two-Dimensional Summation Method Compared to Magnetic Resonance Imaging. (2011). *American Journal of Cardiology*. Vol. 107, No. 3, (February, 2011), pp. 484-89, ISSN: 0002-9149

Nauser TD, Stites SW. Diagnosis and treatment of pulmonary hypertension. (2001). *American Family Physician*. Vol. 63, No. 9, (May, 2001), pp. 1789–1798, ISSN: 0002-838X

Pearl RG. Perioperative management of PH: covering all aspects from risk assessment to postoperative considerations. (2005). *Advances in Pulmonary Hypertension*. Vol. 4, No. 4, (Winter, 2005), pp. 6–15, ISSN: 1933-088X

Pedoto A and Amar D. Right heart function in thoracic surgery: role of echocardiography. (2009). *Current Opinion in Anaesthesiology*. Vol. 22, No. 1, (Februar,y 2009). pp. 44-49, ISSN: 0952-7907

Petros AJ, Turner SC, Nunn AJ. Cost implications of using inhaled nitric oxide compared with epoprostenol for pulmonary hypertension. (1995). *Journal of Pharmacy Technology*. Vol. 11, No. 4, (July, 1995), pp. 163–166, ISSN: 8755-1225

Phillips BG, Norkiewk K, Perck CA, et al. Effects of obstructive sleep apnea on endothelin-1 and blood pressure. (1999). Journal of Hypertension.Vol. 17,No. 1, (January, 1999), pp. 61–66. ISSN: 0263-6352

Ramakrishna G, Sprung J, Ravi BS, et al. Impact of pulmonary hypertension on the outcomes of noncardiac surgery: predictors of perioperative morbidity and mortality. (2005). *Journal of the American College of Cardiology*. Vol. 45, No. 10, (May, 2005), pp. 1691–1699, ISSSN: 0735-1097

Rich GF, Roos CM, Anderson SM, et al. Direct effects of intravenous anesthetics on pulmonary vascular resistance in the isolated rat lung. (1994). *Anesthesia and Analgesia*. Vol. 78, No. 5, (May ,1994):961–966, ISSN: 0003-2999

Roberts NV, Keast PJ. Pulmonary hypertension and pregnancy: a lethal combination. (1993). *Anaesth Intensive Care.*Vol. 18, No. 3, (August, 1993), pp. 366–374, ISSN: 1472-0299

Rodriguez RM, Pearl RG. Pulmonary hypertension and major surgery. (1998). *Anesthesia and Analgesia.* Vol. 87, No. 4, (October, 1998), pp. 812–815, ISSN: 0003-2999

Ross AF, Ueda K. Pulmonary hypertension in thoracic surgical patients. (2010). *Current Opinion in Anaesthesiolology.* Vol. 23, No. 1, (February, 2010), pp. 25–33, ISSN: 0952-7907

Schulte-Sasse U, Hess W, Tarnow J. Pulmonary vascular responses to nitrous oxide in patients with normal and high pulmonary vascular resistance. (1982). *Anesthesiology.* Vol. 57, No. 1, (July, 1982), pp. 9–13, ISSN: 0003-3022

Sciomer S, Magri D, Badagliacca R. Non-invasive assessment of pulmonary hypertension: Doppler-echocardiography. (2007). *Pulmonary Pharmacology and Therapeutics.* Vol. 20, No. 2, pp. 135-40, ISSN: 1522-9629.

Subramaniam K, Yared JP. Management of pulmonary hypertension in the operating room. (2007). *Seminars in Cardiothoracic and Vascular Anesthesia.* Vol. 11, No. 2, (June, 2007), pp. 119–136, ISSN: 1089-2532

Tan HP, Markowitz JS, Montgomery RA, et al. Liver transplantation in patients with severe portopulmonary hypertension treated with preoperative chronic intravenous epoprostenol. (2001). *Liver Transplantation.* Vol. 7, No. 8, (August, 2001), pp. 745–749, ISSN: 1527-6465

Tanake H, Tajimi K, Moritsune O, et al. Effects of milrinone on pulmonary vasculature in normal dogs and dogs with pulmonary hypertension. (1991). *Critial Care Medicine.* Vol 19, No. 1, (January 1991), pp. 68–74, ISSN: 0090-3493

Tay SM, Ong BC, Tan SA. Cesarean section in a mother with uncorrected congenital coronary to pulmonary artery fistula. (1999). *Canandian Journal of Anaesthesia.* Vol. 46, No. 4, (April, 1999), pp. 368–371, ISSN: 0832-610X

Tuder RM, Cool CD, Yeager M, et al. The pathobiology of pulmonary hypertension: endothelium.(2001). *Clinics in Chest Medicine.* Vol. 22, No. 3, (September, 2001), pp. 405–418, ISSN: 0272-5231

Weimann J, Ullrich R, Hromi J, et al. Sildenafil is a pulmonary vasodilator in awake lambs with acute pulmonary hypertension. (2000). *Anesthesiology.* Vol. 92, No. 6, (June, 2000), pp. 1702–1712, ISSN: 0003-3022

Weiss BM, Atanassoff PG. Cyanotic congenital heart disease and pregnancy: natural selection, pulmonary hypertension, and anesthesia. (1993). *Journal of Clinical Anesthesia.* Vol. 5, No. 4, (July, 1993), pp. 332–341, ISSN: 0952-8180

Weiss BM, Maggiorini M, Jeni R, et al. Pregnant patient with primary pulmonary hypertension: inhaled pulmonary vasodilators and epidural anesthesia for cesarean delivery. (2000). *Anesthesiology.* Vol. 92, No. 4, (April, 2000), pp. 1191–1194, ISSN: 0003-3022

Wilkens H, Guth A, Konig J, et al. Effect of inhaled iloprost plus oral sildenafil in patients with primary pulmonary hypertension. (2001). *Circulation.* Vol. 104, No. 11, (September, 2001), pp. 1218–1222, ISSN: 0009-7322

17

Pulmonary Hypertension in the Critically Ill

Michelle S. Chew[1], Anders Åneman[2],
John F. Fraser[3] and Anthony S. McLean[4]
[1]Department of Intensive Care Medicine,
Skåne University Hospital Malmö, Lund University,
[2]Intensive Care Unit, Liverpool Hospital, Sydney,
[3]Critical Care Research Group, The Prince Charles Hospital, Brisbane,
[4]Intensive Care Unit, Nepean Hospital, Sydney University,
[1]Sweden
[2,3,4]Australia

1. Introduction

Pulmonary hypertension (PHT) is frequently seen in the critically ill patient. PHT is defined as a mean pulmonary arterial pressure (MPAP) >25mmHG at rest (Farber and Loscalzo, 2004; Task Force for the Diagnosis and Treatment of Pulmonary Hypertension of the European Society of Cardiology (ESC) and the European Respiratory Society (ERS), endorsed by the International Society of Heart and Lung Transplantation (ISHLT), 2009). The updated clinical classification (Dana Point 2008) describes pulmonary hypertension according to arterial or venous aetiology, as well as those associated with heart, respiratory and thromboembolic diseases (Table 1) (Task Force for the Diagnosis and Treatment of Pulmonary Hypertension of the European Society of Cardiology (ESC) and the European Respiratory Society (ERS), endorsed by the International Society of Heart and Lung Transplantation (ISHLT), 2009).

PHT is inextricably linked to respiratory and right ventricular (RV) function. Increased pulmonary vascular resistance increases the afterload of the right ventricle, eventually leading to RV dysfunction and failure. This is reflected clinically as systemic venous hypertension with the classical signs of distended neck veins, pulsatile hepatomegaly and peripheral oedema. A vicious cycle is set up as elevated right ventricular end-diastolic pressures worsens tricuspid insufficiency, which in turn aggravates splanchnic and peripheral venous engorgement, leading to organ failure by reducing the perfusion pressure within these organs (Figure 1). Due to ventricular interdependence, left sided filling and contractility also becomes impaired, further contributing to systemic hypotension and organ hypoperfusion. It is therefore not surprising that the presence of PHT and RV failure is associated with a poorer clinical outcome in ICU patients (Moloney et al., 2003; Osman et al., 2008; Ribiero et al., 1997; Viellard Baron et al., 2001).

ICU patients are at particular risk for developing PHT and RV failure for a number of reasons. Firstly, the presence of mechanical ventilation may impose an additional load on the RV. Secondly, ARDS inevitably increases pulmonary vascular resistance due to the presence of pulmonary vasoconstriction, which in turn may be triggered by hypoxia and the release of vasoconstrictive mediators. Thirdly, endothelial dysfunction and high risk for pulmonary vascular occlusion also contribute to increased pulmonary vascular resistance. It is estimated that approximately 25% of patients with ARDS have right ventricular dysfunction and pulmonary hypertension (Viellard Baron et al., 2001) .

1	**Pulmonary arterial hypertension (PAH)**
1.1	Idiopathic
1.2	Heritable
1.2.1	BMPR2
1.2.2	ALK1, endoglin (with or without hereditary haemorrhagic telangiectasia)
1.2.3	Unknown
1.3	Drugs and toxins induced
1.4	Associated with (APAH)
1.4.1	Connective tissue diseases
1.4.2	HIV infection
1.4.3	Portal hypertension
1.4.4	Congenital heart disease
1.4.5	Schistosomiasis
1.4.6	Chronic haemolytic anaemia
1.5	Persistent pulmonary hypertension of the newborn
1'	**Pulmonary veno-occlusive disease and/or pulmonary capillary haemangiomatosis**
2	**Pulmonary hypertension due to left heart disease**
2.1	Systolic dysfunction
2.2	Diastolic dysfunction
2.3	Valvular disease
3	**Pulmonary hypertension due to lung diseases and/or hypoxia**
3.1	Chronic obstructive pulmonary disease
3.2	Interstitial lung disease
3.3	Other pulmonary diseases with mixed restrictive and obstructive pattern
3.4	Sleep-disordered breathing
3.5	Alveolar hypoventilation disorders
3.6	Chronic exposure to high altitude
3.7	Developmental abnormalities
4	**Chronic thromboembolic pulmonary hypertension**
5	**PH with unclear and/or multifactorial mechanisms**
5.1	Haematological disorders: myeloproliferative disorders, splenectomy.
5.2	Systemic disorders: sarcoidosis, pulmonary Langerhans cell histiocytosis, lymphangioleiomyomatosis, neurofibromatosis, vasculitis
5.3	Metabolic disorders: glycogen storage disease, Gaucher disease, thyroid disorders
5.4	Others: tumoural obstruction, fibrosing mediastinitis, chronic renal failure on dialysis

ALK-1 = activin receptor-like kinase 1 gene; APAH = associated pulmonary arterial hypertension; BMPR2 = bone morphogenetic protein receptor, type 2; HIV = human immunodeficiency virus; PAH = pulmonary arterial hypertension.

Table 1. Updated clinical classification of pulmonary hypertension (Dana Point 2008). Reprinted from the Task Force for the Diagnosis and Treatment of Pulmonary Hypertension of the European Society of Cardiology (ESC) and the European Respiratory Society (ERS), endorsed by the International Society of Heart and Lung Transplantation (ISHLT), 2009 with permission from Oxford University Press.

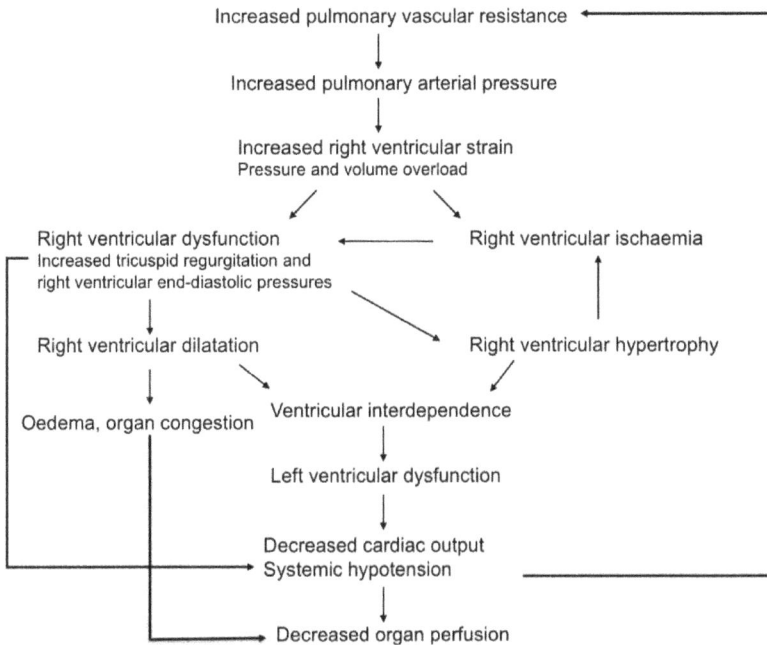

Fig. 1. Increased pulmonary vascular pressures lead to right ventricular dysfunction, impaired left sided filling and contractility, systemic hypotension and organ hypoperfusion.

Management of pulmonary hypertension in this group of patients is complex, given that the critically ill are often haemodynamically unstable, have varying responses to loading conditions on the heart, and are commonly mechanically ventilated. There is a complex interaction between the left and right ventricles, and management strategies that apply to non-ventilated inpatients or outpatients do not necessarily apply in the ICU setting.

In this paper we review the pathophysiology, diagnostic possibilities and discuss management strategies of PHT in the critically ill.

2. Pathophysiology

The molecular pathophysiology of pulmonary hypertension is complex and probably varies depending on causative factors. In general however, pulmonary hypertension may be regarded as an imbalance between vasodilatory and vasoconstrictive forces leading to abnormal vascular reactivity in the pulmonary vascular bed predisposing to vasoconstriction. Several molecular mechanisms have been implicated in the pathogenesis of pulmonary hypertension and the reader is referred to Farber & Localzo, 2004 and Mandegar et al., 2004 for in-depth reviews. There are numerous experimental and clinical data demonstrating the importance of pulmonary vasocontrictors such as endothelin-1 (ET-1), serotonin, thromboxane and leukotrienes, acting against vasodilators such as adrenomedullin, nitric oxide (NO) and prostacyclin via second messengers such as cAMP and cGMP (Berkenbosch et al., 2000; Chew et al., 2008; Farber & Localzo, 2004; Giaid et al., 1993; Giaid and Saleh, 1995; Moloney et al., 2003; Steudel et al., 1997; Zhao et al., 2003). Neurohormonal factors such as atrial and brain natriuretic peptides seem not only to be markers of disease severity, but play an active role by promoting cGMP mediated pulmonary vasodilation (Zhao et al., 2003). Hypoxic pulmonary vasoconstriction, a normally adaptive mechanism directing blood away from poorly ventilated areas may become maladaptive when sustained, contributing to increased pulmonary vascular resistance. At the cellular level, a number of mechanisms including potassium channel downregulation contribute to pathological intracellular calcium handling and homeostatis. The end result is smooth muscle proliferation, vascular remodelling and vasocontriction. Finally, genetic factors also play a role in the development of pulmonary hypertension. For example, an imbalance between apoptosis and proliferation is thought to occur as a result of mutations in bone morphogenetic receptor type II (BMP-R2) and polymorphisms in the serotonin receptor transporter (Mandegar et al., 2004; Newman et al., 2001) have been described.

3. Diagnosis and haemodynamic monitoring of pulmonary hypertension

3.1 Monitoring

The definition of to monitor is 'to watch over somebody or something, especially to ensure that good order or proper conduct is obtained'. The three components of monitoring are the subject matter, parameters measured, and periodicity chosen. Pulmonary hypertension being the subject matter leads to a number of parameters that should be considered for measurement including central venous pressure/right atrial pressure (CVP/RAP), pulmonary artery pressures (systolic, mean, diastolic), mixed venous oxygen saturation (SvO$_2$), cardiac output (CO), right ventricular systolic function, and left ventricular end diastolic pressure or left atrial pressure (LAP). Periodicity will vary according to the clinical objectives, although in the critically ill patient parameters are likely to measured continuously, over hours or sometimes over days.

Two modalities are available to the physician managing the critically ill patient with PHT are (1) right heart catherization using the pulmonary artery catheter and (2) echoDoppler (ED) assessment.

3.1.1 Pulmonary Artery Catheter

Right heart catheterization using the pulmonary artery catheter (PAC) is the gold standard in the confirming the diagnosis and accurately monitoring the haemodynamic abnormalities on a minute-to-minute basis in PHT. PAH is defined by a MPAP ≥25 mm Hg at rest and by a pulmonary vascular resistance (PVR) > 3 mm Hg/l (Wood units) (Task Force for the Diagnosis and Treatment of Pulmonary Hypertension of the European Society of Cardiology (ESC) and the European Respiratory Society (ERS), endorsed by the International Society of Heart and Lung Transplantation (ISHLT), 2009), with further subclassification into precapillary or postcapillary PHT determined by the pulmonary capillary wedge pressure (PCWP) and transpulmonary gradient (TPG = MPAP – PCWP). In addition to the benefit of RHC in obtaining an accurate PAP measurement, it should be utilized where rapid assessment of responses to intravenous or nebulised therapy is required. Although the emphasis may be on the PAP, including the systolic (SPAP), mean (MPAP) and diastolic (DPAP) pulmonary arterial pressures, other parameters including cardiac output, pulmonary vascular resistance, mixed venous oxygen saturation and the PCWP may contribute to the evaluation. These should be measured in conjunction with systemic circulation parameters including arterial oxygen saturation and blood pressure.

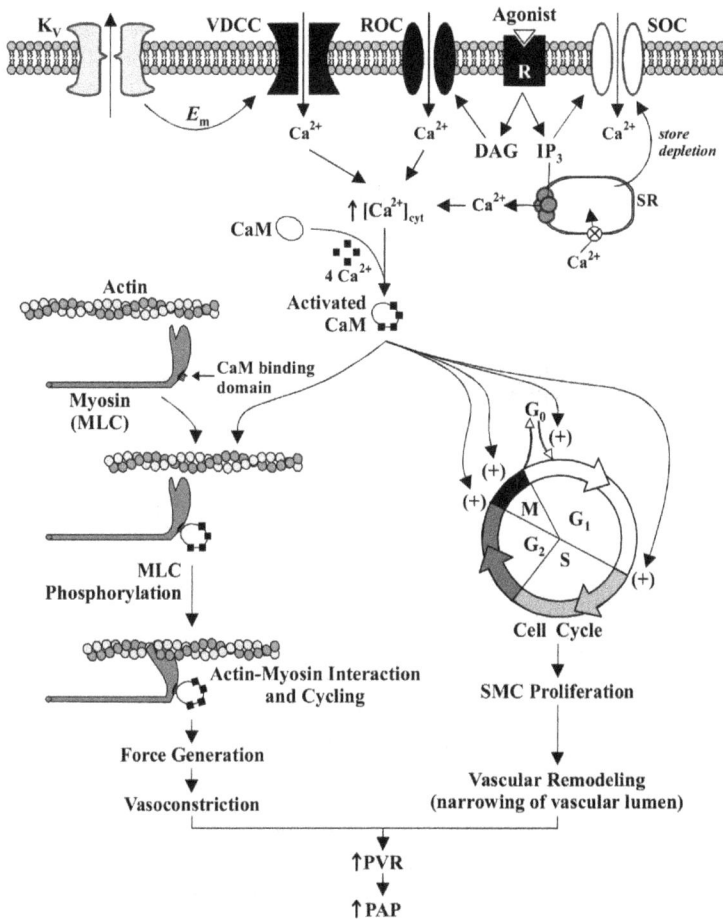

Fig. 2. Increased intracellular calcium [Ca²⁺]cyt triggers pulmonary vasoconstriction and promotes pulmonary vascular remodeling via several mechanisms: 1. Decreased activity of voltage-gated K⁺ channel (Kv) leading to opening of voltage dependent Ca²⁺ channels (VDCC), 2. Activation of receptors (R), such as G-protein coupled receptors leading to the production of second messengers such as diacylglycerol (DAG) and inositol 1,4,5 triphosphate (IP3), which mobilizes intracellular Ca²⁺, 3. Activation of receptor operated Ca²⁺ channels (ROC), 4. Opening of store-operated Ca²⁺ channels (SOC) by store depletion inducing Ca²⁺ mobilization from the sarcoplasmic reticulum (SR). Ca²⁺ binds to Calmomodulin (CaM), and the Ca²⁺/CaM complex activates myosin light chain kinase, phosphorylating the myosin light chain (MLC). This leads to crossbridge formation with actin filaments. The Ca²⁺/CaM complex also activates steps in the cell cycle propelling quiescent cells into mitosis (M) and cellular proliferation (+). The end result is vasoconstriction, smooth muscle proliferation and vascular remodelling leading to sustained elevations in pulmonary vascular resistance. Reprinted from Mandegar et al. (2004) with permission from Elsevier.

Testing acute vasodilator responses using short-acting agents such as intravenous adenosine and prostacyclin, or inhaled nitric oxide, should be undertaken in a systematic and careful manner. A positive vasoreactive response is defined as a reduction of MPAP mean PAP ≥ 10 mmHg to reach a MPAP mean PAP ≤ 40 mm Hg with an increased or unchanged CO (Galie et al., 1995). While the RHC has clear advantages over ED for precise PAP, SvO_2 and minute-to-minute monitoring, it carries the disadvantage of being invasive and having limited ability to assess other relevant parameters such as RV function and size, left heart function and the presence of confounding pathologies like intercardiac shunts and significant valvular dysfunction.

3.1.2 Doppler echocardiography

Doppler echocardiographic monitoring of PAP began over 30 years ago when Hatle and colleagues applied Doppler ultrasound to calculate the time difference between PV closure and TV opening to estimate SPAP, basing the approach on earlier work by Burstin (Burstin, 1967; Hatle et al., 1981).

Not only is PAP obtainable noninvasively in the great majority of patients, but important associated right and left heart evaluations can be made and repeated when desired. An example would be where the PHT is secondary to pulmonary embolic disease and assessment of right heart structure and function to evaluate chronicity can be undertaken. The presence of significant RV wall hypertrophy indicates longstanding pathology; alternatively in the setting of acute PE the SPAP is unlikely to rise beyond 40 mm Hg (McIntyre & Sasahara, 1971; Fisher et al., 2009). Guidelines recommend the subcostal (SC) 4-chamber view for measurements of RV wall thickness, which correlates with RV systolic pressure (Lang et al., 2005).

Parameters measured directly or indirectly in PHT by ED include CVP/RAP, SPAP, DPAP, MPAP, RV systolic function, CO, and LAP.

3.1.2.1 Right atrial pressure

The calculation of this specific parameter using echocardiography has been established in haemodynamically stable, supine, spontaneously ventilated patients for many years using IVC diameter (D) changes, determined from the SC view, throughout the respiratory cycle (Brennan et al., 2007). A large IVC diameter (>21mm) with <35% collapsibility index ($D_{expiration} - D_{inspiration} / D_{inspiration}$ X 100%) gives an RAP of 10-20 mmHg, 35-50% an RAP 10-15 mm Hg, >55% an RAP 0-10 mm Hg. A smaller IVC (<21mm) with a collapsibility index of 35-55% gives a RAP 0-10 mm Hg, >55% 0-5 mm Hg. Unfortunately the relationship doesn't hold for critically ill positive pressure ventilated patients when attempting to obtain a static RAP measurement. It does have value in determining fluid responsiveness in patients on controlled ventilation using the Distensibility Index or IVC variability index, but for the purposes of calculating a PAP a static measurement is required (Barbier et al., 2004; Feissel et al., 2004). Since many of these patients will have a central line in-situ it is recommended that the invasively obtained CVP be added to the ED derived RV-RA gradients.

3.1.2.2 Pulmonary artery pressures

(i) Systolic pulmonary artery pressure (SPAP)

The tricuspid regurgitant (TR) jet method is the most commonly used method in clinical practice. It is operator dependent and this factor alone could explain the modest sensitivity and specificity identified in a recent metanalysis (Janda et al., 2011). The preferred approach is to apply the continuous wave spectral Doppler across the tricuspid valve from either the apical 4 chamber (A4C) and/or parasternal short axis (PSAX) view, with careful attention to the angle of insonation to obtain the maximal regurgitant velocity. The modified Bernoulli equation is applied to calculate the RV-RA gradient, with subsequent addition of the RAP to calculate the SPAP. If an adequate TR jet is obtained the correlation with RHC-obtained SPAP measurements is very good (Janda et al., 2011). An experienced operator will take time to optimize the Doppler signal, especially when confounding factors such as minimal TR is present, the jet is eccentric, or there is poor coaptation of the tricuspid valve leaflets resulting in a broad turbulent jet.

Diagnosis in the absence of tricuspid regurgitation: Nepean Index

Using a combination of tissue Doppler velocity (TDI) of the lateral tricuspid annulus and the RV enddiastolic diameter (RVD), the ratio of RVD/T_{peak} (where T_{peak}=duration of TDI from the start of isovolumic contraction to peak systole) of > 22 cm/sec, predicted the presence of PHT, diagnosed as SPAP > 35 mm Hg, with 80% sensitivity and 83% specificity in patients with or without RV dysfunction (McLean et al., 2007).

(ii) Mean pressure

The diagnosis of pulmonary hypertension is based on the MPAP as measured by high-fidelity RHC measurements where the MPAP is measured as the area under the pressure curve divided by the pulse interval (Badesch et al., 2009; McGoon et al., 2004).

In clinical practice a flotation pulmonary artery catheter is generally utilized, which estimates the MPAP by the formula MPAP= 2/3DPAP+ 1/3SPAP. An extension therefore is to calculate the MPAP in a similar fashion utilizing ED derived SPAP and DPAP. Interestingly, further analysis indicates that SPAP is responsible for 98% of MPAP variability and therefore the use of the single parameter SPAP should be sufficient to accurately measure MPAP (Chemla et al., 2009). In investigating 2 separate formulae, the Chemla and Syyed formulae, where only the SPAP and not the DPAP is used, Aduen and colleagues demonstrated similar accuracy and precision to RHC-obtained measurements by ED derived measurements, indicating they were suitable for clinical use (Aduen et al., 2011)[30].

Chemla formula: MPAP = 0.61 x SPAP + 2 mm Hg
Syyed formula: MPAP = 0.65 x SPAP + 0.55 mm Hg

It has also been shown that the relationship between SPAP and MPAP remains linear during activity and change in posture (Syyed et al., 2008).

(iii) Pulmonary artery diastolic pressure

DPAP can be estimated using the pulmonary regurgitant jet. The velocity at end diastole is calculated and the modified Bernoulli equation is used.

eg.   DPAP = 4 x (pulmonary regurgitant end diastolic velocity)^2 + RAP

3.1.2.3 Cardiac output

This parameter can be obtained using the Simpsons Method from analysis of the left ventricular dimensions in the A4C and A2C views. Measurement of both left ventricular end diastolic and end systolic volumes is undertaken. The ultrasound machine has inbuilt software that utilizes division into multiple discs and a resultant summation in the overall volume leading to a simple method of calculating CO. This along with the left ventricular outflow tract (LVOT) Doppler method of calculating the cardiac output has been validated in the critically ill population (McLean et al., 1997).

The latter method is more reliable but does require more experience because continuous wave (CW) Doppler is involved. The more experienced operator should adopt the latter approach. The right ventricular outflow can also used in preference to the LVOT if desired.

3.1.2.4 RV systolic function

Assessment of right ventricular contraction on a regular basis in a critically ill patient with PHT is absolutely essential. Prognosis depends on the ability of the RV to adapt to elevated PAP, and being a thinned wall chamber its ability to adapt to systolic demands is limited. RV contractility can be monitored subjectively or objectively.

The subjective assessment of RV contraction relies upon both chamber sizes and visual 'eyeballing ' of the RV free wall. Dilatation of the RV is a guide to pulmonary pressure and/or fluid status. The relative area or volume of the RV to the LV as seen in the A4C view using transthoracic echocardiography or mid-oesphageal view using transoesophageal echocardiography should be <0.6, with a ratio of >1.0 indicating marked RV dilatation and 0.6-1.0 moderate dilatation. Paradoxical septal motion, usually best seen in the parasternal short axis view, adds to the evaluation with abnormal systolic motion indicating pressure overload and abnormal diastolic motion indicating RV fluid overload. The free wall of the RV is best viewed in the SC and A4C views although may be visualized in other views. Particular attention to RV wall thickness should be taken to assist in determining the chronicity of the PHT.

A number of parameters have been used in the evaluation of RV systolic function but most studies have demonstrated the clinical value of Right ventricular Myocardial performance index (RV MPI), tricuspid annulus plane systolic excursion (TAPSE), fractional area change (FAC) and S′ of the tricuspid annulus (Rudski et al., 2010).

i) Right Ventricular Myocardial Performance Index

The Myocardial Performance Index or 'Tei Index' was initially validated as a index of global left ve ntricular function but became adapted to the right heart (Karnati et al., 2008). RV MPI requires PW or CW Doppler recordings of the TV inflow and RV outflow. RV MPI is calculated from the isovolumic contraction time, isovolumic relaxation time and ejection time. A RV MPI >0.40 indicates global RV dysfunction. If tissue Doppler of the lateral tricuspid annulus is used, then global RV dysfunction is present if the RV MPI >0.55. The latter avoids errors related to variability in heart rate although both are less accurate with increasing RA pressures because of a decrease in the IVRT.

ii) TAPSE

The tricuspid annulus plane systolic excursion (TAPSE), otherwise known as the Tricuspid Annulus Displacement (TAD), is a parameter obtained by placing the M-mode cursor over the lateral tricuspid annulus. Although only one small part of RV motion is evaluated, this single simple measurement has been demonstrated to be a relatively reliable guide in both diagnostic and prognostic studies. A TAPSE of 16 mm or less implies RV contractile impairment (Forfia et al., 2006; Rudski et al., 2010).

iii) Right Ventricular Fractional Area Change

RV FAC is defined as (enddiastolic area –endsystolic area)/enddiastolic area x 100 and correlates with MRI evaluation of RV systolic function (Anavekar et al., 2007). Measurements of FAC are taken in the A4C view with the RV cavity area traced from the tricuspid annulus along the free wall and back down the ventricular septum, in both systole and diastole. A normal RV FAC is >35%.

iv) S' obtained by Tissue Doppler Imaging

From the A4C view the tricuspid annulus and basal free wall segments of the right ventricle can be assessed by either pulsed tissue Doppler or colour tissue Doppler to measure longitudinal velocity excursion. The S' velocity of the basal free wall measured by pulsed wave Doppler is the recommended value to measure (Rudski et al., 2010). Population studies give normal values of 15 cm/sec at the annulus and basal free wall. The lower limit of normal can be taken as 10 cm/sec (Lindqvist et al., 2005).

This is a simple and reproducible parameter with a S' <10 cm/s indicating abnormal RV systolic function in adult patients.

3.1.2.5 Left atrial pressure

Either direct measurement of the LAP, or a surrogate, is essential when monitoring PHT. The contribution of left heart dysfunction, or lack thereof, needs to be established. Also, over time an elevated PAP needs to be continually assessed, particularly in a patient with underlying PHT who is failing to improve and where LV dysfunction or elevated LAP develops during the ICU stay. A subjective view of the left heart may identify contractile dysfunction or significant left ventricular wall hypertrophy suggesting the presence of clinically relevant diastolic dysfunction. A number of methods including analysis of the mitral inflow wave form, pulmonary venous waveform, and M-Mode colour Doppler across the mitral inflow have been used historically for diastolic assessment, as a guide to elevated LAP. However, today the application of TDI makes the situation easier, particularly when combined with a dilated left atrium. The E/E' is of proven value in identifying elevated left atrial pressure, particularly when combined with a dilated left atrium.

3.2 Periodicity of measurements

The third component of the monitoring triad is that of periodicity and this may dictate which technique should be chosen in a particular patient. If daily assessment of the selected parameters is sought then ED in the majority of patients is sufficient. Where minute-to-minute monitoring is required and the parameters are limited to PAP and CO then the RHC should be considered. Where parameters are to be measured every few hours than the choice may depend on the availability and expertise present in the ICU. A word of caution is that if the RHC is chosen, then an ED should also be undertaken at some stage allowing for a better overall assessment of cardiovascular status. Conversely if very precise PAP measurements are required then a RHC should be chosen. Table 2 summarizes the main characteristics, advantages and disadvantages of the two modes of monitoring.

	Pulmonary Artery Catheter	Echo Doppler
Ease of use	Requires training	Requires training
Portability	No	Yes
User dependence	No, but data interpretation requires training	Yes, for data acquisition and interpretation
Continuous measurement	Yes	No
Invasive	Yes	No
CO measurement	Yes	Yes
Pressure measurements	Direct	Indirect, pressure are calculated
Evaluation of RV function	No	Yes

Table 2. Characteristics of PAC and ED monitoring

4. Heart-lung interactions and mechanical ventilation

Mechanical interactions between the respiratory and circulatory systems are produced by changes in the intrathoracic pressure (ITP) and changes in the lung volume. The institution of positive pressure ventilation (PPV) profoundly affects both ITP and lung volumes. To add further complexity, these effects may vary considerably between the healthy state and during disease, particularly in acute respiratory failure (ALI/ARDS). Pulmonary hypertension (PHT) is a notable feature of ALI/ARDS.

The heart and lungs are anatomically linked by their shared position in the thorax, with the vascular compartments acting like pressure chambers within a pressure chamber during PPV. This has important implications for the heart-lung interactions. The serial vascular arrangement of the heart and lungs means that any changes of right ventricular (RV) function will change pulmonary perfusion that in turn will change left ventricular (LV) function (Figure 3).

The venous return determines RV and LV output that must remain equal albeit small variations occur from heartbeat to heartbeat. Furthermore, the right and left ventricles of the heart are linked to each other by common myocardial tissue, the septal wall and the enclosure in the fibrous, non-compliant pericardial sac. These features result in ventricular interdependence, i.e. forces are transmitted from one ventricle to the other (Bove & Santamore, 1981). Diastolic ventricular interdependence means that increased volume-pressure in one ventricle will shift the compliance curve of the other ventricle to the left and upward (Weber et al., 1981). Diastolic interdependence is present during physiological conditions and is accentuated by PPV. Conditions involving the pericardium, e.g. cardiac tamponade and constrictive pericarditis, further accentuate diastolic ventricular interdependence. Systolic ventricular interdependence occurs as a physiological phenomenon and experimental data suggest that 20-40% of right ventricular systolic pressure result from left ventricular contraction (Damiano et al., 1991). The greater part of ventricular interdependence occurs through the septum although the ventricular free wall is also involved. Conditions that decrease the relative compliance of the septum, such as volume overload, increase ventricular interdependence as does increased stiffening of the right ventricle, for example by PHT (Santamore & Dell'Italia, 1998).

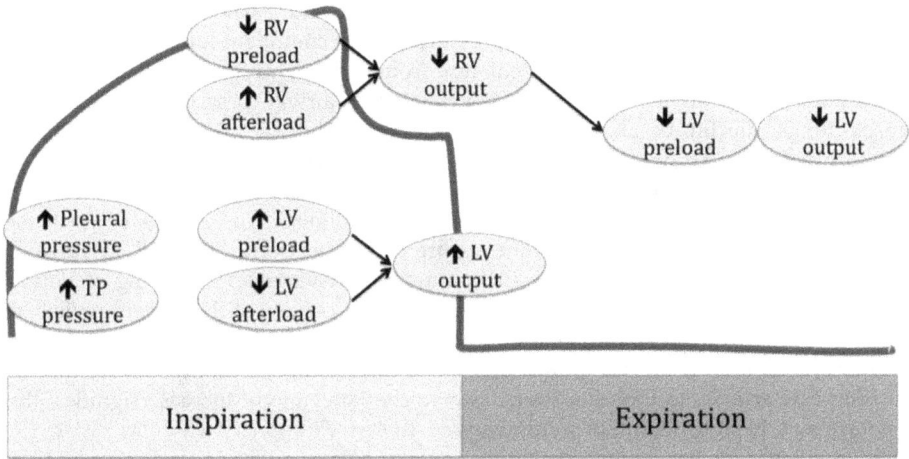

Fig. 3. Heart-lung interactions - effects of mechanical ventilation. Increased transpulmonary pressure due to positive pressure ventilation increases RV afterload, whilst RV preload is decreased due to the decreased venous return. During the inspiratory phase, LV preload is transiently increased due to a 'squeezing' effect from pulmonary vasculature into the left atrium. Ultimately however, the decrease in RV filling leads to decreased LV filling and output. TP=transpulmonary pressure=alveolar-pleural pressure. Adapted from Michard & Teboul (2000).

The RV preload is determined by the venous return, governed by the pressure gradient between mean systemic pressure and right atrial pressure, as well as caval size and collapsibility. Increased ITP generated by PPV may thus reduce venous return by decreasing the mean systemic to right atrial pressure gradient and by compressing the cavae, limiting flow (Michard & Teboul, 2000; Shekerdemian & Bohn, 1999). These effects can be offset by intravascular volume loading to increase mean systemic pressure, by increasing the extrathoracic pressure on large vessels, e.g. increasing intraabdominal pressure to increase mean systemic pressure, or by increasing venous vascular tone (through sympathetic activation or drugs). The classical effects of PEEP originally described by the two Nobel laureates Cournand and Richards (Cournand et al., 1948) are clinically not as prominent probably related to increased intraabdominal pressure by the diaphragmatic descent produced by PEEP and by sympathetic activation. Normally RV diastolic compliance is so high that RAP changes largely reflects changes in pericardial pressure rather than RV filling per se. Hence RAP is a poor indicator of RV end-diastolic filling. In patients with decreased RV compliance, such as in PHT, the dissociation between RAP and RV end-diastolic filling is lost.

LV function is influenced by PPV via the effects on RV function, thus governing LV filling, and by reduction of thoracic aortic transmural pressure leading to increased compliance and hence reduced LV afterload. Reduction of LV transmural pressure, and as a result LV mural tension, decreases oxygen consumption and forms the rationale for using PPV in patients with acute heart failure (Räsänen et al., 1985).

The ITP and airway pressures influence vascular pressures, but the extent and regional distribution of this effect may differ considerably in ALI/ARDS due to the uneven distribution of lung volume and alveolar pressure. Poorly compliant lungs, characteristic of ALI/ARDS, generally "protect" the vasculature from high airway pressures, meaning that PHT in this setting might not be as closely related to airway pressures as seen in less diseased lungs (Jardin et al., 1985). More precisely, the ITP significantly influences transmural pressure, i.e. the intravascular to ITP difference. This needs to be considered when assessing cardiac filling pressures as well as pulmonary vascular resistance (PVR). Increased ITP during PPV will decrease RV and LV filling in the setting of unchanged chamber pressures, since the transmural pressure decreases, even if RV and LV functional characteristics remain unchanged. The PVR is a complex variable, consisting of Poiseulle and Starling resistors, the details of which are beyond the context of the present review, and should not be viewed in the simplistic "Ohmic" manner typically applied to the systemic circulation (Versprille, 1984). The pulmonary blood is the sum of RV output and shunt flow from bronchial arteries to the pulmonary artery. The latter might increase significantly in RV failure and PHT to maintain pulmonary perfusion. Pulmonary vascular resistance is equally divided between pulmonary arteries/arterioles, capillaries and venules/veins. Active neurogenic and humoral vasoconstriction plays a minor role to control resistance and as a consequence regional distribution of pulmonary flow depends on other factors including gravity and hypoxic pulmonary vasoconstriction.

Oesophageal pressure can be used to estimate the ITP, and thus to work out vascular transmural pressures. Similarly, the transpulmonary pressure can be assessed, determining the stretch of the lungs. The caveat of airway pressure not being uniformly transmitted onto intrathoracic structures, including the oesphagus, must be kept in mind (Jardin et al., 1985).

Mechanical ventilation has complex effects on (PVR). In respiratory failure PPV can reduce PVR by increasing oxygenation above above 60 mm Hg to alleviate hypoxic pulmonary vasoconstriction (HPV). Furthermore, sympathetic outflow can be diminished by reducing work of breathing and by increasing alveolar ventilation to attenuate respiratory acidosis. The relationship between lung volume and PVR is U-shaped with increased PVR occuring at low lung volumes (due to increased resistance in extra-alveolar vessels and alveolar collapse increasing HPV) and at high lung volumes (due to hyperinflation and increased alveolar pressure compressing alveolar vessels) (Whittenberger et al., 1960). PVR is lowest at FRC that is typically reduced in ALI. The effects of PEEP on PVR are highly dependent on the intravascular volume status. Increased intravascular filling mitigates the potential of raised ITP to transfer lung areas from West zone 3 to zones 1 or 2 (Fourgéres et al., 2010).

Ventilator settings for patients with PHT with incipient or manifest RV failure should be tailored to minimize inspiratory swings in ITP, i.e. small tidal volumes (6 ml/kg) delivered with a slow rise to peak inspiratory pressure. The expiratory drop in ITP should be rapid with the expiratory time set to minimize intrinsic PEEP, usually meaning expiratory time should at least equal the inspiratory time.

Severely increased PVR either acutely or added onto pre-existing PHT, for example by mechanical ventilation, can precipitate acute cor pulmonale with RV distension, septal flattening and leftward displacement with impaired LV filling and rapid haemodynamic deterioration. Fluid administration in this setting can further worsen RV failure and the use of extracorporeal circulation might be the only therapeutic option for the acutely pressure- and volume-overloaded RV (Höhn et al., 1999).

5. Current therapeutic strategies

Pharmacological management of right heart failure and pulmonary vascular disease in the intensive care is dependent on its aetiology. While pulmonary hypertension may be due to left heart and/or underlying lung disease, its ultimate effects on the right heart are considered to be particularly deleterious. There are many components that can be related to the clinical syndrome of right heart failure seen in the critical care patient. This includes hypoxic pulmonary vasoconstriction, microvascular thromboses, increase or decrease of the permeability of the pulmonary vasculature and endothelial dysfunction. Further, changes in the lungs may precipitate right ventricular failure. RV failure may be primarily be related to RV function – for example due to ischemia of the right ventricle, volume overload or sepsis – or be secondary to LV failure. The management protocol of right ventricular dysfunction is dependent on the aetiology of the disease process, and these must be addressed prior to the isolated management of RV dysfunction. We will concentrate on specific management of RV dysfunction from this point onwards.

Management of RV dysfunction can be separated into surgical and pharmacological.

5.1 Surgical management

5.1.1 Intra Aortic Balloon Pump (IABP)

IABPs can support LV dysfunction but is of limited use in RV dysfunction. This is due to the differences in timing of coronary arterial filling of left and right coronary arteries. As the IABP inflates during diastole , it substantially augments left coronary filling. However the right coronary artery fills throughout systole and diastole, hence any diastolic augmentation of coronary filling is relatively small in the RV. Equally, IABP decreases the afterload for the left ventricle, but this does not affect right ventricular afterload. Right coronary perfusion is affected by the gradient between the intra ventricular pressure in the right ventricle and the coronary perfusion pressure – so the RV pressure must also be optimized, as too high an RV pressure will induce RV ischaemia. Pulmonary arterial pressures are raised by positive pressure ventilation hence all efforts should be made to move as rapidly as possible to negative pressure ventilation. Many centers will tracheostomise patients for this process. Equally if there is a risk of hypoxic pulmonary vasoconstriction, optimisation and maintaining a PO2 >100mmHg may reduce any pulmonary arterial vasoconstriction and hence decrease RV afterload.

5.1.2 Assist devices

Mechanical assist devices have been developed specifically with left ventricular support in mind. First generation ventricular assist devices such as Thoratec PVAD™ (Pleasanton, California, USA) and Abiomed BV5000™ (Massachusetts, **USA**) can be used in the biventricular setting. However this limits mobilization of the patient. A short-term device such as Levotronix™ (Massachusetts, USA) , or extracorporeal membrane oxygenation

(ECMO) can improve RV dysfunction in the acute setting but again limits the mobility of the patient and the ability to move from intensive care. In the setting of long term mechanical RV support, work is ongoing regarding the development of an implantable biventricular devices/total artificial heart , and using two rotary pumps in series, (Timms et al., 2008) - one for left and one for right ventricular support (Gregory et al., 2011). This necessitates either changing pump speeds or crimping the outflow of the VAD placed in the right heart to decrease pressures consistent with pulmonary arterial pressure (Timms et al., 2011). This would only be used in the chronic setting which is refractory to medical management. Whilst laboratory research has not been completed, some centres have already used this technique clinically (Strueber et al., 2010).

5.2 Pharmacological management

The pharmacological management of right ventricular dysfunction should aim at:

1. Prevention of right ventricular ischemia;
2. Improving right ventricular cardiac output;
3. Reducing pulmonary vascular resistance to a greater degree than systemic vascular resistance.

5.2.1 Prevention of right ventricular ischemia

Right ventricular ischaemia is clearly associated with increased mortality (Jacobs AK et al., 2003). Since the right coronary artery is filled through both systole and diastole with the majority of flow occurring through systole, the aortic root pressure is a key determinant of right coronary filling. Adequate systolic pressure is therefore required to optimize right ventricular oxygenation and this may necessitate vasopressor support. Vasopressors should be used carefully since they may increase left ventricular afterload, resulting in a shift of the intraventricular septum towards the right ventricle and reducing its output (see Section 4). Vasopressors which increase systemic systolic pressure may also increase pulmonary vascular pressure and the resistance which the failing right ventricle has to oppose. Therefore there is a trade-off between increasing right coronary perfusion pressures and increasing left and right ventricular afterload. Phenylephrine is well recognised to worsen right ventricular function. The data for Adrenaline and Noradrenaline are less clear. Increased, unchanged or decreased pulmonary vascular resistance (PVR) have been documented (Ghighone et al., 1984; Hirsch et al., 1991; Le Tulzo et al., 1997)

Vasopressin has some attributes suggesting it may be useful in patients with pulmonary vascular disease and RV dysfunction. In conscious animal models, vasopressin induces reversed drug induced vasoconstriction and induced pulmonary vasodilation (Trempy et al., 1994). In an ex-vivo model Evora et al describe how Vasopressin induces pulmonary vasodilatation due to a release of nitric oxide whilst simultaneously inducing systemic vasoconstriction. (Evora et al., 1993). The data in humans is much less clear. When Vasopressin and Noradrenalin were used to mitigate the hypotension associated with Milrinone Jeon et al noted that Vasopressin induced differential effects in the systemic and pulmonary vasculature, with a beneficial reduction in the PVR/SVR ratio following vasopressin only (Jeon et al., 2006). As has been described, maintenance of systemic pressure to optimize right coronary filling, with minimal or no simultaneous increase in PVR are ideal attributes in patients with the failing right ventricle.

Hence, data is clear that Phenylephrine seems to be deleterious in the face of right ventricular dysfunction; Noradrenalin improves coronary filling and may improve cardiac output, while animal and limited human data suggest that Vasopressin increases systemic pressure with minimal adverse effects on the pulmonary circulation.

5.2.2 Improving right ventricular cardiac output

Vasopressors may improve cardiac output through increasing coronary filling. However, there is more data to support the use of inotropic agents such as Levosimendan, Dobutamine, Milrinone and Adrenaline in right ventricular failure although Noradrenaline should not be entirely dismissed. Inodilators such as Dobutamine have a number of properties that make it ideal in the face of pressure overload of the RV. In causing systemic vasodilation it reduces the preload to the right ventricle and improves right ventricular contractility with minimal effect on pulmonary vascular resistance. (Pagnamenta et al., 2003). Some data support the use of Levosimendan in the similar situation, where it increases in cardiac output by increasing right ventricular contractility, decreasing pulmonary vascular resistance and improving RV-PA coupling (Kerbaul et al., 2006). Of note, there are few studies of Levosimendan for the treatment of sepsis-induced cardiomyopathy and pulmonary hypertension.

The phosphodiesterase-3 (PDE3) inhibitors improve cardiac output through improved contractility and reduction in both systemic and pulmonary arterial pressure. Milrinone is the most commonly used drug of this family at present. However in patients with severe right ventricular dysfunction an associated renal failure, drug accumulation may be a difficulty. There is minimal data on its clearance during continuous renal replacement therapy. Milrinone is most commonly administered intravenously but there are interesting reports of substantial benefits using the inhalational route. This is presumed to be due to a direct delivery to the pulmonary circulation with avoidance of systemic effects such as hypotension. A number of studies confirm the reduction in pulmonary arterial pressure and pulmonary artery resistance with maintenance of systemic pressure, especially in combination with vasopressors (Jeon et al., 2006). An additional benefit is an improvement of PaO2/FiO2 ratio, due to optimization of ventilation/perfusion by the selective action on Milrinone delivery to only aerated alveoli. This improvement in oxygenation may further assist the right ventricle and decrease pulmonary arterial pressure by attenuating hypoxic pulmonary vasoconstriction (Wang et al., 2009).

5.2.3 Pulmonary vasodilatation

Increased pulmonary vascular resistance is often associated with, and worsens right ventricular dysfunction. Therefore another strategy for improving right ventricular function is to reduce pulmonary vascular resistance, thereby decreasing RV afterload. Nitric oxide (NO) can be easily administered and measured, and reduces pulmonary vascular resistance. It is commonly used after mitral valve and congenital heart surgery where right ventricular failure is a common occurence. Contrary to the evidence in ARDS where NO has no beneficial affect on clinical outcome, it is clear that NO reduces pulmonary vascular resistance in patients with idiopathic pulmonary arterial hypertension, and has a proven role in this situation. Prostacyclin may be nebulised or given intravenously. It is derived from pulmonary endothelial cells, and is used in the stable chronic pulmonary hypertensive patients in an intravenous form with good effect (Benedict et al., 2007). However in the critically ill population, significant systemic vasodilation limits the usefulness of intravenously administered Prostacyclin. Moreover, its effect on platelet aggregation precludes its use in patients at risk of bleeding. Nebulised Prostacyclin however avoids these risks and has a very short half-life. It may be given up to three hourly, and can be useful for extubating patients requiring NO, who frequently become unstable when removing the last 1-2 parts per million. Nebulised drugs such as NO, Prostacyclin and Milrinone will not only reduce pulmonary vascular resistance but also optimize the ventilation-perfusion ratio since the drug is only delivered to aerated alveoli. Iloprost is an analogue of Prostacyclin with a much longer half-life of thirty minutes and a clinical activity of approximately sixty minutes. This makes it more practical to use in a critical care environment. These inhaled agents may be combined for improve synergistic affect. Research has been conducted investigating synergisitic combinations of Sildenafil and NO, Iloprost and NO, nebulised Milrinone and Prostacyclin, and Iloprost and Sildenafil, as well as the use of Sildenafil to allow safe weaning from NO (Huang J et al., 2011; Kumar et al., 2010; Lakshminrusimha et al., 2009; Lee et al., 2008; Winterhalter et al., 2010).

Oral Sildenafil has been used for the treatment of pulmonary hypertension in the critically ill for some time, and more recently has become available as an intravenous form. This phosphodiesterase type 5 inhibitor substantially decreases the pulmonary vascular resistance although a smaller reduction in systemic pressure also occurs. There is limited experience with intravenous sildenafil but this preparation would potentially be beneficial in patients who have inadequate gastric absorption due to splanchnic venous hypertension, a condition seen very frequently seen in patients with right ventricular dysfunction (Abrams et al., 2000; Barst et al., 1996; Prasad et al., 2000; Zhao et al., 2001)

Goal	Drug	Route	Mechanism
Prevention of RV ischaemia	Noradrenaline	i.v.	Increases systemic (=aortic root) pressure ⇒ improves right coronary arterial filling
	Adrenaline	i.v.	
	Vasopressin	i.v.	
Improve RV output	Dobutamine	i.v.	Increases RV contractility Inodilation ⇒ reduces PVR ⇒ decreases RV afterload
	Adrenaline	i.v.	
	Levosimendan	i.v.	
	PDE3 inhibitors eg. Milrinone	i.v., inhaled	
Pulmonary vasodilation	Nitric Oxide	inhaled	Dilates pulmonary vascular bed ⇒ reduces PVR ⇒ decreases RV afterload Improves V/Q matching
	Prostacyclin	i.v., inhaled	
	Iloprost	i.v.	
	Milrinone	i.v., inhaled	
	PDE5 inhibitors eg. Sildenafil	i.v., p.o.	
	ET-receptor antagonists eg. Bosentan	p.o.	

Table 3. Medical management of pulmonary hypertension

Endothelin antagonists such as Bosentan have minimal role in the critical care patient population as they take between three and six months to cause any effect. If they have been administered chronically to a patient, they should not be ceased acutely in ICU as this may induce rebound pulmonary hypertensive crisis. Care must be taken specifically with liver dysfunction.

Finally, some inotropic agents such as Milrinone, Dobutamine, Adrenaline and Levosimendan may have dual actions of improving cardiac output as well as reducing pulmonary vascular resistance (Chew et al., 2008; Jeon et al., 2006; Kerbaul et al., 2006; Le Tulza et al., 1997; Pagnamenta et al., 2003; Price et al., 2010;). A clinically useful systematic review with GRADE recommendations for the management of pulmonary vascular and right ventricular dysfunction may be found in Price et al (2010).

Regardless of drug and mechanical assistance to the patient with the failing right ventricle, there must be close and effective observation to assess response to therapy. Similarly, whilst volume challenges have a role in right ventricular failure, these should be small, with repeated assessment of adequacy of response, due to the impaired Frank-Starling mechanism.

6. Conclusion

Pulmonary hypertension occurs commonly in the critically ill population. The aetiology of this disease is varied and it is often associated with right ventricular failure. The presence of the latter increases mortality therefore treatment strategies for pulmonary hypertension also involve improving right ventricular function. The mainstay of therapy is pharmacological, and is aimed at reducing pulmonary vascular resistance, improving ventilation-perfusion matching and improving RV function. Commonly used therapies in critical care such as fluid loading, mechanical ventilation and vasopressor therapy have a place but must be used judiciously since they may worsen pulmonary vascular resistance and right ventricular function. Monitoring is essential in this population and a combination of right heart catheterization and Echo Doppler methods may be used. This paper provides an up-to-date review on the pathophysiology, monitoring and clinical management of pulmonary hypertension in critically ill adults.

7. Acknowledgements

MC was supported by the Acta Foundation, Region Skåne County Council (ALF), Lund University and the Anna Lisa and Sven Erik Lundgren's Foundation. AÅ has received research grants from the ALF-project at Sahlgrenska University Hospital. JF declares that he is Chief Medical Officer at Bivacor TM.

8. References

Abrams, D., Schulze-Neick, I., & Magee AG. (2000). Sildenafil as a selective pulmonary vasodilator in childhood primary pulmonary hypertension. *Heart*, 84(2), pp.E4
Aduen, JF., Castello, R., Daniels, JT., Diaz, JA., Safford, RE., Heckman, MG., Crook, JE., & Burger, CD. (2011). Accuracy and precision of three echocardiographic methods for estimating mean pulmonary artery pressure. *Chest*, 139(2), pp.347–52

Anavekar, NS., Gerson, D., Skali, H., Kwong, RY., Yucerl, K., & Solomon SD. (2007). Two-dimensional assessment of right ventricular function:an echocardiographic –MRI correlative study. *Echocardiography*, 24, pp.452-6

Badesch, DB., Champion, HC., Sanchez, MA., Hoeper, MM., Loyd, JE., Manes, A., McGoon, M., Naeije, R., Olchewski, H., Oudiz, RJ., & Torbicki A. (2009). Diagnosis and assessment of pulmonary arterial hypertension. *J Am Coll Cardiol*, 54(1 Suppl), pp.S55 - S66

Barbier, C., Loubières, Y., Schmit, C., Hayon, J., Ricome, JL., Jardin, F., & Viellard Baron A. (2004). Respiratory changes in inferior vena cava diameter are helpful in predicting fluid responsiveness in ventilated septic patients. *Intensive Care Med*, 30, pp.1740-46

Barst, RJ., Rubin, LJ., Long, WA., McGoon, MD., Rich, S., Badesch, DB., Groves, BM., Tapson, VF., Bourge ,RC., Brundage, BH., & et al. (1996). A comparison of continuous intravenous epoprostenol (prostacyclin) with conventional therapy for primary pulmonary hypertension. The Primary Pulmonary Hypertension Study Group. *N Engl J Med*, 334(5):296-302

Benedict, N., Seybert, A., & Mathier, MA. (2007). Evidence-based pharmacologic management of pulmonary arterial hypertension. *Clin Ther*, 29(10), pp.2134-53

Berkenbosch, JW., Baribeau, J., & Perreault T. (2000). Decreased synthesis and vasodilatation to nitric oxide in piglets with hypoxia-induced pulmonary hypertension. *Am J Physiol Lung Cell. Mol Physiol*, 278, pp.L276-L283

Bove, AA. & Santamore, WP. (1981). Ventricular interdependence. *Prog Cardiovasc Dis*, 23, pp.365-88

Brennan, JM., Blair, JE., Goonewardera, S., Ronan, A., Shah, D., Vasaiwala, S., Kirkpatrick, JN., & Spencer KT. (2007). Reappraisal of the use of IVC for estimating RAP. *J Am Soc Echocardiography*, 20, pp.857-61

Burstin L. (1967). Determination of pressure in the pulmonary artery by external graphic recordings. *Br Heart J*, 29, pp.396-404

Chemla, D., Castelain, V., Provencher, S., Humbert, M., Simonneau, G., & Hervé, P. (2009). Evaluation of various empirical formulas for estimating mean pulmonary artery pressure by using systolic pulmonary artery pressure in adults. *Chest*, 135(3), pp.760-8

Chew, MS., Bergenzaun, L., Öhlin, H., & Ersson A. (2008). Pulmonary hypertension in the critically ill. *Current Hypertension Reviews*, 4, pp.150-60

Cournand, A., Motley, HL., Werkö, L., & Richards DW Jr. (1948). Physiological studies of the effects of intermittent positive pressure breathing on cardiac output in man. *Am J Physiol*,152, pp.162-74

Damiano, RJ. Jr., La Follette, P. Jr., Cox, JL., Lowe, JE., & Santamore WP. (1991). Significant left ventricular contribution to right ventricular systolic function. *Am J Physiol*, 261, pp.1514-24

Evora, PR., Pearson, PJ., & Schaff, HV. (1993). Arginine vasopressin induces endothelium-dependent vasodilatation of the pulmonary artery. V1-receptor-mediated production of nitric oxide. *Chest*, 103(4), pp.1241-5

Farber, HW. & Loscalzo, J. (2004). Pulmonary arterial hypertension. *New Engl J Med*, 351, pp. 1655-65

Feissel, M., Michard, F., Faller, JP., & Teboul, JL. (2004). The respiratory variation in inferior vena cava diameter as a guide to fluid therapy. *Intensive Care Med*, 30, pp.1834-37

Fisher, MR., Forfia, PR., Chamera, E., Housten-Harris, T., Champion, HC., Girgis, RE., Corretti, MC., & Hassoun, PM. (2009). Accuracy of Doppler echocardiography in the hemodynamic assessment of pulmonary hypertension. *Am J Resp Crit Care Med*, 179, pp.615–21

Forfia, PR., Fisher, MR., Mathai, SC., Housten-Harris, T., Hemnes, AR., Borlaug, BA., Chamera, E., Corretti, MC., Champion, HC., Abraham, TP., Girgis, RE., & Hassoun PM. (2006). Tricuspid annular displacement predicts survival in pulmonary hypertension. *Am J Resp Crit Care Med*, 174(9), pp.1034-41

Fougères, E., Teboul, JL., Richard, C., Osman, D., Chemla, D., & Monnet, X. (2010). Hemodynamic impact of a positive end-expiratory pressure setting in acute respiratory distress syndrome: importance of the volume status. *Crit Care Med*, 38, pp.802-7

Galie, N., Ussia, G., Passarelli, P., Parlangeli, R., Branzi, A., & Mangani, B. (1995). Role of Pharmacologic tests in the treatment of primary pulmonary hypertension. *Am J Cardiol*, 75, pp.55A-62A

Ghighone, M., Girling, L., & Prewitt, RM. (1984). Volume expansion versus norepinephrine in treatment of low cardiac output complicating an acute increase in right ventricular after load in dogs. *Anesthesiology*, 60(2), 132-5

Giaid, A., Yanagisawa, M., Langleben, D., Michel, RP., Levy, R., Shennib, H., Kimura, S., Masaki, T., Duguid, WP., & Stewart, DJ. (1993). Expression of endothelin-1 in the lungs of patients with pulmonary hypertension. *N Engl J Med*, 328, pp.1732-9

Giaid, A. & Saleh, D. Reduced expression of endothelial nitric oxide synthase in the lungs of patients with pulmonary hypertension. (1995). *New Engl J Med*, 333, pp.214-21

Gregory, SD., Timms, D., Gaddum, N., Mason, DG., & Fraser, JF. (2011). Biventricular Assist Devices: A Technical Review. *Ann Biomed Eng*. Jul 8. [Epub ahead of print]

Hatle, L., Angelsen, BAJ., & Tromsdal, A. (1981). Non-invasive estimation of pulmonary artery systolic pressure with Doppler ultrasound. *Br Heart J*, 45, pp.157-65

Hirsch, LJ., Rooney, MW., Wat, SS., Kleinmann, B., & Mathru, M. (1991). Norepinephrine and Phenelephrine affects on right ventricular function in experimental canine pulmonary embolism. *Chest*, 100(3), pp.796-801

Höhn, L., Schweizer, A., Morel, DR., Spiliopoulos, A., & Licker, M. (1999). Circulatory failure after anesthesia induction in a patient with severe primary pulmonary hypertension. *Anesthesiology*, 91, pp.1943-5

Huang, J., Bouvette, MJ., & Zhou, J. (2010). Simultaneous delivery of inhaled prostacyclin and milrinone through a double nebulizer system. *J Cardiothorac Vasc Anesth*, 25(3), pp.590-1

Jacobs, AK., Leopold, JA., Bates, E., Mendes, LA., Sleeper, LA., White, H., Davidoff, R., Boland, J., Modur, S., Forman, R., & Hochman, JS. (2003). Cardiogenic shock caused by right ventricular infarction: a report from the SHOCK registry. *J Am Coll Cardiol*, 241(8), pp.1273-9

Janda, S., Shahidi, N., Gin, K., & Swiston, J. (2011). Diagnostic accuracy of echocardiography for pulmonary hypertension: a systematic review and meta-analysis. *Heart*, 97, pp.612-22

Jardin, F., Genevray, B., Brun-Ney, D., & Bourdarias, JP. (1985). Influence of lung and chest wall compliance on transmission of airway pressure to the pleural space in critically ill patients. *Chest*, 88, pp.653-8

Jeon, Y., Ryum JH., Lim, YJ., Kim, CS., Bahk, JH., Yoon, SZ., & Choi, JY. (2006). Comparative hemodynamic effects of vasopressin and norepinephrine after milrinone-induced hypotension in off-pump coronary artery bypass surgical patients. *Eur J Cardiothorac Surg*, 29(6), pp.952-6.

Karnati, PK., El-Hajjar, M., Torosoff, M., & Fein, SA. (2008). Myocardial performance index correlates with right ventricular ejection fraction measured by nuclear ventriculography. *Echocardiography*, 25, pp.381-5

Kumar, VH., Swartz, DD., Rashid, N., Lakshminrusimha, S., Ma, C., Ryan, RM., & Morin, FC. 3rd. (2010). Prostacyclin and milrinone by aerosolization improve pulmonary hemodynamics in newborn lambs with experimental pulmonary hypertension. *J Appl Physiol*,109(3), pp.677-84

Kerbaul, F., Rondelet, B., Demester, JP., Fesler, P., Huez, S., Naeije, R., & Brimioulle, S. Effects of levosimendan versus dobutamine on pressure load-induced right ventricular failure. *Crit Care Med*, 34(11), pp.2814-9.

Lakshminrusimha, S., Porta, NF., Farrow, KN., Chen, B., Gugino, SF., Kumar, VH., Russell, JA., & Steinhorn, RH. (2009). Milrinone enhances relaxation to prostacyclin and iloprost in pulmonary arteries isolated from lambs with persistent pulmonary hypertension of the newborn. *Pediatr Crit Care Med*,10(1), pp.106-12

Lang, RM., Bierig, M., Devereux, RB., Flachskampf, FA., Foster, E., Pellikka, PA., Pikard, MH., Roman, MJ., Seward, J., Shanewise, JS., Solomon, SD., Spencer, KT., Sutton, MS., & Stewart, MJ. Chamber Quantification Writing Group; American Society of Echocardiography's Guidelines and Standards Committee; European Association of Echocardiography . (2005). Recommendations for Chamber Quantification: a report from the American Society of Echocardiography's Guidelines and Standards Committee and the Chamber Quantification Writing Group, developed in conjunction with the European Association of Echocardiography, a branch of the European Society of Cardiology. *J Am Soc Echo*, 18, 1440-63

Lee, JE., Hillier, SC., & Knoderer, CA. (2008). Use of sildenafil to facilitate weaning from inhaled nitric oxide in children with pulmonary hypertension following surgery for congenital heart disease. *J Intensive Care Med*, 23(5), pp.329-34

Le Tulzo, Y., Seguin, P., Gacouin, A., Camus, C., Suprin, E., Jouannic, I., & Thomas, R. (1997). Effects of epinephrine on right ventricular function in patients with severe septic shock and right ventricular failure: a preliminary descriptive study. *Intensive Care Med*, 23(6), pp.664-70.

Lindqvist, P., Waldenstrom, A., Henein, M., Morner, S., & Kazzam, E. (2005). Regional and global right ventricular function in healthy individuals aged 20-90 years: a pulsed Doppler tissue imaging study:Umea General Population Heart Study. *Echocardiography*, 22, pp.305-14

Mandegar, M., Fung, Y-C B., Huang, W., Remillard, CV., Rubin, LJ., & Yuan, J X-J. (2004). Cellular and molecular mechanisms of pulmonary vascular remodeling: role in the development of pulmonary hypertension. *Microvasc Res*, 68, pp.75-103

McGoon, M,. Gutterman, D., Steen, V., Barst, R., McCrory, DC., Fortinm TA., & Loyd, JE; American College of Chest Physicians. (2004). Screening, early detection, and diagnosis of pulmonary arterial hypertension: ACCP evidence-based clinical practice guidelines. *Chest*, 126(1 Suppl), pp.14S- 34S

McIntyre, KM. & Sasahara, AA. (1971). The hemodynamic response to pulmonary embolism in patients without prior cardiopulmonary disease. *Am J Cardiol*, 28, pp.288-93

McLean, AS., Needham, A., Stewart, D., & Parkin, R. (1997). Estimation of Cardiac Output in a critically ill subject by noninvasive echocardiographic techniques. *Anaesthetics and Intensive Care* 25(3), pp.250-4

McLean ,AS., Ting, I., Huang, SJ., & Wesley, S. (2007). The use of the right ventricular diameter and tricuspid annular tissue Doppler velocity parameter to predict the presence of pulmonary hypertension. *Eur J Echo*, 8, pp.128-36

Michard, F. & Teboul, JL. (2000). Using heart-lung interactions to assess fluid responsiveness during mechanical ventilation. *Crit Care*, 4, pp.282-9

Moloney, ED. & Evans, TW. (2003). Pathophysiology and pharmacological treatment of pulmonary hypertension in acute respiratory distress syndrome. *Eur Resp J*, 21, pp.720-7

Newman, JH., Wheeler, L., Lane, KB., Loyd, E., Gaddipati, R., Phillips, JA. 3rd., & Loyd, JE. (2001). Mutation in the gene for bone morphogenetic protein receptor II as a cause of primary pulmonary hypertension in a large kindred. *N Engl J Med*,345,pp-319-24

Osman, D., Monnet, X., Castelain, V., Anguel, N., Warszawski, J., Teboul, JL., & Richard, C. (2008). Incidence and prognostic value of right ventricular failure in acute respiratory distress syndrome. *Int Care Med*, 34, pp.873-80

Pagnamenta, A., Fesler, P., Vandinivit, A., Brimioulle, S., & Naeije, R. (2003). Pulmonary vascular effects of dobutamine in experimental pulmonary hypertension. *Crit Care Med*, 31(4):1140-6

Prasad, S., Wilkinson, J., & Gatzoulis, MA. Sildenafil in primary pulmonary hypertension. (2000). *N Engl J Med*, 2000;343(18), p.1342

Price, LC., Wort, SJ., Marino, PS., & Brett, SJ. (2010). Pulmonary vascular and right ventricular dysfunction in critical care: current and emerging options for management: a systematic literature review. *Crit Care*, 14, pp.R169

Räsänen, J., Väisänen, IT., Heikkilä, J., & Nikki, P. (1985). Acute myocardial infarction complicated by left ventricular dysfunction and respiratory failure: the effects of continuous positive airway pressure. *Chest*, 87, pp.158-62

Ribeiro, A., Lindmarker, P., Juhlin-Dannfelt, A., Johnsson, H., & Jorfeldt, L. (1997). Echocardiography Doppler in pulmonary embolism: right ventricular dysfunction as a predictor of mortality rate. *Am Heart J*, 134, pp.479-87

Rudski, LG., Lai, WW., Afilalo, J., Hua, L., Handschumacher, MD., Chandreasekaran, K., Solomon, SD., Louie, EK., & Schiller, NB. (2010). Guidelines for the Echocardiographic Assessment of the Right Heart in Adults: A Report from the American Society of Echocardiography endorsed by the European Association of Echocardiography, a registered branch of the European Society of Cardiology, and the Canadian Society of Echocardiography. *J Am Soc Echo*, 23, pp.685-713

Santamore, WP. & Dell'Italia, LJ. (1998). Ventricular interdependence: Significant left ventricular contributions to right ventricular systolic function. *Prog Cardiovasc Dis*, 40, pp.289-308

Shekerdemian, L. & Bohn, D. (1999). Cardiovascular effects of mechanical ventilation. *Arch Dis Child*, 80, pp.475-80

Steudel, W., Ichinose, F., Huang, PL., Hurford, WE., Jones, RC., Bevan, JA., Fishman, MC., & Zapol, WM. (1997). Pulmonary vasoconstriction and hypertension in mice with targeted disruption of endothelial nitric oxide synthase (NOS3) gene. *Circ Res*, 81, pp.34-41

Strueber, M., Meyer, AL., Malehsa, D., & Haverich, AE. (2010). Successful use of the HeartWare HVAD rotary blood pump for biventricular support. *J Thorac Cardiovasc Surg* 140(4), pp.936-7.

Syyed, R., Reeves, JT., Welsh, D., Raeside, D., Johnson, MK., & Peacock, AJ. (2008). The relationship between the components of pulmonary artery pressure remains constant under all conditions in both health and disease. *Chest,*133, pp.633–9

The Task Force for the Diagnosis and Treatment of Pulmonary Hypertension of the European Society of Cardiology (ESC) and the European Respiratory Society (ERS), endorsed by the International Society of Heart and Lung Transplantation (ISHLT). (2009). Guidelines for the diagnosis and treatment of pulmonary hypertension. *Eur Heart J,* 30, pp.2493–537

Timms, D., Fraser, J., Hayne, M., Dunning, J., McNeil, K., & Pearcy, M. (2008). The BiVACOR rotary biventricular assist device: concept and in vitro investigation. *Artif Organs,* 32(10), pp.816-9

Timms, D., Gude, E., Gaddum, N., Lim, E., Greatrex, N., Wong, K., Steinseifer, U., Lovell, N., Fraser, J., & Fiane, A. 2011. Assessment of Right Pump Outflow Banding and Speed Changes on Pulmonary Hemodynamics During Biventricular Support With Two Rotary Left Ventricular Assist Devices. *Artif Organs,* Jul 5. doi: 10.1111/j.1525-1594.2011.01283.x. [Epub ahead of print]

Trempy, GA., Nyhan, DP., & Murray, PA. (1994). Pulmonary vasoregulation by arginine vasopressin in conscious, dhalothane-anesthetized, and pentobarbital-anesthetized dogs with increased vasomotor tone. *Anesthesiology* 81(3), pp.632-40.

Versprille, A. (1984). Pulmonary vascular resistance. A meaningless variable. *Intensive Care Med,*10, pp.51-3

Viellard Baron, A., Schmitt, J., Augarde, R., Fellahi, JL., Prin, S., Page, B., Beauchet, A., & Jardin, F. (2001). Acute cor pulmonale in acute respiratory distress syndrome submitted to protective ventilation: Incidence, clinical implications and prognosis. *Crit Care Med,* 29(8), pp.1551-5

Wang, H., Gong, M., Zhou, B., & Dai, A. (2009). Comparison of inhaled and intravenous Milrinone in patients with pulmonary hypertension undergoing mitral valve surgery. Adv Ther, 26(4), pp.462-468.

Weber, KT., Janicki, JS., Shroff, S., & Fishman, AP. (1981). Contractile mechanisms and interaction of the right and left ventricles. *American Journal of Cardiology,* 47, pp.686-95

Whittenberger, JL., McGregor, M., Berglund, E., & Borst, HG. (1960). Influence of state of inflation of the lung on pulmonary vascular resistance. *J Appl Physiol,*15, pp.878-82.

Winterhalter, M., Antoniou, T., & Loukanov, T. (2010). Management of adult patients with perioperative pulmonary hypertension: technical aspects and therapeutic options. *Cardiology,* 116(1), pp.3-9

Zhao, L., Mason, NA., Morrell, NW., Kojonazarov, B., Sadykov, A., Maripov, A, Mirrakhimov, MM., Aldashev, A., & Wilkins, MR. (2001). Sildenafil inhibits hypoxia-induced pulmonary hypertension. *Circulation,* 104(4), pp.424–8

Zhao, L., Mason, NA., Strange, JW., Walker, H., & Wilkins, MR. (2003). Beneficial effects of phosphodiesterase 5 inhibition in pulmonary hypertension are influenced by natriuretic peptide activity. *Circulation,*107:234-7

Permissions

The contributors of this book come from diverse backgrounds, making this book a truly international effort. This book will bring forth new frontiers with its revolutionizing research information and detailed analysis of the nascent developments around the world.

We would like to thank Dr. Roxana Sulica, for lending her expertise to make the book truly unique. She has played a crucial role in the development of this book. Without her invaluable contribution this book wouldn't have been possible. She has made vital efforts to compile up to date information on the varied aspects of this subject to make this book a valuable addition to the collection of many professionals and students.

This book was conceptualized with the vision of imparting up-to-date information and advanced data in this field. To ensure the same, a matchless editorial board was set up. Every individual on the board went through rigorous rounds of assessment to prove their worth. After which they invested a large part of their time researching and compiling the most relevant data for our readers. Conferences and sessions were held from time to time between the editorial board and the contributing authors to present the data in the most comprehensible form. The editorial team has worked tirelessly to provide valuable and valid information to help people across the globe.

Every chapter published in this book has been scrutinized by our experts. Their significance has been extensively debated. The topics covered herein carry significant findings which will fuel the growth of the discipline. They may even be implemented as practical applications or may be referred to as a beginning point for another development. Chapters in this book were first published by InTech; hereby published with permission under the Creative Commons Attribution License or equivalent.

The editorial board has been involved in producing this book since its inception. They have spent rigorous hours researching and exploring the diverse topics which have resulted in the successful publishing of this book. They have passed on their knowledge of decades through this book. To expedite this challenging task, the publisher supported the team at every step. A small team of assistant editors was also appointed to further simplify the editing procedure and attain best results for the readers.

Our editorial team has been hand-picked from every corner of the world. Their multi-ethnicity adds dynamic inputs to the discussions which result in innovative outcomes. These outcomes are then further discussed with the researchers and contributors who give their valuable feedback and opinion regarding the same. The feedback is then collaborated with the researches and they are edited in a comprehensive manner to aid the understanding of the subject.

Apart from the editorial board, the designing team has also invested a significant amount of their time in understanding the subject and creating the most relevant covers. They scrutinized every image to scout for the most suitable representation of the subject and create an appropriate cover for the book.

The publishing team has been involved in this book since its early stages. They were actively engaged in every process, be it collecting the data, connecting with the contributors or procuring relevant information. The team has been an ardent support to the editorial, designing and production team. Their endless efforts to recruit the best for this project, has resulted in the accomplishment of this book. They are a veteran in the field of academics and their pool of knowledge is as vast as their experience in printing. Their expertise and guidance has proved useful at every step. Their uncompromising quality standards have made this book an exceptional effort. Their encouragement from time to time has been an inspiration for everyone.

The publisher and the editorial board hope that this book will prove to be a valuable piece of knowledge for researchers, students, practitioners and scholars across the globe.

List of Contributors

Rajamma Mathew
Dept of Pediatrics, Maria Fareri Children's Hospital at Westchester Medical Center, New York Medical College, Dept. of Physiology, New York Medical College, Valhalla, NY, USA

Christophe Guignabert
INSERM UMR 999, "Pulmonary Hypertension:, Physiopathology and Novel Therapies", Le Plessis-Robinson, France

Enrique Arciniegas
Instituto de Biomedicina, Facultad de Medicina, Universidad Central de Venezuela, Venezuela

José Cardier
Instituto Venezolano de Investigaciones Científicas, Centro de Medicina Experimental, Venezuela

Héctor Rojas
Instituto de Inmunología, Facultad de Medicina, Universidad Central de Venezuela, Venezuela

Luz Marina Carrillo
Servicio Autónomo Instituto de Biomedicina, Venezuela

Caroline Morin
Department of Physiology and Biophysics, Université de Sherbrooke, Sherbrooke, Québec, Canada
SCF-Pharma, Ste-Luce, Québec, Canada

Christelle Guibert
Centre de Recherche Cardio-Thoracique de Bordeaux, INSERM U1045, Université Bordeaux Segalen, France

Éric Rousseau
Department of Physiology and Biophysics, Université de Sherbrooke, Sherbrooke, Québec, Canada

Samuel Fortin
SCF-Pharma, Ste-Luce, Québec, Canada

Miriam de Boeck and Peter ten Dijke
Department of Molecular Cell Biology and Centre for Biomedical Genetics, Leiden University Medical Center, The Netherlands

Aureliano Hernández and Martha de Sandino
Universidad Nacional de Colombia, Facultad de Medicina Veterinaria y de Zootecnia, Bogotá, Colombia

B. J. van Beek-Harmsen, H. M. Feenstra and W. J. van der Laarse
Department of Physiology, Institute for Cardiovascular Research, VU University Medical Center Amsterdam, The Netherlands

Dimitar Sajkov, Karen Latimer and Nikolai Petrovsky
Australian Respiratory and Sleep Medicine Institute (ARASMI), Flinders Medical Centre and Flinders University, Flinders Drive, Bedford Park, Australia

Enric Domingo
Area del Cor, Hospital Universitari Vall d'Hebron, Spain
Dept Physiology, Universitat Autonoma Barcelona, Spain

Antonio Roman
Servei de Pneumologia i CIBERES, Hospital Universitari Vall d'Hebron, Spain

Juan Grignola
Dept Pathophysiology, Hospital de Clínicas, Universidad de la República, Uruguay

Rio Aguilar-Torres
Dept Physiology, Universitat Autonoma Barcelona, Spain
Unit of Cardiac Image, Hospital Universitario Bellvitge, Spain

Chin-Chang Cheng and Chien-Wei Hsu
Kaohsiung Veterans General Hospital, Taiwan

Muhammad Ishaq Ghauri
Department of Medicine, Jinnah Medical College Hospital, Pakistan

Kamran Hameed
Department of Medicine, Ziauddin Medical University, Karachi, Pakistan

Jibran Sualeh Muhammad
Department of Biological and Biomedical Sciences, Aga Khan University, Pakistan

Veronica Palmero, Phillip Factor and Roxana Sulica
Albert Einstein College of Medicine, Beth Israel Medical Center, New York, United States of America

Jae H. Kim and Anup Katheria
Division of Neonatal-Perinatal Medicine, Department of Pediatrics, University of California San Diego, United States of America

Alessandro Domenici, Remo Luciani, Francesco Principe, Francesco Paneni, Giuseppino Massimo Ciavarella and Luciano De Biase
Department of Cardiovascular, Renal and Pulmonary Diseases, Sant'Andrea Hospital, Sapienza University of Rome, Italy

Jean M. Elwing and Ralph J. Panos
Pulmonary, Critical Care, and Sleep Division, Department of Internal Medicine, University of Cincinnati, School of Medicine, Cincinnati Veterans Administration Hospital, Cincinnati, OH, USA

Philip L. Kalarickal, Sabrina T. Bent, Michael J. Yarborough, Kavitha A. Mathew and Charles Fox
Department of Anesthesiology, Tulane University School of Medicine, New Orleans, LA, United States of America

Michelle S. Chew
Department of Intensive Care Medicine, Skåne University Hospital Malmö, Lund University, Sweden

Anthony S. McLean
Intensive Care Unit, Nepean Hospital, Sydney University, Australia

John F. Fraser
Critical Care Research Group, The Prince Charles Hospital, Brisbane, Australia

Anders Åneman
Intensive Care Unit, Liverpool Hospital, Sydney, Australia